Oxford Clinical Practice Series

HANDBOOK OF ORAL DISEASES
FOR MEDICAL PRACTICE

W0234601

The Oxford Clinical Practice series covers an array of resources providing essential evidence-based, up-to-date information and key clinical references that will enhance the clinical knowledge of healthcare practitioners and medical students across the globe.

Oxford Clinical Practice Series

HANDBOOK OF ORAL DISEASES
FOR MEDICAL PRACTICE

Edited by
S. R. Prabhu
BDS, MDS, FDS RCS (Edin), FDS RCS (Eng),
FDS RCPS (Glasg), FFD RCS Ire (Oral Med),
M O Med RCS (Edin), FFGDP RCS (U.K.), FICD

School of Dentistry and Health Sciences, Charles Sturt University,
Orange, New South Wales, Australia, and Adjunct Visiting Professor,
Manipal University College of Dentistry, Manipal, India

Formerly at dental schools in Manipal, Nairobi,
Khartoum, Adelaide, Trinidad and Tobago, Kuala Lumpur,
Riyadh and Ras Al Khaimah

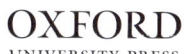

OXFORD
UNIVERSITY PRESS

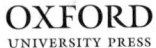
OXFORD
UNIVERSITY PRESS

Oxford University Press is a department of the University of Oxford.
It furthers the University's objective of excellence in research, scholarship,
and education by publishing worldwide. Oxford is a registered trademark of
Oxford University Press in the UK and in certain other countries.

Published in India by
Oxford University Press
YMCA Library Building, 1 Jai Singh Road, New Delhi 110 001, India

© Oxford University Press 2016

The moral rights of the authors have been asserted.

First Edition published in 2016

ISBN-13: 978-0-19-946819-5
ISBN-10: 0-19-946819-2

Typeset in Helvetica Neue LT Std 7.5/9.5
by Tranistics Data Technologies, Kolkata 700 091
Printed in India by Multivista Global Ltd., Chennai

Contents

vii

Foreword

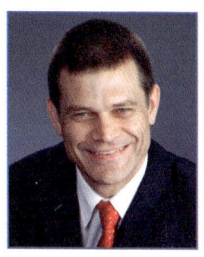

Charles Sturt University is an institution that is committed to the well-being of its communities. It has also had a long tradition of encouraging interprofessional practice and motivating practitioners to think broadly about problems rather than considering them within their own specialties. *Handbook of Oral Diseases for Medical Practice*, edited by S. R. Prabhu, is a great example of this philosophy. From rural and regional communities, we know that oral and dental health is an important indicator of general health. We also know that, if neglected, oral health issues can go on to cause significant general health problems. It is, therefore, essential that a handbook that provides guidance to medical and health professionals more generally is made available by dental specialists. I am particularly pleased that the collation of this handbook has come from our dental school, when it is still relatively young. It features contributions from across the globe and, in turn, I hope that the advice contained in this book helps to improve outcomes for all patients worldwide.

Andrew Vann, BEng (Hons), PhD,
Grad Cert Bus Ad, FAIM, GAICD, FIEAust
Vice Chancellor and President,
Charles Sturt University,
Bathurst, New South Wales
Australia

Preface

The public at large and a vast majority of medical and health professionals generally hold the view that dentists diagnose and treat only tooth-related problems. Among other factors, this view is one of the reasons why many patients with oral soft tissue and jaw bone-related conditions frequently seek consultation and treatment from medical practitioners. To date, very little information is available on dental and oral diseases targeted at medical students and practitioners and other health professionals. *Handbook of Oral Diseases for Medical Practice* aims to fulfil this need. The main goal of this book is to provide short and objective approach to the diagnosis and management of oral diseases that are likely to be encountered by medical and other health professionals.

This handbook is divided into four parts. Part 1 deals with basic diagnostic methods used in medical and dental practice. In Parts 2 and 3, a symptom-based approach has been used and Part 4 is predominantly disease-oriented. Essential information offered in each chapter includes a definition (or brief description), causes, clinical features, diagnostic steps and principles of management of oral diseases.

I hope that medical students, medical practitioners, specialists and other health professionals find this book useful.

Acknowledgements

First of all, I wish to thank Professor Andrew Vann, Vice Chancellor and President, Charles Sturt University, Australia, for recognising the potential contribution of this book to overall health through oral health and for writing a foreword. I also acknowledge those distinguished contributors who have made this work possible. I am grateful to the national and international colleagues and publishers who provided me with permission to use their clinical material.

Thanks to Oxford University Press for the excellent quality of production. My wife Uma deserves special thanks for her continuing support throughout this project.

Editor and Contributors

S. R. Prabhu, BDS, MDS, FDS RCS (Edin), FDS RCS (Eng), FDS RCPS (Glasg), FFD RCS Ire (Oral Med), M O Med RCS (Edin), FFGDP RCS (U.K.), FICD
School of Dentistry and Health Sciences, Charles Sturt University, Australia, and Adjunct Visiting Professor, Manipal University, India

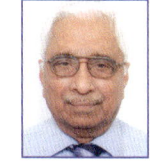

Paul Abbott, BDS, PhD, FRACDS
Winthrop Professor of Clinical Dentistry, School of Dentistry, The University of Western Australia, Australia

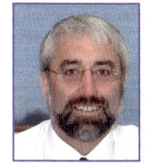

Haytham Al Bayaty, BDS, MDSc, PhD, FDS RCS (Edin)
Senior Lecturer, School of Dentistry, University of the West Indies, Trinidad and Tobago

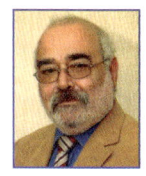

Ramesh Balasubramaniam, BSc, BDSc (UWA), MS, Cert Orofacial Pain (UKy), Cert Oral Medicine (UPenn), ABOP, FOMAA, FADI, FPFA, FICD
Clinical Associate Professor, School of Dentistry, Perth Oral Medicine & Dental Sleep Centre, University of Western Australia, Australia

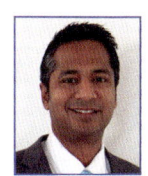

H. M. H. N. Bandara, BDS (Hons), PhD
Senior Postdoctoral Research Fellow, Department of Health and Behavioral Sciences, School of Dentistry, University of Queensland, Australia

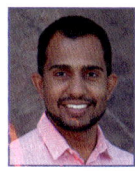

David H. Felix, BDS, MB ChB, FDS RCS (Eng), FDS RCPS (Glasg), FDSRCS (Edin), FRCP (Edin)
Dean, Postgraduate Dental Education, NHS Education for Scotland, United Kingdom

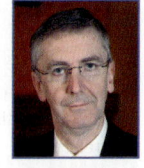

Jeffrey Hill, DMD
Professor, School of Dentistry, University of Alabama in Birmingham, United States of America

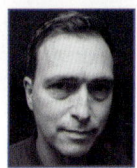

Newell Johnson, CMG, FMedSci, MDSc, PhD, FDSRCS (Eng), FRACDS, FRCPAth (U.K.), FFOP (RCPA), FHEA (U.K.), FICD
Emeritus Professor of Dental Research, Griffith University, Australia

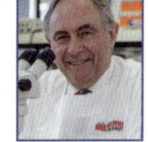

Sabrina Manickam, BDS, FICD
Senior Lecturer, Restorative Dentistry, School of Dentistry and Health Sciences, Charles Sturt University, Australia

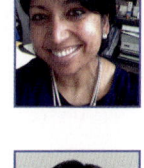

Nagamani Narayana, DMD, MS
Associate Professor of Oral Medicine, School of Dentistry, University of Nebraska Medical Centre, United States of America

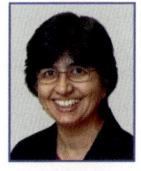

Atieh Sadr, DDS, MS
Lecturer, Restorative Dentistry (Endodontics), School of Dentistry and Health Sciences, Charles Sturt University, Australia

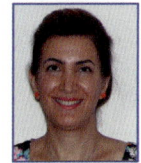

Lakshman Samaranayake, DSc, DDS (Glasg), FRCPath, FDSRCS (Edin), FRACDS (Hons), FHKCPath, FCDSHK, FICD
Professor of Oral Microbiomics and Infection, School of Dentistry, University of Queensland, Australia

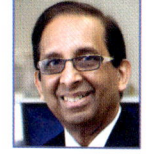

Valerie G. A. Suter, Dr. Med. Dent.
Head of Section Dental Radiology and Stomatology, Department of Oral Surgery and Stomatology, University of Bern, Switzerland

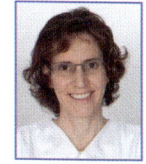

Kobkan Thongprasom, B.Sc. (Hons), D.D.S (Hons), M.Sc.
Professor of Oral Medicine, Faculty of Dentistry, Chulalongkorn University, Thailand

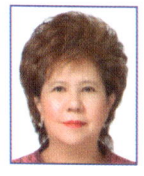

Saman Warnakulasuriya, OBE
BDS, FDSRCS, Dip Oral Med, PhD, DSc
Professor of Oral Medicine & Experimental Pathology, King's College, London, United Kingdom

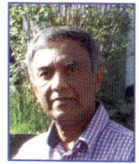

David F. Wilson, BDS, MDS, FFOP (RCPA), FDS RCPS (Glasg)
Professor of Oral and Maxillofacial Pathology, School of Dentistry and Health Sciences, Charles Sturt University, Australia

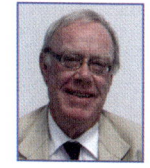

Sue Yeoh, BDS, FRACDS (Oral Med)
Oral Medicine Specialist, Baulkham Hills, NSW, Australia

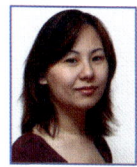

Abbreviations

AFP	Atypical facial pain
AI	Amelogenesis imperfecta
AIDS	Acquired immunodeficiency syndrome
ATN	Atypical trigeminal neuralgia
BANA	Benzoyl-arginine naphthylamide
BMS	Burning mouth syndrome
BONJ	Bisphosphonate-associated osteonecrosis of the jaw
CMV	Cytomegalovirus
CPAP	Continuous positive airway pressure
CT	Computed tomography
DLE	Discoid lupus erythematosus
EBV	Epstein-Barr virus
EFGR	Epidermal growth factor receptor
EM	Erythema multiforme
FBC	Full blood count
FD	Fibrous dysplasia
FDA	Food and Drug Administration
FDI	Federation Dentaire International
GP	Gutta-percha
GVHD	Graft-versus-host disease
HAART	Highly active antiretroviral therapy
HHT	Hereditary haemorrhagic telangiectasia
HHV-8	Human herpesvirus 8
HIV	Human immunodeficiency virus
HPV	Human papillomavirus
HSV	Herpes simplex virus
KS	Kaposi's sarcoma
LA	Local anaesthesia
LE	Lupus erythematosus
LGE	Linear gingival erythema
LP	Lichen planus
MAD	Mandibular advancement device
MAS	McCune-Albright syndrome
MG	Myasthenia gravis
MRI	Magnetic resonance imaging
MRONJ	Medication-related osteonecrosis of the jaw
MS	Multiple sclerosis
NHL	Non-Hodgkin's lymphoma
NSAIDs	Nonsteroidal anti-inflammatory drugs
NUG	Necrotising ulcerative gingivitis
NUP	Necrotising ulcerative periodontitis
OFG	Orofacial granulomatosis

OHL	Oral hairy leukoplakia
OLL	Oral lichenoid lesion
OLP	Oral lichen planus
OLR	Oral lichenoid reaction
OPMD	Oral potentially malignant disorders
OPVL	Oral proliferative verrucous leukoplakia
ORN	Osteoradionecrosis
OSA	Obstructive sleep apnoea
OSCC	Oral squamous cell carcinoma
PGCG	Peripheral giant cell granuloma
PHN	Postherpetic neuralgia
POF	Peripheral ossifying fibroma
RAU	Recurrent aphthous ulcers
SB	Sleep bruxism
SCC	Squamous cell carcinoma
SLE	Systemic lupus erythematosus
ST	Smokeless tobacco
TB	Tuberculosis
TMJ	Temporomandibular joint
TMJD	Temporomandibular joint disorder
TPPA	*Treponema pallidum* particle agglutination assay
TRD	Tongue-retaining devices
VDRL	Venereal Disease Research Laboratory
VZV	Varicella-zoster virus
WHO	World Health Organization

Part I

Basic diagnostic approaches

Chapter 1

Examination of the mouth and the teeth

S. R. Prabhu

SEQUENCE OF ORAL SOFT TISSUE EXAMINATION

Examination of the mouth and the teeth should be carried out in a systematic order. Starting with the lips, the following sequence is recommended for oral examination:

Labial mucosa → Cheek (buccal) mucosa → Floor of the mouth → Ventral surface of the tongue → Dorsal surface of the tongue → Hard and soft palates → Gingivae and the teeth.

Examination of the Labial Mucosa

Lips are gently everted to examine the labial mucosa.

- Labial mucosa is normally pink in colour.
- The inner surface of each lip is connected in the middle line to the corresponding gum by a fold of mucous membrane known as the labial frenulum.
- Palpation reveals nodular consistency of the lips. This is because of the presence of minor salivary glands.

Examination of the Cheek (Buccal) Mucosa

Inspection of the check (buccal) mucosa is conducted with mouth half open.

- Cheek mucosa is pink in colour.
- Parotid duct (Stenson's duct) opening is seen as a small nodular projection located opposite to the left and right second maxillary molars. This is called parotid papilla (Figure 1.1).
- Parotid papilla should not be mistaken for a pathological nodular lesion.
- Granular spots of yellowish-white colour are commonly seen on the buccal mucosa. These are called Fordyce granules. Fordyce granules should not to be mistaken for pathological conditions.

Examination of the Floor of the Mouth and the Ventral Surface of the Tongue

These areas are best examined when the patient raises the tongue, which also raises the floor of the mouth for examination.

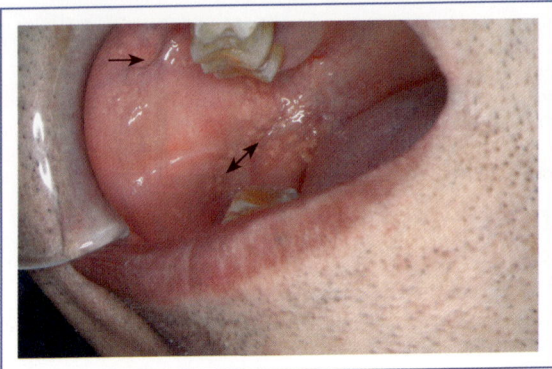

Figure 1.1 Parotid papilla (arrow) on the buccal mucosa; also seen are the yellowish granules called Fordyce granules (double arrow), which are considered as normal structures.
Courtesy: Nagamani Narayana.

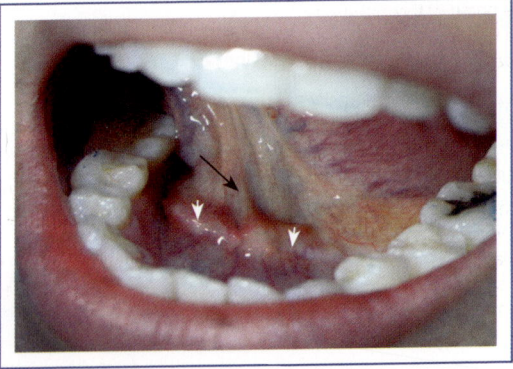

Figure 1.2 Lingual frenum (black arrow) and sublingual caruncle (white arrows).
Reproduced with permission from: Clarence Da Cruz and Cheng Zhang.

Anatomical features of the floor of the mouth and the ventral surface of the tongue include the following:

- Lingual frenulum or lingual frenum: It is a fold of tissue in the midline between the ventral surface of the tongue and the floor of the mouth.
- Sublingual caruncles: These are two small, raised folds of tissue found on either side of the lingual frenum (Figure 1.2). Each sublingual caruncle contains a salivary duct opening for submandibular salivary gland (Wharton duct).

- Sublingual folds: These are the folds of tissue that begin at the sublingual caruncles on either side of the lingual frenum and run posteriorly toward the base of the tongue. Sublingual folds contain multiple ducts from the sublingual salivary gland.
- Other normal structures include tortuous purple-coloured lingual veins, visible on either side of the lingual frenum. These veins are prominent in the elderly.

Examination of the Dorsum of the Tongue

The examiner can grasp the tongue with a sterile gauze and examine the dorsum of the tongue when the tongue is protruded.

- Large 8 to 10 circumvallate papillae separate the anterior two-thirds of the tongue from its posterior one-third.
- Large lymphoid masses are located behind the circumvallate papillae. These are the lingual tonsils.
- Many filiform papillae and a few fungiform papillae are located on the anterior two-thirds of the dorsum of the tongue.
- An inverted V-shaped groove called sulcus terminalis runs laterally and anteriorward from a small pit called the foramen cecum. Sulcus terminalis forms the boundary between the anterior two-thirds and the posterior one-third of the tongue. The foramen cecum indicates the origin of the embryonic thyroglossal duct.
- On the posterolateral borders of the tongue, leaf-like structures are located. These are the foliate papillae.

Examination of the Hard Palate

Palatal mucosa is pink and firmly attached to the mucoperiosteum.

- Anteriorly, hard palate shows transverse ridges called rugae on either side of the incisive papilla.
- Several minor salivary glands are located in the posterior hard palate.
- In some individuals, bony lumps may be seen on the posterior centre of the palatal vault. These are tori and should not be mistaken for tumours.

Examination of the Soft Palate, Uvula and Fauces

By using a mouth mirror, soft palate is examined for its movements when the patient says 'aah'. This allows the inspection of the posterior part of the tongue and pharynx.

- Movable part of the palate is the soft palate, which ends in uvula.
- The soft palate is continuous laterally with two folds — the palato-glossal and palatopharyngeal arches (Figure 1.3).
- The space between the oral cavity and the pharynx, bounded by the soft palate and the base of the tongue, is called fauces.

Examination of the Gingivae

- Gingivae are pale pink and firm, with stippled surface.
- In between the teeth, the gingivae form interdental gingival papillae.

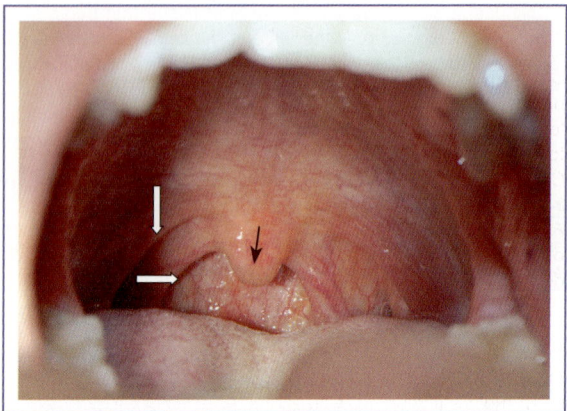

Figure 1.3 Soft palate and uvula (black arrow), palatopharyngeal arch (horizontal white arrow) and palatoglossal arch (vertical white arrow). Reproduced with permission from: Clarence Da Cruz and Cheng Zhang.

- The attached gingiva is pale pink and keratinised. This is demarcated from the alveolar mucosa, which is nonkeratinised.
- The junction between the alveolar mucosa and the attached gingiva is called the mucogingival junction.
- The part of the gingiva that surrounds a tooth and is not directly attached to the tooth surface is called the marginal gingiva.

Examination of the Teeth

A medically trained clinician should be familiar with the basic examination procedures of the teeth and dentition and with the general principles of inspection, palpation and percussion.

The basic examination of the teeth includes the following steps:

- **Inspection:** Clinician should look for developmental tooth abnormalities in number, size, shape, colour and structure and for acquired disorders, such as dental caries, retained roots, periodontal disease and tooth mobility.
- **Palpation:** Clinician should palpate for the tenderness, consistency and texture of any swellings derived from periapical dental infections, cysts and tumours.
- **Percussion:** When the dental pulp, periodontal tissue, or periapical tissue are inflamed, the clinician can gently percuss the suspicious tooth by using the handle of a dental mirror and elicit tenderness. Patient must be warned before this procedure.
- **Probing:** The clinician can place a fine blunt dental probe gently into the gingival sulcus that surrounds the tooth to examine the health of the gingival tissues. Bleeding and/or sulcus depth greater than 3 to 4 mm is an indication of gum disease.

- **Mobility test:** The clinician can test the mobility of a tooth by holding it between the fingers (from the buccal and lingual sides). A mobility of 0.5 mm is considered normal.
- Other procedure that can be useful is the vitality testing of the suspicious tooth. Application of hot (melting gutta-percha) or cold (ethyl chloride on a cotton bud) stimuli provides information on the tooth vitality. Nonvital teeth do not present any symptoms.
- Checking occlusion of the teeth is important if fracture of the jaw is suspected.
- **Radiographic examination:** Obtaining periapical views of the offending tooth or an orthopantamograph of the jaws is helpful in detecting dental and jaw bone pathology.

IDENTIFICATION OF THE TEETH

An adult has 32 permanent teeth: 8 incisors, 4 canines, 8 premolars and 12 molars (including wisdom teeth), whereas a child has 20 deciduous teeth: 8 incisors, 4 canines and 8 molars.

Numbering System for Identification of the Teeth

To simplify the identification of permanent and deciduous teeth, numbering systems have been used in dental practice. The three systems used are as follows:

1. The American Dental Association's sequential numbering system (also called the Universal Numbering System)
2. The Zsigmondy-Palmer system
3. The Federation Dentaire Internationale (FDI) system (also called international system)

The FDI system recommended by the World Health Organization is widely used (Table 1.1).

The FDI system uses two-digit numbers to identify each tooth. Some of the aspects of this system are described as follows:

- The first number denotes the quadrant and the second number denotes the specific tooth in that quadrant.

Table 1.1 FDI's two-digit notation

Permanent teeth															
Patient's upper right								Patient's upper left							
18	17	16	15	14	13	12	11	21	22	23	24	25	26	27	28
48	47	46	45	44	43	42	41	31	32	33	34	35	36	37	38
Patient's lower right								Patient's lower left							

Deciduous teeth									
Upper right					Upper left				
55	54	53	52	51	61	62	63	64	65
85	84	83	82	81	71	72	73	74	75
Lower right					Lower left				

- The quadrant numbers are 1, 2, 3 and 4 for permanent teeth and 5, 6, 7 and 8 for deciduous teeth.
- For permanent teeth, quadrant number 1 refers to the maxillary right quadrant, 2 to the maxillary left quadrant, 3 to the mandibular left quadrant and 4 to the mandibular right quadrant.
- For deciduous teeth, quadrant number 5 refers to the maxillary right quadrant, 6 to the maxillary left quadrant, 7 to the mandibular left quadrant and 8 to the mandibular right quadrant.
- Permanent teeth in the maxillary right quadrant are recorded as 11 to 18, in the maxillary left quadrant as 21 to 28, in the mandibular left quadrant as 31 to 38 and in the mandibular right quadrant as 41 to 48. For deciduous teeth, the notation is 51 to 55, 61 to 65, 71 to 75 and 81 to 85, respectively.

Specific examples of permanent teeth are as follows:

- Maxillary left second molar: 27 (pronounced as 'two-seven')
- Mandibular right first molar: 46 (pronounced as 'four-six')
- Maxillary right deciduous first molar: 54 (pronounced as 'five-four')

Specific examples of deciduous teeth are as follows:

- Maxillary left second deciduous molar: 65 (pronounced as 'six-five')
- Mandibular right first deciduous molar: 84 (pronounced as 'eight-four')

The FDI system has been designed for the computer use.

Tooth Eruption and Exfoliation Schedule for Deciduous Teeth

Tooth eruption and exfoliation schedule for deciduous teeth is represented in Box 1.1.

- Deciduous teeth appear in the mouth between the ages of 6 months and 2.5 years.

Box 1.1 Eruption and exfoliation dates of deciduous teeth

Tooth	Eruption date (months)	Exfoliation date (years)
Maxillary		
Central incisor	6–10	6–7
Lateral incisor	9–12	7–8
First molar	12–18	9–11
Canine	16–22	10–12
Second molar	24–32	10–12
Mandibular		
Central incisor	6–10	6–7
Lateral incisor	7–10	7–8
First molar	12–18	9–11
Canine	16–22	9–12
Second molar	20–32	10–12

Box 1.2 Eruption dates of permanent teeth

Tooth	Eruption date (years)
Maxillary	
First molar	6–7
Central incisor	7–8
Lateral incisor	8–9
First premolar	10–11
Second premolar	11–12
Canine	11–12
Second molar	12–13
Third molar	17–21
Mandibular	
First molar	6–7
Central incisor	6–7
Lateral incisor	7–8
First premolar	9–10
Second premolar	10–11
Canine	11–12
Second molar	11–13
Third molar	17–21

- The first teeth that erupt are the mandibular central incisors, at about 6 months.
- All deciduous teeth are shed by about 12 years.

Tooth Eruption Schedule for Permanent Teeth

Tooth eruption schedule for permanent teeth is represented in Box 1.2.

- Permanent teeth begin to appear in the oral cavity at the age of about 6 years. By the age of 12 years, permanent teeth generally replace all deciduous teeth.
- The first tooth to erupt is the first molar, at about 6 to 7 years of age (also called 6-year molar); the second molar erupts at about 12 years of age (the 12-year molar); and the third molar may erupt any time between 17 years and 21 years of age. Congenital absence of third molars can occur frequently.
- Delay in eruption dates can occur due to local or systemic factors. Details are provided in Chapter 12 (Delay and failure of tooth eruption).
- It is advisable to display the tooth eruption and shedding charts in the medical practitioner's clinics. Eruption delays of more than two years should be investigated. Such patients should be referred to dentists.

STRUCTURE OF THE TOOTH

The structure of the tooth is shown in Figure 1.4.

- A tooth consists of a crown and single or multiple roots.

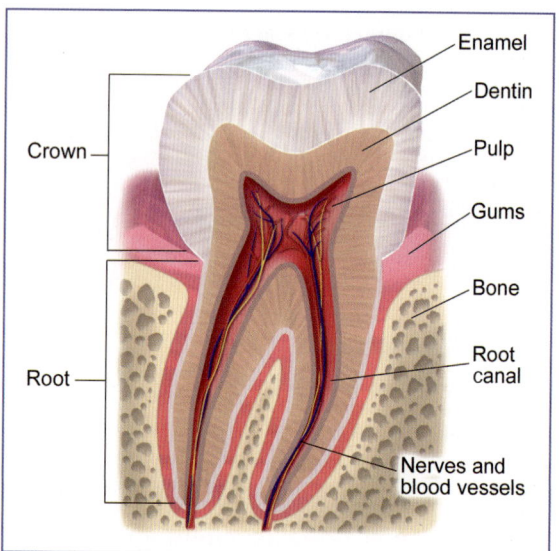

Figure 1.4 Anatomy of the tooth.
Reproduced with permission from: Blausen.com staff. Blausen gallery 2014. *Wikiversity Journal of Medicine*. doi:10.15347/wjm/2014.010. ISSN 20018762.

- The junction between the crown and root is called the cervical margin.
- Tooth comprises three hard tissues, namely enamel, dentine and cementum. Dental soft tissue is called dental pulp.
- Enamel, the hardest tissue in the body, is the visible part of the tooth in the mouth.
- Tooth enamel is avascular and nonsensitive. Dentin forms the main bulk of the tooth, which is present in both the crown and root(s) of the tooth.
- Dental pulp is located centrally in the pulp cavity (chamber) and in the root canals carrying neurovascular supply.
- Dentin and pulp make one functional unit and form the sensitive part of the tooth. Tooth root is covered by cementum.
- The root is anchored to the alveolar bone of the tooth socket by means of fibrous connective tissue called periodontal ligament.
- The alveolar bone is the part of the jaw that accommodates tooth sockets.

DESCRIPTIVE TERMINOLOGY USED FOR THE DIFFERENT ANATOMIC SURFACES OF THE TEETH

- Labial surface refers to the surface of the teeth (incisors and canines) that is closer to the lips.

- Buccal surface refers to the surface of the teeth (premolars and molars) that is closer to the cheek.
- Facial surface is a general term that collectively refers to both the buccal and labial surfaces.
- Lingual surface refers to the surface of the mandibular teeth that faces the tongue.
- Palatal surface of the tooth refers to the surface of the maxillary teeth that faces the palate.
- Interproximal surface refers to the contacting surfaces between two adjacent teeth.
- Mesial surface refers to the interproximal surface closest to the midline.
- Distal surface refers to the interproximal surface away from the midline.
- Occlusal surface refers to the chewing surface of the posterior teeth.
- Incisal surface refers to the biting surface of the anterior teeth.
- Apical means toward the root.
- Coronal means toward the crown of the tooth.

SUGGESTED READINGS

Prabhu SR. Intraoral clinical examination. In: Prabhu SR, editor. *Textbook of Oral Diagnosis*. New Delhi, India: Oxford University Press; 2007. pp. 42–58 and 78–94.

World Health Organization. *Oral Health Surveys: Basic Methods*. 5th ed. Geneva, Switzerland: World Health Organization; 2013.

Medscape [Internet]. Atlanta (GA): WebMD LLC; c2005-2016. *Mouth Anatomy: Overview*; 2015 [updated 2015 Sept 11]. Available from: http://emedicine.medscape.com/article/1899122-overview

Wikipedia [Internet]. San Francisco, (CA): Wikimedia Foundation Inc. *FDI World Dental Federation Notation*; 2015 [updated 2015 Nov 24]. Available from: https://en.wikipedia.org/wiki/FDI_World_Dental_Federation_notation

Chapter 2

Diagnostic approaches to common oral and dental symptoms

S. R. Prabhu

HISTORY OF PAIN, SWELLINGS AND ULCERS

Pain is an unpleasant sensation of varying intensity and is a symptom. Tenderness is a sign of pain.

Pain History

Pain history is recorded by using the following features:

- Site of pain: Superficial/deep/diffuse/localised.
- Time and mode of onset of pain: Whether pain began suddenly or insidiously.
- Severity of pain: Pain can be expressed as mild, moderate or severe. Use a pain scale ranging 0–10, where 0 indicates no pain and 10 indicates very severe pain.
- Nature of pain: Aching (chronic), stabbing (sudden, severe and sharp), burning, throbbing (acute abscess), electric-like (neuralgic), gripping, gnawing, etc.
- Frequency of pain: How often? Is there any trigger?
- Progression of pain: Severe at the beginning and may remain or disappear after a while or may increase in severity.
- Duration of pain: Time elapsed since the onset of pain.
- Relieving factors: What relieves pain? Posture? Hot or cold drink?
- Factors exacerbating pain: What makes pain worse — lying down or bending over?
- Radiation of pain to other site: For example, cardiac pain that radiates to the jaw.

History of Swellings

History of a swelling is recorded by probing the following features:

- When was the swelling first noticed?
- What made the patient notice the swelling?
- Is the swelling painful?
- Is the swelling interfering with normal functions?
- Has the swelling changed its size since it was first noticed?
- Does the swelling ever change its size during normal activity?
- Has the patient ever had any other swellings?
- Has the patient had any other associated symptom?
- What according to the patient caused the swelling?

History of Ulcers

History of ulcers is recorded by probing the following features:

- Where was the ulcer first noticed?
- What made the patient notice the ulcer?
- Is the ulcer painful?
- Is the ulcer interfering with normal functions?
- Has the ulcer changed since it was first noticed?
- Has the patient ever had any other ulcers?
- Has the patient had any other associated local or systemic symptoms?
- What according to the patient caused the ulcer?
- Is the ulcer persistent or recurrent?

EXAMINATION OF SWELLINGS AND ULCERS

Examination of the Swelling

- Inspection and palpation:
  - Location
  - Size
  - Shape
  - Colour and temperature
  - Pain and tenderness
  - Crepitus
  - Movement
  - Surface texture
  - Margin
  - Associated swellings

Examination of an Ulcer

- Inspection:
  - Size and shape (Is the ulcer variable, oval or linear?)
  - Number (Is the ulcer single or multiple in number?)
  - Position/location (Is the ulcer present at the site of injury, nonkeratinised regions, keratinised regions or gingival papillae?)
  - Edge of the ulcer (Is the edge of the ulcer undermined, raised, punched out, everted or sloping?)
  - Floor of the ulcer (Is the floor of the ulcer granulation tissue, black, yellowish or yellowish white?)
  - Discharge, if any (Does the ulcer have any purulent discharge?)
  - Surrounding area (Is the surrounding area of the ulcer a red halo, glossy or oedematous?)
- Palpation:
  - Tenderness
  - Margin and edges of an ulcer (raised/everted/firm)
  - Base of the ulcer
  - Depth of the ulcer
  - Bleeding in the ulcer
  - Relationship of ulcer with deeper structures
  - Surrounding skin or mucous membrane
  - Association with regional lymph nodes

Descriptive Terms Used for Oral Mucosal Pathology

- Lesion: A lesion is a general term used for a single, small area of skin or mucosal disease.
- Macule: An area of colour change that is 1.5 cm or less in diameter. This is a flat lesion.
- Patch: An area of colour change that is larger than 1.5 cm in diameter. This is nonpalpable.
- Papule: A small palpable lesion that is 1.5 cm or less in diameter.
- Plaque: A palpable lesion that is larger than 5 mm in diameter.
- Nodule: A spherical solid lesion that is larger than 5 mm in diameter.
- Vesicle: A fluid-filled elevation that is less than 5 mm in diameter.
- Pustule: Accumulation of pus in a skin/mucosal vesicle.
- Bulla: A fluid-filled elevation that is larger than 5 mm in diameter.
- Erosion: Loss of epithelium or epidermis.
- Ulcer: Loss of epidermis/epithelium and dermis/corium.
- Petechia: A small (<2 mm) haemorrhagic papule.
- Scale: Dry and flat flake of keratin.
- Stria: A linear elevation.
- Tumour: Any localised tissue enlargement (interchangeably used for neoplastic growth).
- Atrophy: Thinning of the skin/mucosa.
- Fissure: A linear slit.
- Crust: Dried blood covering an ulcerated area of the skin. It is also called scab.
- Pseudomembrane: A crust in a moist area.
- Scar: Permanent replacement of lost normal tissue by fibrous tissue.
- Fistula: An abnormal passage between two epithelium-lined structures (e.g., oroantral fistula).
- Sinus: Blind-ended track (e.g., a dental abscess opening into the vestibule).

Diagnostic Tests Used in Dental Practice

- Thermal and electrical tooth vitality tests
- Percussion of teeth for tenderness
- Tooth mobility tests
- Transillumination test for tooth cracks and interproximal caries
- Magnification loupe or video camera for the detection of caries and restoration cracks
- Clinical photography for recording, follow-up and medico-legal purposes
- Clinical methods: Inspection and palpation for swellings, growth of mucosal lesions and temporomandibular joint (TMJ) pathology
- Auscultation of the TMJ for TMJ pathology
- Radiography (conventional) for tooth and jaw bone structures and pathology
- Diagnostic local anaesthesia test to localise dental pain
- Biopsy (e.g., excision, incision, needle and aspiration) for soft and hard tissue lesions
- Toluidine blue staining for screening oral dysplastic lesions

- Microbiology for microbe identification, culture studies and antibiotic sensitivity tests for infectious oral diseases (samples: swabs/smears)
- Haematology: Full blood count, differential count, platelet count, haemoglobin, ferritin and erythrocyte sedimentation rate and other relevant haematological investigations, as required
- Coagulation screening (international normalised ratio/prothrombin time, activated partial thromboplastin time, factor VIII, fibrinogen level, etc.) for dental patients with blood coagulation defects
- Blood film for abnormalities of red blood cell morphology (for different types of anaemia)
- Blood chemistry for estimation of acid phosphatase, alkaline phosphatase, calcium, phosphate and glucose for patients with endocrine and metabolic diseases presenting with oral manifestations
- Immunological tests for immune-related diseases (e.g., Sjögren's syndrome) and immunohistochemistry for patients with pemphigus and pemphigoid presenting with oral manifestations
- Urinalysis for urinary sugar, albumin, bilirubin, red blood cells and casts

Radiographic Views Used in Dentistry

Intraoral Views

- Periapical radiographs
- Bitewing radiographs
- Occlusal radiographs

Extraoral Views

- Lateral oblique view
- Occipitomental view
- Posteroanterior view of the skull
- Posteroanterior view of the mandible
- Reverse Towne's projection
- Submentovertex projection
- Lateral cephalometric view
- Pantomographic view (orthopantomograph)

Indications for pantomographic views

- To obtain a broad view of both the maxillary and mandibular teeth and their supporting structures
- To evaluate eruption patterns, growth and development
- To detect diseases and lesions affecting the teeth and jaw bones
- To evaluate trauma such as tooth or jaw fractures
- Assessment of the TMJ, tooth impactions and periodontal disease
- Assessment of the floor, posterior wall and anterior wall of the maxillary sinus

Advanced Imaging Tests

- Computed tomography for major salivary gland disease, sinus pathology, etc.

- Magnetic resonance imaging for major salivary gland diseases
- Sialography for major salivary gland diseases

Details of the above-listed tests are beyond the scope of this chapter.

Patients with systemic diseases with oral manifestations often seek medical consultation before consulting dentists. A close interdisciplinary consultation with the help of relevant test results is necessary in these circumstances.

SUGGESTED READINGS

Cawson RA, Odell EW. Principles of investigation and diagnosis. In: Cawson RA, Odell EW, editors. *Cawson's Essentials of Oral Pathology and Oral Medicine*. 8th ed. Edinburgh, Scotland: Churchill Livingstone; 2008. pp. 1–17.

Prabhu SR. Diagnostic approaches to common oral symptoms. In: Prabhu SR, editor. *Textbook of Oral Medicine*. New Delhi, India: Oxford University Press; 2004. pp. 1–11.

Birnbaum W, Dunne SM. In: Birnbaum W, Dunne SM, editors. *Oral Diagnosis: The Clinician's Guide*. Oxford, U.K.: Wright; 2000. pp. 33–71.

Chapter 3

Anatomical variants and normal structures often mistaken as pathological lesions

S. R. Prabhu

FORDYCE GRANULES

Definition/Description

- Fordyce granules are whitish granular lesions located superficially in the labial and buccal mucosae.

Cause

- Ectopic collection of sebaceous glands.

Clinical Features

- Visible as white or cream spots on the labial or buccal mucosa. These are asymptomatic.
- An image of Fordyce granules is shown in Chapter 1 (Figure 1.1).

Diagnosis

- Clinical grounds.

Management

- No treatment is required.

FOLIATE PAPILLAE

Definition/Description

- The foliate papillae are vertical folds and grooves located on the posterolateral surfaces of the tongue.

Cause

- Normal anatomical structures.

Clinical Features

- Seen as vertical folds located on the posterolateral surfaces of the tongue. These are occasionally mistaken for inflammatory diseases. Foliate papillae have taste buds located on their walls.

Diagnosis

• Clinical grounds.

Management

• No treatment is required.

LINGUAL TONSILS

Definition/Description

• Rounded masses of dense, nodular lymphatic tissue that cover the dorsal surface at the base of the tongue posterior to circumvallate papillae.

Cause

• Normal structures.

Clinical Features

• Usually asymptomatic but may enlarge with viral infections. Unilateral lingual tonsils are sometimes mistaken for carcinomas.

Diagnosis

• Clinical grounds.

Management

• No treatment is necessary.

LYMPHOID AGGREGATES

Definition/Description

• Lymphoid aggregates are collection of normal or hyperplastic lymphoid tissues located anywhere in the oral cavity but are more commonly seen on the lateral surface of the tongue, oropharynx and soft palate.

Cause

• Normal structures.

Clinical Features

• Hyperplastic lymphoid tissues on the posterolateral surface of the tongue (Figure 3.1). When inflamed due to bacterial or viral infections, lymphoid aggregates may become symptomatic. Occasionally, hyperplastic lymphoid aggregates are mistaken for carcinomas or lymphomas.

Diagnosis

• Clinical grounds.

Management

• No treatment is required.

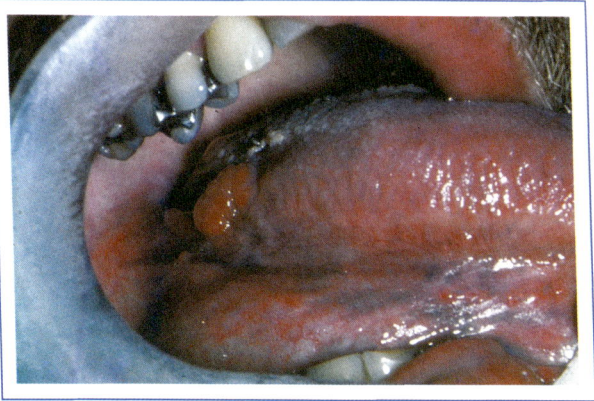

Figure 3.1 Lymphoid aggregate located on the posterolateral surface of the tongue. This may often be misdiagnosed as cancerous growth. *Courtesy*: S. R. Prabhu.

CIRCUMVALLATE PAPILLAE

Definition/Description

- The circumvallate papillae are 8 to 12 dome-shaped structures situated on the dorsum of the tongue immediately in front of the foramen caecum and sulcus terminalis.

Cause

- Normal structures.

Clinical Features

- Eight to twelve dome-shaped structures on the posterior part of the dorsum of the tongue (Figure 3.2). Sometimes, these may become prominent and may be mistaken as disease.

Diagnosis

- Clinical grounds.

Management

- No treatment is required.

PAROTID PAPILLA

Definition/Description

- Parotid papilla is the projection seen at the oral opening of the duct of the parotid salivary gland located in the buccal mucosa, opposite to the second upper-left and -right molar teeth.

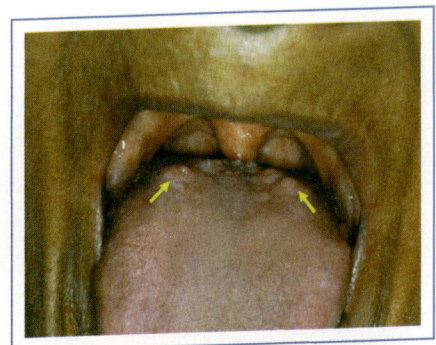

Figure 3.2 Circumvallate papillae (arrows) at the junction of the anterior two-thirds and posterior one-third of the dorsum of the tongue. Reproduced with permission from: Ramadas K, Lucas E, Thomas G, et al. *A Digital Manual for the Early Diagnosis of Oral Neoplasia*. IARC, Lyon, 2008. Available from: http://screening.iarc.fr/atlasoral.php?lang=1

Cause
- Normal structure.

Clinical Features
- Small asymptomatic mucosal projections of normal colour on the buccal mucosa, opposite to the maxillary second molars.

Diagnosis
- Clinical grounds.

Management
- No treatment is required.

HAIRY TONGUE

Definition/Description
- Elongated, hair-like white or black structures on the dorsum of the tongue.

Cause
- Accumulation of excess keratin on the filiform papillae of the dorsal surface of the tongue leads to the formation of elongated strands that resemble hair.

Clinical Features
- The colour of the hair-like projections on the tongue can range from white or tan to black (Figure 3.3). Hairy tongue is associated with smoking, poor oral hygiene and the use of tobacco, coffee and

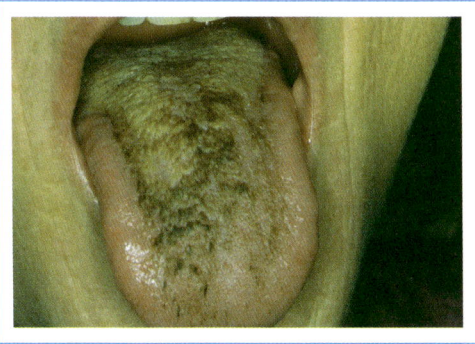

Figure 3.3 Hairy tongue. Brown or black colour may be due to coffee or tobacco stains.
Courtesy: Nagamani Narayana.

certain antibiotics. Most patients are asymptomatic, but some complain of halitosis or abnormal taste.

Diagnosis

• Clinical appearance.

Management

• No treatment is required. Patient should be advised to carry out gentle daily debridement with a 'tongue scraper' or soft toothbrush.

FISSURED TONGUE (SCROTAL TONGUE)

Definition/Description

• Fissured tongue is also known as scrotal tongue or lingua plicata. It is characterised by the presence of fissures on the dorsum of the tongue.

Cause

• Unknown. Heredity may play a role.

Clinical Features

• Fissured tongue can be found in healthy individuals. It is characterised by the presence of fissures on the dorsum of tongue, which extend from the midline to the sides (Figure 3.4).
• In majority of patients, fissured tongue is asymptomatic. Occasionally, tongue may become sore because of the food particles lodging in the fissures.

Diagnosis

• Clinical grounds.

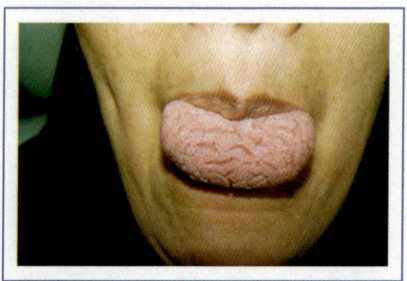

Figure 3.4 Fissured tongue.
Courtesy: David Wilson.

Management

- No treatment is required.

VARICOSITIES

Definition/Description

- Oral varicosities refer to abnormally dilated veins.

Cause

- Possibly due to the weakening of the vessel walls in the elderly.

Clinical Features

- Purple-coloured dots, nodules or tortuous veins are usually seen in the elderly on the ventral surface of the tongue (Figure 3.5). Labial and buccal mucosae may also be involved. On the lips, varicosities may resemble mucocoeles.

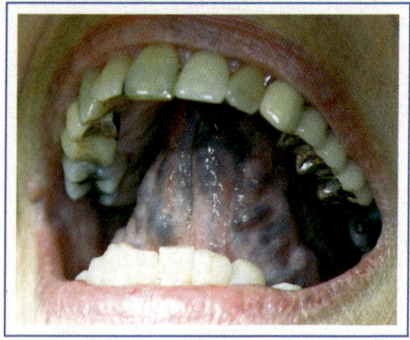

Figure 3.5 Lingual varicosities on the ventral surface of the tongue.
Courtesy: Nagamani Narayana.

Diagnosis

- Clinical appearance.

Management

- Treatment is not required.

LEUKOEDEMA

Definition/Description

- Leukoedema refers to a bilateral diffuse milky-white translucent whitening of the buccal mucosa, commonly seen in black races.

Cause

- Unknown. The collection of intercellular oedema in the spinous layer is responsible for the whitish translucency.

Clinical Features

- Buccal mucosa has a diffuse cloudy translucent appearance (Figure 3.6). Soft palate, tongue and floor of the mouth may also be involved. Commonly seen in persons of African origin.

Diagnosis

- Clinical examination. Translucency usually disappears or fades on stretching the mucosa.

Management

- No treatment is necessary.

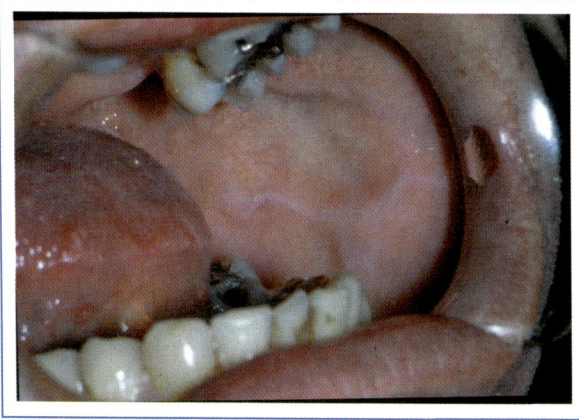

Figure 3.6   Leukoedema seen as a milky-white translucent film on the buccal mucosa.
Courtesy: David Wilson.

TORI OF THE PALATE AND MANDIBLE (TORUS PALATINUS AND TORUS MANDIBULARIS)

Definition/Description

- Tori are exostoses located in the midline of the palate (torus palatinus) or in the lingual alveolus in the premolar region of the mandible (torus mandibularis).

Cause

- Unknown. Genetic factors may play a role.

Clinical Features

- Palatal tori are usually located in the midline of the palate. They may be seen as a single nodule or may appear lobulated (Figure 3.7 A). Occasionally, exostoses can also be seen over the maxillary canine and premolar root region on the facial surfaces. Mandibular tori are located above the attachment of mylohyoid muscle (Figure 3.7 B). Tori are subjected to trauma, which may cause mucosal ulceration or infection.

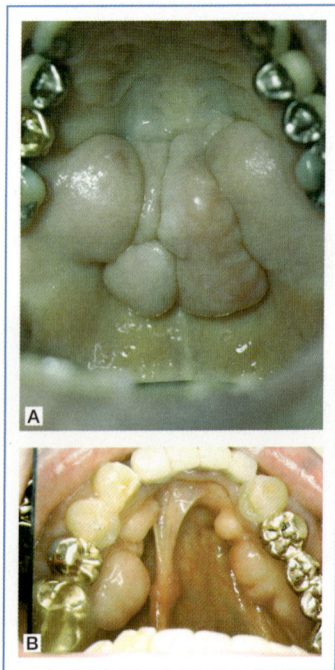

Figure 3.7   (A) Torus palatinus and (B) Torus mandibularis.
Courtesy: Nagamani Narayana.

Diagnosis

- Clinical grounds.

Management

- Tori usually do not require any treatment. However, when fabrication of lower dentures pose problems, surgical removal may be necessary.

RACIAL PIGMENTATION

Definition/Description

- Racial pigmentation, also known as physiological pigmentation, is commonly seen in individuals of African origin.

Cause

- A normal physiological process.

Clinical Features

- Pigmented patches of the gingiva and oral mucosa are brown to black in colour (Figure 3.8) and often mimic the pigmentation of Addison's disease, smoker's melanosis and drug-related pigmentation. Pigmentation is usually diffuse and symmetrical.

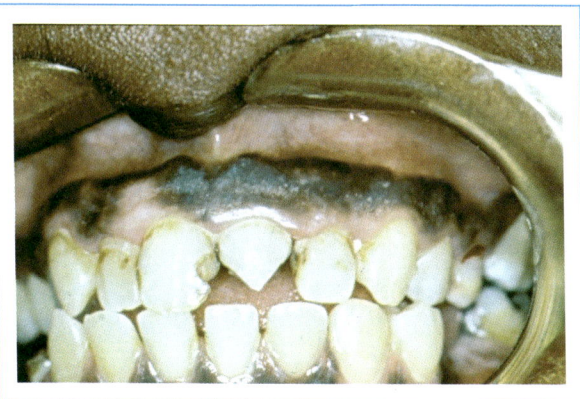

Figure 3.8 Physiological (racial) pigmentation of the gingiva. *Courtesy*: S. R. Prabhu.

Diagnosis

- Clinical grounds.

Management

- No treatment is required.

SUGGESTED READINGS

Migliorati CA, Panagakos FS, editors. *Diagnosis and Management of Oral Lesions and Conditions: A Resource Handbook for the Clinician.* Rijeka, Croatia: InTech; 2014 [cited 2015 Jan 03]. Available from: http://dx.doi.org/10.5772/57597

Dunlap CL, Barker BF. *A Guide to Common Oral Lesions.* Kansas City, MO: UMKC School of Dentistry; 2003 [2015 Mar 13]. Available from: http://dentistry.umkc.edu/Practicing_Communities/asset/OralLesions.pdf

Part II

Presenting complaints related to the teeth, jaws and temporomandibular joint

Chapter 4

Orofacial pain of dental origin

A. Sadr, S. Manickam and S. R. Prabhu

GENERAL CONSIDERATIONS

History and Examination

- In majority of patients with orofacial pain, the cause is local. Most problems are identified by history and clinical examination.
- Key points to remember while taking history of orofacial pain include the following:
  - ◆ **Location of the pain:** Is the pain localised or diffuse? If the patient points to the location of pain with one finger, the cause of pain may be of dental origin or of neuralgic type. Pain in such circumstances does not cross the midline. On the contrary, diffuse pain may be a feature of atypical facial pain that often crosses the midline.
  - ◆ **Character of the pain:** Is the pain 'sharp', 'dull', 'aching', 'throbbing' or 'shooting'? Pain severity should be rated by the patient on a scale of zero (no pain) to ten (most severe pain that the patient has ever experienced).
  - ◆ **Duration of the pain:** Information on the duration of pain is useful in the diagnostic workup. Transient pain lasting only a few seconds is a feature of dentin sensitivity due to exposed dentin, whereas the pain from dental pulp lasts longer. Neuralgic pain is of short duration and lasts only a few seconds, and the patient is generally free from pain in between attacks. Atypical facial pain is persistent.
  - ◆ **Frequency and periodicity of the pain:** Patient should be asked whether the pain occurs at specific times or with events. Pain of the temporomandibular joint disorder is severe in the morning on waking. The pain of maxillary sinusitis aggravates by lying down. Pain of salivary stone in the duct increases in intensity during mealtime, when saliva is stimulated.
  - ◆ **Precipitating and relieving factors:** Heat is known to aggravate dental pain; touching a trigger zone may precipitate pain of neuralgia; stress may worsen atypical facial pain and alcohol may precipitate migrainous neuralgia.
  - ◆ **Associated features:** If jaw swelling is associated with the pain, dental abscess should be suspected. In migraine, patient may complain of nausea and vomiting.

Characteristics of Dental Pain and Its Possible Causes

- *Sharp, short and shooting pain:* This type of pain may be caused by dental caries, dentin exposure due to attrition, abrasion or erosion, split cusp, fractured restoration or fractured tooth. Patients complain of pain only when a stimulus (hot, cold or sweet) is applied. In majority of cases, the pain is localised. Desensitising toothpaste and fluoride mouth rinses are recommended for these patients.
- *Dull, throbbing and persistent dental pain:* This type of pain is caused by several conditions. Examples include dental caries with or without existing restoration, fracture of the tooth involving the pulp, periapical inflammation (apical periodontitis), food impaction and pericoronitis. Pain aggravates by lying down. Heat makes the dental pain worse, whereas cold may alleviate the pain. Recommended treatment includes root canal treatment or extraction of the offending tooth.
  - ◆ Acute pain is the most common form of symptom, which in most cases is of dental origin and is easy to diagnose and manage, provided that appropriate diagnostic steps are followed by the clinician.
  - ◆ Chronic pain can be neuropathic, psychogenic or somatic in origin, which can be difficult to diagnose. Chronic pain of nonodontogenic source can often mimic toothache and pose diagnostic difficulty.

Examinations and Tests Used for the Diagnosis of Pain of Dental Origin

- *Pulp sensitivity tests:* An ice stick or dry ice or electric pulp tester can be placed on the cervical third of the tooth crown. Carbon dioxide snow test and heat test are the other methods used for thermal testing in dental clinic. A response to the stimulus indicates that the pulpal tissue is capable of transmitting nerve impulses. No response indicates pulp necrosis.
- *Percussion test:* By using the handle of an instrument, the tooth is tapped in the longitudinal axis. A painful response indicates possible periapical inflammation.
- *Probing:* Placing a fine, blunt probe gently into the gingival sulcus surrounding the tooth enables the assessment of the gingival health. Sulcus depth greater than 3 to 4 mm indicates gum disease.
- *Tooth mobility test:* Holding a tooth firmly between fingers from the buccal and lingual sides and gently moving it in both directions enables the mobility of the tooth to be assessed. Mobility less than 0.5 mm is normal. Visible movement indicates loss of bone support around the root of the tooth.
- *Palpation:* Gentle palpation around the area of concern may elicit tenderness and help in identifying the type and extent of swelling.
- *Radiographical examination:* Radiographical findings can assist the clinician to localise the cause of dental pain, for example, a tooth with caries or periapical pathology.

Special note:

Effective pain management begins with an accurate diagnosis and an appropriate plan using the principles of the '3Ds' — diagnosis, dental treatment and drugs.

Diagnosis: First, the disease and its cause must always be determined.

Dental treatment: Once the diagnosis has been reached, the appropriate dental treatment should be provided.

Drugs: The final consideration is whether any drugs are required. This decision should be deferred until the response to the dental treatment has been reviewed.

COMMON CONDITIONS AETIOLOGICALLY ASSOCIATED WITH PAIN OF DENTAL ORIGIN

Dentin Hypersensitivity

Definition/Description

- Dentin hypersensitivity is a painful response to hot and cold stimuli. It results from the exposed dentin.

Cause

- Dental (dentin) caries, faulty tooth brushing/flossing resulting in tooth abrasion, fracture of the tooth, defective restoration with leaky margins, gingival recession, recent metal restoration without a lining, acid erosion due to gastroesophageal reflux disease, eating disorders, chronic alcoholism and consumption of acidic beverages. Stimulus promotes sensitivity by causing the movement of fluid in the dentinal tubules, which in turn affects odontoblasts and the accompanying nerve endings, thereby causing pain.

Clinical Features

- Sharp pain related to hot, cold, sweet, sour or touches.
- When stimuli are absent, pain is not felt.
- Pain is localised.
- Examination may reveal gingival recession, fractured tooth, leaky margins of the restoration and tooth wear (attrition, abrasion or erosion).
- Tooth brushing or scratching with an instrument may cause sensitivity in the tooth.

Diagnosis

- A dental history to identify the local cause.
- Medical history to rule out (or confirm) acid reflux disease. This condition can cause erosions of the palatal surfaces of maxillary anterior teeth.
- Radiographs are helpful in detecting the local cause.
- Identifying the offending tooth/teeth: Isolate teeth by using cotton rolls. Blow cold air, use ethyl chloride on a cotton bud or apply hot gutta-percha (GP) to the tooth/teeth. These tests yield positive results.
- Electric pulp test is within normal limits.
- Percussion test is within normal limits.

Management

- Advise the patient to avoid food and drinks that provoke sensitivity.
- Antibiotics are not required.
- Advise the patient to use toothpastes that contain 5% potassium. If the pain is very severe, local anaesthetic (LA) administration will help in providing temporary relief.
- Refer the patient to a dentist. Dentists may carry out mechanical or chemical obstruction of dentinal tubules by using potassium oxalate, strontium chloride and sodium fluoride or stannous fluoride applications.
- The pulp condition in dentin hypersensitivity is reversible.

Reversible Pulpitis (Hyperaemia of the Dental Pulp)

Definition/Description

- Reversible pulpitis refers to mild inflammation of the dental pulp and is characterised by pain that lasts for a short period of time and disappears after the stimulus is removed.
- Reversible pulpitis is also called hyperaemia of the dental pulp.

Cause

- Large coronal restorations or carious lesions that are close to the pulp.

Clinical Features

- The pain is intense, unilateral and of immediate onset to thermal changes, especially to cold or sweet stimuli. Pain may remain for 5 to 10 minutes but mostly disappears on withdrawal of the irritant.
- Affected tooth responds to the stimulation of the electric pulp tester at low level of current, indicating a low pain threshold.
- The tooth may show a deep carious lesion, large restoration or restoration with defective margins.

Diagnosis

- Look for faulty restorations or caries.
- Air blast or application of cold may give rise to sensitivity.
- Percussion of the offending tooth does not elicit tenderness.
- Vitality (thermal) tests present exaggerated response in the affected tooth in comparison with the adjacent normal tooth.
- Tooth is of normal colour.
- Radiographs may show extensive caries or large restorations close to the dental pulp. No periapical changes are seen in X-rays.
- Both clinical and radiographical evidences of periapical involvement are absent.

Management

- The condition is reversible if the irritant is removed before the pulp is severely damaged.
- Advise the patient to avoid food and drinks that provoke sensitivity.
- Antibiotics are not required.

- Administer LA if the pain is severe.
- Dressing of the carious lesion with a sedative filling, such as zinc oxide eugenol paste, is effective. This is possible in the medical clinic setting.
- Refer the patient to a dental practitioner, who may choose to dress the deep cavities by using a calcium hydroxide lining and a sedative filling.
- If primary cause is not corrected, extensive pulpitis may result in death of the pulp.
- Dentist may choose restorative/endodontic treatment, depending on the extent of the pulpal involvement.

Acute Pulpitis (Symptomatic Irreversible Pulpitis)

Definition/Description

- Acute pulpitis refers to inflammation of the pulp, which results in severe pain in the tooth.
- Symptoms and signs of acute pulpitis (symptomatic irreversible pulpitis) indicate that the vital inflamed pulp is incapable of healing.

Cause

- Large restorations, extensive carious lesions and tooth fracture.

Clinical Features

- Sharp pain, which may be spasmodic and may become dull with time.
- Pain is poorly localised.
- Initial involvement elicits exaggerated response to hot stimulus (food/drinks), which may last for 15 seconds or more even after the removal of the stimulus.
- Patient may or may not have pain on percussion or palpation.
- Application of cold may provide temporary relief.
- Pain is worst at night and on lying down.

Diagnosis

- Vitality test: Initially exaggerated response to heat and electric pulp test. This test is usually carried out by dentists.
- Radiography: No periapical changes are noticed. Occasionally, condensing osteitis may be seen.
- A diagnostic LA administration is helpful to locate the offending tooth.

Management

- Use of painkillers: Sedative dressing may be helpful.
- Advise the patient to avoid food and drinks that provoke pain.
- Antibiotics are not required.
- Administer LA if the pain is severe.
- Dressing of the carious lesion with a sedative filling, such as zinc oxide eugenol paste, is effective. This is possible in the medical clinic setting.

- Refer the patient to a dental practitioner, who may choose to carry out restorative treatment.
- If carious exposure has occurred, dentist may decide to perform pulpotomy, pulpectomy or extraction of the tooth, depending on the extent of caries.

Chronic Pulpitis (Asymptomatic Irreversible Pulpitis)

Definition/Description

- Chronic pulpitis is the chronic inflammation of the dental pulp, resulting in irreversible pulpitis.

Cause

- Large amalgam restorations, broken restorations or recurrent caries under a restoration. Chronic pulpitis may also develop as a sequel of acute pulpitis.

Clinical Features

- Pain is not a prominent feature. Mild, dull intermittent ache may occur.
- The tooth is not tender to percussion unless the pulpal inflammation has spread beyond the root apex into the periapical tissues.
- Patients with chronic pulpitis can withstand pain for weeks or months.
- Pain may aggravate on changing the position, such as bending over or lying down.
- Pain is diffuse and can cause referred pain.
- Chronic pulpitis can cause abscess formation in the pulp or at the periapical area.

Diagnosis

- Pulp vitality test and radiographs are useful diagnostic tools for chronic pulpitis.
- Electric pulp tester requires maximum electrical discharge to elicit pain or discomfort because of degeneration of the nerves.
- Hot drinks may increase the discomfort.
- Radiographs are useful in revealing interproximal or recurrent caries under a restoration.
- Radiographs may show no periapical changes or may reveal a radiopacity because of condensing osteitis (sclerosed bone) in the cancellous bone surrounding the roots of the offending tooth. This may be due to chronic low-grade infection derived from the pulp.

Management

- Analgesics are effective for pain relief.
- Refer the patient to a dentist. Dental treatment includes pulp extirpation and endodontic therapy or extraction of the offending tooth.

Pulp Polyp (Chronic Hyperplastic Pulpitis)

Definition/Description

- Pulp polyp, also known as chronic hyperplastic pulpitis, is characterised by the presence of hyperplastic pulp tissue in the form of a polyp in a large tooth cavity derived from grossly carious tooth. The condition is an example of chronic inflammation of the pulp that leads to the formation of granulation tissue.
- It is a persistent inflammatory reaction in the pulp, with little or no constitutional symptoms.

Cause

- Chronic caries with an open cavity, exposing the chronically inflamed and hyperplastic pulp tissue to the oral cavity. This mostly occurs in children and young adults with high degree of tissue resistance and blood supply.

Clinical Features

- Common in primary molars.
- Patients generally do not complain of pain. However, sometimes, mild pain or discomfort in the offending tooth may be present.
- Patients complain of a soft pinkish-red mass of tissue protruding from the open carious occlusal surface of the tooth (Figure 4.1). The soft tissue mass shows a tendency to bleed when accidentally traumatised.
- Pulp polyp is not sensitive to touch because hyperplastic tissue lacks nerve endings.
- Pulp polyp should not be confused with hyperplastic gingiva that extends into the carious cavity.

Diagnosis

- Clinical examination.
- Radiographs will confirm the extent of the carious lesion.
- Generally, the apical foramen is large, allowing a good blood flow to the pulp.

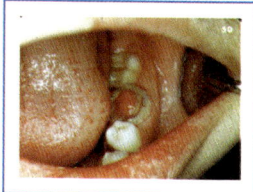

Figure 4.1   Chronic hyperplastic pulpitis presenting as a pink fleshy mass (pulp polyp) in the centre of a grossly carious lower first molar.
Courtesy: Atieh Sadr.

Management

- Refer the patient to a dental practitioner.
- Dental practitioners may choose to remove the polyp and carry out root canal therapy or extract the offending tooth.

Cracked Tooth Syndrome

Definition/Description

- Cracked tooth syndrome may involve cracks in different parts of the tooth, such as enamel only; enamel and dentin only; enamel, dentin and pulp; root; or crown and root.

Cause

- Cracks in the teeth occur as a result of an unexpected encounter with a hard object during mastication (such as a piece of bone) or from a blow to the chin.
- Large metallic mesio-occluso-distal restorations may cause crack in the tooth because of their expansion during mastication.

Clinical Features

- Sharp localised pain on biting food.
- Because the pain is intermittent, patient may not seek treatment for a considerable time.
- Pain on release of the biting force is worse than the pain on application of the biting force (rebound phenomenon).
- Sensitivity to cold and heat may occur due to stimulation of pulp through the fracture line. If cracked tooth involves pulp, symptoms are severe. This may lead to reversible or irreversible pulpitis.

Diagnosis

- Biting on cotton wool or a wooden spatula elicits pain.
- Painting the tooth with a dye (methylene blue or tincture of iodine) and washing it will retain the dye in the crack (diagnostic).
- Radiographs generally do not reveal cracks. If pulpitis is suspected, pulp vitality tests need to be conducted.

Management

- History is important to identify the cause.
- Advise the patient to avoid foods that provoke pain.
- Appropriate analgesics are recommended for pain relief. Antibiotics are not required.
- If the pain is very severe, LA administration may be necessary.
- Refer the patient to a dentist.
- Dentists may prefer to use a full crown if pulp is not involved. If dental pulp is involved, endodontic therapy and preparation of full crown are carried out.
- Extraction of the tooth may be necessary if the involvement of the crack is extensive.

A detailed discussion on tooth fracture and its management is provided in Chapter 30 (Oral and dental trauma).

Acute Apical Periodontitis (Symptomatic Apical Periodontitis)

Definition/Description

- Acute apical periodontitis is the inflammation of the periodontal tissues, causing painful response to biting, percussion or palpation.

Cause

- Infection from the dental pulp, severe trauma of the periodontal tissues, large restorations or carious lesions.

Clinical Features

- History of pain on biting.
- Excruciating pain lasting for a few days.
- Pain is localised and the patient is able to identify the offending tooth.
- Tooth is very tender to touch.
- Constant throbbing or pounding pain.
- Tooth may be in supraoccclusion.

Diagnosis

- Tender tooth on percussion (apical direction).
- Depending on the stage of the disease, radiographs may or may not show any changes in the width of the periodontal ligament.

Management

- Systemic anti-inflammatory medications and analgesics are effective in relieving symptoms.
- Under LA, correction of occlusion may become necessary.
- Root canal treatment of the offending tooth is necessary for majority of cases.

Chronic Apical Periodontitis (Asymptomatic Apical Periodontitis)

Definition/Description

- Chronic apical periodontitis occurs as a result of pulpal necrosis and leads to asymptomatic inflammation of apical periodontium.

Cause

- Large restorations, defective root canal treatment and pulp necrosis.

Clinical Features

- None to mild pain on percussion.
- Radiographs show periapical radiolucency (indicating a periapical granuloma or a cyst).
- Tooth may be discoloured due to pulp necrosis.

Diagnosis

- Percussion: Mild tenderness and a dull percussion note.
- Vitality: Usually negative. Heat may cause a mild response (by expansion of gases in the pulp chamber).

- Radiographs: Periapical radiolucency is present. Large restoration or inadequate root filling may be evident and thin radiopaque line or zone of sclerotic bone is sometimes seen outlining the radiolucent lesion.
- Long-standing lesion may show varying degrees of root resorption.

Management

- Refer the patient to a dentist, who would perform endodontic treatment. If conventional endodontic treatment has failed or cannot be attempted, retreatment or apical surgery is indicated.

Acute Apical Abscess

Definition/Description

- Acute apical abscess is an acute inflammatory response to pulpal infection, resulting in pus formation and swelling.

Cause

- Infection and necrosis of the dental pulp, traumatic injury or irritation of periapical tissues due to endodontic procedure.

Clinical Features

- Spontaneous pain of rapid onset and swelling.
- Extreme tenderness of the tooth to pressure and percussion.
- Pus formation and swelling of the associated tissues.
- Occasional cervical lymphadenopathy and fever.

Diagnosis

- Thermal testing is negative, indicating pulp necrosis.
- Radiography: Widened periodontal space may be seen at the time of presentation.

Management

- Systemic antibiotics and analgesics are necessary.
- Refer the patient to a dentist. Establishment of drainage either through root canal or by incision and drainage of the fluctuant abscess is necessary.
- Depending on the extent of the abscess, root canal treatment or extraction of the offending tooth is necessary.

Chronic Apical Abscess (Suppurative Apical Periodontitis or Phoenix Abscess)

Definition/Description

- Chronic apical abscess is the chronic inflammatory response to pulpal infection and necrosis and is characterised by intermittent discharge of pus through an associated sinus tract.

Cause

- Extensive bridgework or old restorations, pulpal necrosis and rapid production of pus.

Clinical Features

- Pain may be absent or mild.
- Draining sinus is present. This can be traced by inserting a GP point.
- Pulp vitality: Negative.
- Percussion: Not sensitive.

Diagnosis

- Clinical examination.
- Radiography: Usually a radiolucent periapical lesion is present.
- If a sinus track is present, dentist uses a #25 GP point into the sinus track and takes a periapical radiograph. The radiograph reveals the extent of the sinus track.

Management

- Refer the patient to a dentist, who would offer endodontic therapy or extraction of the involved tooth.

Condensing Osteitis

Definition/Description

- Condensing osteitis is a diffuse radiopaque periapical lesion that represents a localised bony reaction to a low-grade inflammatory stimulus.

Cause

- Low-grade pulpal or periodontal inflammation.

Clinical Features

- Symptoms vary depending on the pulpal or periapical status.
- Mild response or no response to pulp vitality tests (depending on the pulp status).
- Usually, pulp is nonvital.
- May elicit mild tenderness on percussion.

Diagnosis

- Radiograph shows increased trabecular bone density at the apex of tooth.
- Large restoration or carious lesion is seen on radiographs.

Management

- Refer the patient to a dentist, who would perform endodontic therapy of the tooth involved. If tooth destruction is extensive, tooth extraction is required.

Pericoronitis (Operculitis)

Definition/Description

- Pericoronitis refers to the inflammation of the soft tissues surrounding the crown of an erupting tooth (commonly a third molar).

Cause

- Accumulation of food debris and the presence of bacterial plaque beneath the gingival tissue that covers the erupting or partially erupting third molar (operculum).
- Trauma from the opposing tooth aggravates the inflammatory process.

Clinical Features

- Most commonly involved tooth is the mandibular third molar.
- Swelling, pain, trismus and tenderness of the soft tissue that covers the erupting tooth are present. Signs of inflammation of soft tissues are present (Figure 4.2).
- Pus may ooze out from beneath the inflamed tissue.
- Patient complains of bad taste and malodour.
- Cervical lymph nodes are enlarged and tender.
- Inability to open the mouth fully (trismus) is common.
- Cellulitis accompanied by fever and malaise can occur in severe infection.

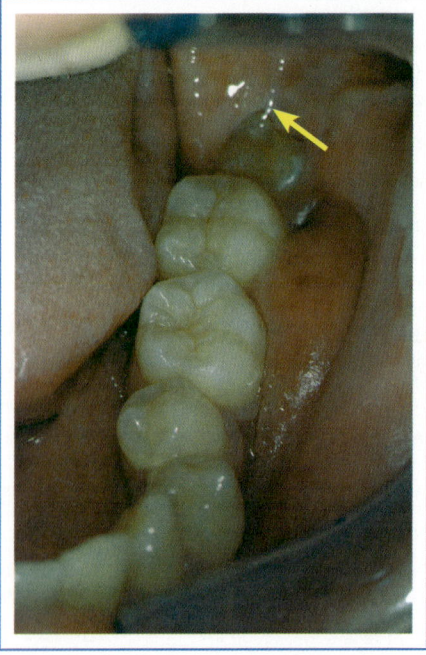

Figure 4.2 Pericoronitis (operculitis). Inflammation surrounding the partially erupted mandibular left third molar is evident (arrow). Inflammation has also spread to the gingival tissues surrounding the first and second molars. Reproduced with permission from: Patnarin Kanjanabuch, Thailand.

Diagnosis

- History and clinical examination.
- Orthopantamograph is an additional useful diagnostic aid.

Management

- For localised pericoronal infection, warm saline mouthwashes and irrigation under the inflamed gingival tissue are adequate. Other solutions that are used may contain hydrogen peroxide, chlorhexidine or other antiseptics.
- For a spreading infection, treatment with antibiotics and analgesics is required. An oral antibiotic with dental follow up in 24 to 48 hours is necessary. Common antibiotics used are phenoxymethylpenicillin or amoxicillin. For patients allergic to penicillin, clindamycin is used. Sometimes, metronidazole (for anaerobes) may be necessary.
- In an emergency, refer the patient to a dentist.
- Dentists decide on whether symptomatic treatment is adequate or surgical removal of the inflamed tissue (operculectomy) or the offending tooth is necessary. In some cases, recontouring the opposing tooth is adequate.

Dry Socket

Definition/Description

- Dry socket, also known as alveolar osteitis, is a painful condition that results from complication of tooth extraction.

Cause

- Reduction of blood supply to the extraction socket.
- Blood clot in the tooth socket is dislodged, usually within two to four days after the extraction.
- Smoking, drinking from a straw and periodontal disease may predispose to a dry socket.
- Infection and trauma of the extraction socket.

Clinical Features

- Lower third molar extraction sockets are most commonly involved in dry socket. This may occur two to four days after the removal of wisdom tooth.
- Pain is rarely relieved with traditional analgesics.
- Dental block provides immediate relief.
- Dull, throbbing, continuous deep-seated pain in the tooth socket.
- Halitosis is common.

Diagnosis

- History of recent extraction and clinical examination of the tooth socket with no blood clot or sign of healing.
- Malodour.
- Inflamed margins of gums around the socket.
- Detection of white dry bone when irrigated with normal saline.

Management

- Removal of food debris from the socket by gently irrigating with normal saline.
- Use of analgesics.
- Dressing the socket with *Alvogyl*™ (Septodont, France). The active ingredients of *Alvogyl*™ include eugenol for analgesic action, butamben for anaesthetic action and iodoform for antimicrobial action.
- Refer the patient to a dentist.

SUGGESTED READINGS

Douglas A, Douglas JM. Common dental emergencies. *Am Fam Physician*. 2003;67:511–7.

Kingon A. Solving dental problems in general practice. *Aust Fam Physician*. 2006;31:211–6.

Klasser G. Management of persistent idiopathic facial pain. *J Can Dent Assoc*. 2013;79:d71.

Wetherell J, Richards L, Sambrook P, Townsend G. Management of acute dental pain: a practical approach for primary health care providers. *Australian Prescriber*. 2001;24:144–8.

Benko K. Acute dental emergencies in emergency medicine. *Emerg Med Pract*. 2003;5:1–24.

Mansour MH, Cox SC. Patients presenting to the general practitioner with pain of dental origin. *Med J Aust*. 2006;185:64–7.

Neville BW, Damm DD, Allan CM, Bougout JE, editors. Pericoronitis. In: *Oral Maxillofacial Pathology*. 3rd ed. Philadelphia, PA: WB Saunders Co; 2009. pp. 171–3.

Abbott PV. Medical management of dental and oral pain. *Australian Prescriber*. 2007;30:77–9.

Prabhu SR, Al Shawaf M. Oro-facial pain. In: Prabhu SR, editor. *Textbook of Oral Medicine*. New Delhi, India: Oxford University Press; 2004. pp. 46–59.

Oral and Dental Expert Group. Post-treatment pain management. In: *Therapeutic Guidelines: Oral and Dental*. Version 2. Melbourne: Therapeutic Guidelines Limited; 2012. pp. 127–36.

Birnbaum W, Dunne SM. Pain of dental origin. In: Birnbaum W, Dunn SM, editors. *Oral Diagnosis: The Clinician's Guide*. Oxford, U.K.: Wright; 2000. pp. 71–123.

Chapter 5

Orofacial pain of nondental origin

S. R. Prabhu

ATYPICAL FACIAL PAIN (PERSISTENT IDIOPATHIC FACIAL PAIN)

Definition/Description

- Atypical facial pain (AFP) is characterised by facial pain that cannot be attributed to any demonstrable organic cause, including dental pain.

Cause

- Cause of AFP is not fully understood. Often, psychogenic factors or depression are associated with this disorder.

Clinical Features

- Malar region, orbit and temple are the common sites of involvement of AFP.
- Pain is deep-seated, severe, continuous and usually throbbing in nature.
- The pain may be bilateral and mainly affects middle-aged women.
- Patients are able to identify the exact location of pain extraorally and/or in the dentoalveolar complex (in a tooth, teeth or edentulous mucosa).

Diagnosis

- A detailed history is important to rule out any known sources of pain.
- Thorough clinical examination of the intraoral and extraoral structures.
- Cranial nerve screening.
- Complete diagnostic imaging, including computed tomography (CT) scans and magnetic resonance imaging (MRI).

Management

- In the absence of an organic cause of facial pain, amitriptyline is effective.
- Analgesics are not recommended.

ATYPICAL ODONTALGIA (PHANTOM TOOTH PAIN)

Definition/Description

- Atypical odontalgia is a subgroup of persistent idiopathic facial pain characterised by persistent facial pain that does not have the characteristics of cranial neuralgias or other orofacial disorders.

Cause

- Cause of atypical odontalgia is not fully understood.
- Factors associated include genetic predisposition, age (middle age to old age) and gender (female preponderance).
- Depression and anxiety are often associated.

Clinical Conditions

- Constant, persistent and unremitting throbbing or aching in a tooth, teeth or extraction site.
- Does not significantly respond to hot or cold food or drink, or to chewing or biting. The intensity of the pain can vary from very mild to very severe.
- Pain often follows or is associated with a history of some type of dental procedure, such as having a root canal or tooth extraction.
- Occasionally, pain can occur without any reason.
- Diagnostic local anaesthetic injections are of no help.
- The patient experiences pain in a tooth or teeth, which continue even after the treatment aimed at alleviating the pain.

Diagnosis

- A detailed history is important to rule out any known sources of pain.
- Thorough clinical examination of the intraoral and extraoral structures.
- Cranial nerve screening.
- Complete diagnostic imaging, including CT scans and MRI.

Management

- Tricyclic antidepressants are useful (e.g., amitriptyline).
- Gabapentin, an anticonvulsant and analgesic agent, is also effective.

TRIGEMINAL NEURALGIA

Definition/Description

- Trigeminal neuralgia is a neuropathic disorder characterised by episodes of intense pain in the face, originating from the trigeminal nerve.

Cause

- It has been suggested that compression of the trigeminal nerve, possibly due to dilated cerebral vessels (aneurysm), can injure the nerve's protective myelin sheath and cause erratic and hyperactive functioning of the nerve.

Clinical Features

- Pain involves the excitation of one or more of the three branches (mandibular, maxillary or ophthalmic) of the trigeminal nerve.
- In most cases, pain is precipitated by touching, eating or talking.
- Pain is unilateral and of sudden onset and short duration. It is sharp, lightning-like or stabbing in nature.

- Repetitive episodes can occur.
- In between the attacks, the area involved generally does not show any signs of pain.
- The pain does not cross to the contralateral side.

Diagnosis

- A detailed history is important to rule out any known sources of pain.
- Thorough clinical examination of the intraoral and extraoral structures.
- Cranial nerve screening.
- Complete diagnostic imaging, including CT scans and MRI.
- Nerve conduction studies (microneurography).

Management

- The anticonvulsant carbamazepine is the first line of treatment. Other medications used include baclofen, lamotrigine, oxcarbazepine, phenytoin, gabapentin, pregabalin and sodium valproate.
- Opioids such as codeine are effective.
- Uncontrolled trials have suggested that clonazepam and lidocaine may also be effective.
- Remissions occur spontaneously and may last for months to years.
- Surgical treatment (section of trigeminal root) is indicated if medical treatments fail.

ATYPICAL TRIGEMINAL NEURALGIA

Definition/Description

- Atypical trigeminal neuralgia (ATN) is characterised by unilateral, constant and severe aching, boring or burning pain.

Cause

- Vascular compression of the trigeminal nerve, infections of teeth or sinuses, physical trauma and past viral infections are the possible causes of ATN.

Clinical Features

- A number of symptoms are found to be associated with ATN.
- The intensity of pain can range from a mild aching to a crushing or burning sensation and may fluctuate.
- The pain can be heavy, aching and burning. Patients suffer from a steady headache similar to migraine and pain in all three branches of the trigeminal nerve.
- The patient experiences ache in teeth and ear; feeling of fullness in sinuses; pain in cheek, forehead, temples, jaws and around the eyes and occasional electric shock-like stabs.
- Patient may experience pain in the back of the scalp and neck in ATN, unlike in typical neuralgia.
- Pain tends to aggravate with talking, with facial expressions, on chewing and on certain sensations such as a cool breeze.

Diagnosis

- History and clinical examination, including cranial nerve screening.
- No specific diagnostic tests are available.
- CT and MRI scans to rule out other causes (such as tumours and multiple sclerosis) of facial pain.
- Nerve conduction studies (microneurography).

Management

- Treatment of ATN is the same as that of trigeminal neuralgia.
- Opioids such as codeine are effective.

OCCIPITAL NEURALGIA

Definition/Description

- Occipital neuralgia refers to chronic pain in the regions of the head supplied by lesser and greater occipital nerves.

Cause

- Damage to the occipital nerves usually due to trauma, physical stress on the nerve or repetitious neck contraction, flexion or extension.

Clinical Features

- An aching, burning and throbbing pain that typically starts at the base of the head and radiates to the scalp.
- Pain on one or both sides of the head.
- Pain behind the eyes.
- Sensitivity to light.
- Tender scalp.
- Pain when moving the neck.

Diagnosis

- History and clinical examination, including cranial nerve screening.
- CT scans and MRI to rule out other causes (such as tumours and multiple sclerosis) of facial pain.
- Nerve conduction studies (microneurography).

Management

- Antidepressants and nerve blocks are effective.
- Opioids such as codeine are also effective.

GLOSSOPHARYNGEAL NEURALGIA

Definition/Description

- Glossopharyngeal neuralgia involves unilateral irritation of the cranial nerve IX, resulting in pain in the throat.

Cause

- The cause is unknown. Abnormally positioned artery that compresses the glossopharyngeal or vagus nerve may cause glossopharyngeal neuralgia.

Clinical Features

- Cutting, stabbing and shooting pain or sharp sensation in the throat.
- Throat pain can last from minutes to hours. Ipsilateral ear sensation of 'fullness' may occur before the beginning of pain episode in the throat.
- The pain is triggered by swallowing, talking, yawning and coughing.
- Activation of the dorsal motor nucleus of the vagus nerve (cranial nerve X) during a glossopharyngeal neuralgia episode may result in bradycardia and syncope.

Diagnosis

- History and clinical examination, including cranial nerve screening.
- CT scan and MRI to rule out other causes (such as tumours and multiple sclerosis) of facial pain.
- Nerve conduction studies (microneurography).

Management

- Antidepressant or anticonvulsant medications are used to treat pain.
- Opioids such as codeine are also effective.

SUPERIOR LARYNGEAL NEURALGIA

Definition/Description

- Superior laryngeal neuralgia is a rare disorder and characterised by severe pain in the lateral aspect of the throat, submandibular region and underneath the ear. The pain is usually initiated by swallowing, shouting or turning the head.

Cause

- The condition is thought to be caused due to compression of the upper fibres of the vagus nerve as they leave the brain stem and traverse the subarachnoid space to the jugular foramen.
- Activation of the superior laryngeal nerve occurs via the general visceral afferent component of the vagus nerve.

Clinical Features

- This syndrome is accompanied by lowered pitch and pain on vocalisation. Lateral throat pain occurs within the submandibular region.
- Pain may also present under the ear. Pain episodes may last from minutes to days.

Diagnosis

- History and clinical examination, including cranial nerve screening.
- CT scan and MRI to rule out other causes (such as tumours and multiple sclerosis) of facial pain.
- Nerve conduction studies (microneurography).

Management

- Antidepressant or anticonvulsant medications are used to treat pain.
- Opioids such as codeine are also effective.

POSTHERPETIC NEURALGIA

Definition/Description

- In postherpetic neuralgia (PHN), nerve damage is caused by the reactivation of varicella-zoster virus. The damaged nerves in the affected dermatomic area of the skin send abnormal electrical signals to the brain. These signals may convey excruciating pain and may persist or recur for months or years, or even for life.

Cause

- With resolution of the herpes zoster (shingles) eruption, the pain that continues for three months or more is defined as PHN.
- Elderly and immunocompromised patients are susceptible.

Clinical Features

- The pain level is variable, from slight discomfort to very severe, and may be described as burning, stabbing or gnawing.
- Area of previous shingles (the side of the face) may show evidence of cutaneous scarring.
- Sensations may be altered over the involved areas in the form of either hypersensitivity or decreased sensation.

Diagnosis

- History and clinical examination.
- CT scan and MRI to rule out other causes (such as tumours and multiple sclerosis) of facial pain. MRI can also detect lesions attributable to zoster infection in the brain stem.
- Serology to detect antibodies to the virus.

Management

Possible options for the management of PHN include the following:

- Antiviral agents such as famciclovir are given at the onset of attacks of herpes zoster virus to shorten the clinical course and to help prevent complications such as PHN.
- Analgesics
  - ◆ Topical agents
    - Aspirin mixed with an appropriate solvent such as diethyl ether may reduce pain.
    - Gallium maltolate in a cream or ointment base has been reported to relieve refractory PHN.
    - Lidocaine skin patches may also be used to relieve the symptoms.
  - ◆ Systemic agents
    - Paracetamol or nonsteroidal anti-inflammatory drugs.
    - Opioids such as codeine, tramadol, morphine and fentanyl.
  - ◆ Antidepressants in smaller doses. Low dosages of tricyclic antidepressants, including amitriptyline.

♦ Anticonvulsants such as phenytoin and carbamazepine can be used for sharp jabbing pain. Newer anticonvulsants include gabapentin and lamotrigine.
♦ Corticosteroids are often used but do not provide much relief.

HEADACHE

Headache is an extremely common complaint. Based on the cause, there are several types of headaches:

• Tension headache
• Migraine
• Cluster headaches
• Headaches associated with disorders of the eye, ear, paranasal sinuses, neuralgias, temporomandibular joint problems, intracranial tumours, infections, increased intracranial pressure and those after head injury
• Drug-induced, such as those associated with glyceryl trinitrate, nifedipine and substance withdrawal

It is important to include the following aspects in the case history when assessing headaches:

Onset
• Sudden onset is due to vascular causes.
• Cluster headaches and migraines intensify in minutes and last for hours.
• Headache due to meningitis lasts for hours and days.
• Headache due to increased intracranial pressure (due to tumour or subdural haemorrhage) is progressive and develops over a period of days or weeks.

Site
• Retro-orbital pain is due to cluster headache.
• Sinus pain is unilateral.
• Pain in the temporal region accompanied by jaw claudication is due to temporal arteritis and ocular pain is due to glaucoma.

Character of pain
• In tension headaches, the pain is described as a tight band around the head.
• In migrainous headaches, the pain is throbbing or dull aching.

Severity of pain
• Headache due to subarachnoid haemorrhage is very severe and is associated with a stiff neck.
• Slow, progressive headache is a feature of slowly evolving intracranial pressure due to tumours.
• In neuralgias, pain is sudden, sharp and severe.

Precipitating factors
• Posture, coughing and sneezing aggravate the headache due to raised intracranial pressure.
• In migraines, photophobia is usually present. Certain foods, such as cheese, may precipitate migraine.

- Common cold can precipitate headache.
- Drugs such as glyceryl trinitrate used for angina can precipitate headaches.
- Associated symptoms: In patients with migraine, flashing lights, and in temporal arteritis, unilateral visual loss may occur. In hydrocephalus with headaches dementia, ataxia and drowsiness may occur.

Diagnosis/Evaluation

- Detailed history of headaches, including a focused physical and neurological examination.
- Evaluation of causes for concern.
- Consideration of secondary headache disorder (e.g., haematoma, metabolic disorder and hydrocephalus).
- Evaluation of the type of primary headache.
- Patient education and lifestyle management.
- Specialty referral, as indicated.
- Diagnostic testing, if indicated.

Treatment/Management

Treatment or management of headaches include the following:
- Triptans
- Adjunctive therapy, including caffeine and metoclopramide
- Dihydroergotamine mesylate
- Chlorpromazine, intravenous valproate sodium, intravenous magnesium sulphate or prochlorperazine
- Opiates
- Dexamethasone
- Inhaled oxygen
- Bridging treatment
  ♦ Corticosteroids
  ♦ Occipital nerve block
- Hormone therapy
- Prophylactic treatment
  ♦ Cyclic prophylaxis
  ♦ Hormone prophylaxis
  ♦ Antiepileptics
  ♦ Beta blockers
  ♦ Calcium channel blockers
  ♦ Tricyclic antidepressants
- Screening for depression and anxiety
- Referral to specialist

MIGRAINE

Definition/Description

- Migraine is a chronic neurological disorder characterised by recurrent moderate to severe headaches.

Cause

- The underlying cause of migraines is unknown; however, they are believed to be related to a mix of environmental and genetic factors.

- In about two-thirds of cases, migraines run in families, and they rarely occur due to a single gene defect.
- Triggers may include cheese, wine and coffee.

Symptoms and Signs

- Typically, headache is unilateral and pulsating or throbbing in nature. It lasts from 2 to 72 hours.
- Associated symptoms may include nausea (in 90% of cases), vomiting (in 30% of cases), photophobia (increased sensitivity to light) and phonophobia (increased sensitivity to sound).
- Pain generally aggravates with physical activity.
- Up to one-third of people with migraines perceive an aura characterised by blurred vision, flashing lights, numbness, tingling sensation and strange smells. Signals such as transient visual, sensory or motor disturbances are an indication that a headache will soon occur.
- Other symptoms may include nasal stuffiness, diarrhoea, frequent urination, pallor or sweating. Swelling or tenderness of the scalp and stiffness in neck may occur.

Diagnosis

- The diagnosis of a migraine is based on signs and symptoms. Imaging tests, including X-ray scans or MRI, are occasionally performed to exclude other causes of headaches.

Management

- Preventive migraine medications are recommended as these help in reducing the frequency or severity of migraine attacks by at least 50%. These include topiramate, propranolol, metoprolol, angiotensin-converting enzyme inhibitors and amitriptyline, which are highly effective and have shown good results.
- Botox® has also been found to be useful in patients who suffer from chronic migraines.

SINUSITIS

Definition/Description

- Sinusitis is the inflammation of the paranasal sinuses. Inflammation of the maxillary sinus causes maxillary sinusitis.

Cause

- Infection by bacteria (such as *Haemophilus influenzae*, *Streptococcus pneumoniae*, *Staphylococcus aureus* and *Moraxella catarrhalis*)
- Allergy
- Systemic autoimmune disorders

Clinical Features

- Headache, facial pain and nasal obstruction. Pain may aggravate when the patient bends over or lie down.

- Thick nasal discharge (usually green in colour), which may contain pus (purulent) and/or blood.
- Halitosis, postnasal drip and cough are present.
- Fullness in the ear and toothache. In rare cases, infection of the eye socket may result in the loss of sight and is accompanied by fever and severe illness.

Diagnosis

- Clinical, sinus tap, lavage and culture methods.
- CT scans may be used to determine the extent of chronic disease.

Management

- Usually self-limiting. Antibiotics are used to speed up recovery.
- Topical decongestants are useful in relieving a stuffy nose.
- Complications may include orbital cellulitis, cavernous sinus thrombosis, meningitis and brain abscesses.

STOMATITIS

Definition/Description

- Stomatitis refers to the inflammation of the oral mucosa. Sometimes, the term 'mucositis' is also used to indicate the inflammation of the oral mucosa (e.g., radiation mucositis).
- Stomatitis may be mild, severe, localised, diffuse, painful or recurrent.

Cause

Local and systemic causes of stomatitis are as follows:

- Trauma from physical agents (e.g., ill-fitting dental appliances) and cheek biting.
- Thermal agents (e.g., pizza burn).
- Chemical burns (e.g., aspirin burn) and tobacco use (smoker's stomatitis).
- Allergic responses to food items (e.g., fish).
- Ingredients of toothpaste, lipstick and chewing gum (e.g., cinnamon, used as flavouring agent).
- Conditions with obscure aetiology that cause stomatitis include lichen planus, burning mouth syndrome and recurrent aphthous stomatitis.
- Local and systemic infections (bacterial, viral and fungal).
- Stomatitis predominantly attributable to local bacterial infections include acute necrotising ulcerative gingivitis (caused by fusospirochetes), streptococcal stomatitis and staphylococcal mucositis. Gonorrhoea (gonococcal stomatitis) and stomatitis due to primary and secondary syphilis are usually caused by systemic infections.
- Viral infections include primary and secondary herpes simplex virus infections (herpetic gingivostomatitis), primary and secondary varicella-zoster virus infections (chickenpox and shingles,

respectively), Epstein-Barr virus infections (infectious mononucle-osis) and Coxsackie virus infections (hand, foot and mouth disease and herpangina).

- Stomatitis caused by *Candida albicans* is particularly common in immunocompromised patients. In denture wearers, candidal infection can cause denture stomatitis, and in those who are on long-term antibiotics, the fungus causes antibiotic sto-matitis. Mucocutaneous candidiasis and stomatitis due to blastomycosis and cryptococcosis are caused by systemic infections.
- Stomatitis predominantly due to systemic causes includes Behcet's disease, coeliac disease, cyclic neutropaenia, ery-thema multiforme, inflammatory bowel disease, iron deficiency (anaemia), leukaemia, mucous membrane pemphigoid, pem-phigus vulgaris, Stevens-Johnson syndrome, thrombocyto-paenic purpura, vitamin B deficiency (pellagra) and vitamin C deficiency (scurvy).
- Radiation damage (radiation mucositis) and chemotherapy.
- Hormonal changes occurring in puberty and pregnancy are also known to cause stomatitis, which is especially confined to the gin-gival tissues.
- Clinical manifestations may differ based on the causes involved. Some present as inflammatory changes with redness, whereas oth-ers may present as erosions or ulcers.
- Pain is a feature in many conditions listed above.

Clinical Features

- Any of the cardinal signs of inflammation of the oral mucosa may be present in patients with stomatitis. Pain is a consistent feature in majority of patients.
- Signs and symptoms depend on the causes, including the un-derlying systemic disorders. Patients may be acutely ill, as in Stevens-Johnson syndrome, or may not exhibit any systemic manifestation if the cause is of local origin. Discussion on symp-toms and signs of all the conditions listed above is beyond the scope of this chapter.

Diagnosis

- A thorough history and clinical examination are of paramount importance for the diagnosis of stomatitis.
- A systemic search for the underlying cause should be carried out if a local cause cannot be found.
- Skin examination is important for mucocutaneous lesions, such as those seen in lichen planus, secondary syphilis or pemphigus.
- Investigations include microscopic examination of the samples obtained from smears, mucosal scrapings, oral rinse and biopsy specimens.
- Conditions of autoimmune background need to be investigated by using immunofluorescence or serological methods.

- When systemic infections are suspected, full blood count, differential count, serology and cultures are recommended. In these circumstances, consultation with a physician is essential.
- Rarely, molecular studies involving polymerase chain reaction methods may become necessary to identify the specific pathogen (e.g., a virus) causing the disease.

Management

- Treatment of stomatitis involves the identification and elimination of the cause. If the cause is local (e.g., physical, thermal and chemical), elimination of the cause and symptomatic treatment and follow-up are adequate.
- Topical local anaesthetic agents may be necessary for pain.
- If stomatitis is caused by local infections, it needs to be managed with topical and/or systemic antibiotics for bacterial infections.
- Topical corticosteroid treatment may be necessary for oral lesions of lichen planus and pemphigus vulgaris.
- The majority of viral infections that cause stomatitis are self-limiting and may not require antiviral medications unless the symptoms are severe.
- Candidal infections can be treated with antifungal agents. Oral and denture hygiene should be emphasised for these patients. Underlying predisposing factors need to be identified, investigated and treated. When systemic causes are suspected (e.g., autoimmune disorders and leukaemia), treatment for stomatitis should be carried out in consultation with the specialist.
- In all cases of stomatitis, maintenance of oral hygiene and symptomatic treatment of oral pain and discomfort are most important.

BURNING MOUTH SYNDROME

Definition/Description

- Burning mouth syndrome, also known as glossopyrosis, glossodynia and stomatodynia, is characterised by a burning sensation in the mouth, where no underlying dental or medical causes or oral signs can be identified. For further details, please refer to Chapter 28 (Oral mucosal burning and burning mouth syndrome).

TEMPOROMADIBULAR JOINT PAIN

Definition/Description

- Temporomandibular joint (TMJ) pain is common. Temporomandibular joint disorders are the major causes of TMJ pain. Temporomandibular joint disorders are broadly divided into inflammatory conditions (capsulitis and synovitis) and internal derangements involving the intra-articular disc. For further details, please refer to Chapter 18 (Temporomandibular joint disorders).

TEMPORAL ARTERITIS (GIANT CELL ARTERITIS)

Definition/Description

- Temporal arteritis, also known as giant cell arteritis, affects the temporal artery in the elderly. This is an autoimmune disorder.

Cause

- Not known. Cellular and humoral immunological systems are implicated.

Clinical Features

- Predominantly present in the elderly Caucasian women.
- Features include scalp tenderness, headaches and thickened and tender temporal arteries.
- Pulseless temporal arteries, ulcers on the scalp and visual disturbances.
- Blindness in advanced cases.

Diagnosis

- Erythrocyte sedimentation rate is elevated.
- C-reactive protein is elevated in active disease.

Management

- Systemic corticosteroids.
- Advanced cases may need immunosuppressants, such as methotrexate and azathioprine.

OTALGIA (EARACHE)

Definition/Description

- Otalgia refers to earache. This is a common condition. Two types of otalgia exist: primary and referred.
- Primary otalgia initiates inside the ear, whereas referred otalgia initiates from the structures outside the ear.

Cause

- External, middle and inner ear diseases.

  External ear pain may be due to the following reasons:

- Mechanical: Trauma and foreign bodies, such as hairs, insects and cotton buds.
- Infective (otitis externa) caused by bacteria, fungi or viruses.

  Middle ear pain may be due to the following reasons:

- Mechanical obstruction of the Eustachian tube.
- Inflammatory/infective: Acute otitis media and mastoiditis.

  Several other conditions that cause earache include impacted teeth, sinus disease, inflamed tonsils, infections in the nose and pharynx and throat cancer.

Clinical Features

- Ear pain may be intermittent or continuous, dull and sharp.
- Patients, particularly children, with ear pain may have fever, cold and runny nose.

Diagnosis

- History and clinical examination of the ear by auroscopy.
- If auroscopy is unremarkable, consider causes of referred ear pain.
- Investigations depend on the suspicion from the history and examination. The following can be performed: Full blood count, thyroid function tests, erythrocyte sedimentation rate, chest X-ray and audiography.

Management

- Treat the underlying cause.
- Medications commonly used to control pain and inflammation in adults with ear pain include the following:
  - ♦ Acetaminophen for pain
  - ♦ Nonsteroidal anti-inflammatory drugs to control inflammation
  - ♦ Narcotic pain medications and antibiotics
  - ♦ Referral to a specialist

CARDIOGENIC JAW PAIN

Definition/Description

- Cardiogenic jaw pain presents in the orofacial and neck region. Commonly involved areas include neck, throat, ear, teeth and mandible.

Cause

- Cardiac ischemia.

Clinical Features

- Pain may last for minutes or hours.
- Pain is precipitated by exertion and is relieved with rest.
- Pain is relieved by the use of sublingual nitroglycerine spray or tablet.

Management

- Nitroglycerine sublingual tablet or spray.
- Oxygen administration.
- Immediate referral to a cardiologist is recommended.

REFERRED PAIN AND RADIATING PAIN

Definition/Description

- Referred or reflective pain is the pain that is experienced at a location other than the site of the painful stimulus.
- For example, when a patient with myocardial infarction experiences pain only in the jaw or the left arm but not in the chest, it is categorised as referred or reflective pain.

- However, in case of radiating pain, the patient with myocardial infarction will experience a pain that radiates from the chest to the left side of the jaw and into the left arm. In this case, pain is present in the chest, the arm and the jaw.

   Detailed discussion on these topics is beyond the scope of this chapter.

SIALOLITHIASIS (SALIVARY CALCULUS)

Definition/Description

- Salivary calculi (stones) in the submandibular duct can cause obstruction to the flow of saliva, resulting in swelling and pain of the submandibular region.

Cause

- Calculi in the submandibular duct.

Clinical Features

- Swelling and pain in the submandibular region usually occur at the time of meals, when salivary flow is stimulated.
- Stone(s) in the duct are palpable and elicit(s) tenderness.
- Radiographical views confirm the presence of salivary stones in the duct.
- Parotid gland sialolythiasis also occurs but is less common.

Diagnosis

- History and clinical examination
- Radiography

Management

- Refer the patient to an oral surgeon.

SUGGESTED READINGS

Douglas A, Douglas JM. Common dental emergencies. *Am Fam Physician*. 2003;67:511–7.

Kingon A. Solving dental problems in general practice. *Aust Fam Physician*. 2006;31:211–6.

Beithon J, Gallenberg M, Johnson K, Kildahl P, Krenik J, Liebow M, et al. *Diagnosis and Treatment of Headache*. Bloomington, MN: Institute for Clinical Systems Improvement; 2011. p. 84.

Scully C. Oral medicine for the general practitioner: pain. *International Dentistry SA*. 2011;13:38–44. Available from: www.moderndentistry-media.com/jan_feb2011/scully.pdf

Klasser G. Persistent idiopathic facial pain. *J Can Dent Assoc*. 2013;79:d71.

Wetherell J, Richards L, Sambrook P. Management of acute dental pain: a practical approach for primary health care providers. *Australian Prescriber*. 2001;24:144–8.

Mansour MH, Cox SC. Patients presenting to the general practitioner with pain of dental origin. *Med J Aust*. 2006;185:64–7.

Abbott PV. Medical management of dental and oral pain. *Australian Prescriber*. 2007;30:77–9.

Balasubramaniam R, Turner L, Fisher D, Klasser GD, Okeson JP. Non-odontogenic toothache revisited. *Open J Stomatol.* 2011;1:92–102.

Prabhu SR, Al Shawaf M. Oro-facial pain. In: Prabhu SR, editor. *Textbook of Oral Medicine*. New Delhi, India: Oxford University Press; 2004. pp. 46–59.

Oral and Dental Expert Group. Post-treatment pain management. In: *Therapeutic Guidelines: Oral and Dental*. Version 1. Melbourne: Therapeutic Guidelines Limited; 2007. pp. 145–55.

Birnbaum W, Dunne SM. Pain of non-dental origin. In: Birnbaum W, Dunn SM, editors. *Oral diagnosis: The Clinician's Guide*. Oxford, U.K.: Wright; 2000. pp. 99–123.

Chapter 6

Dental caries

S. R. Prabhu

Definition/Description

- Dental caries, also known as tooth decay, is the most common dental disease involving teeth. It is characterised by the destruction of dental hard tissues (particularly enamel and dentine) because of the action of acids produced by the oral microorganisms that act on sugar-rich foods.

Cause

- Dental plaque, a complex biofilm that consists of bacteria and their products, must be present for dental carries to develop.
- Acid produced by cariogenic bacteria (mainly *Streptococcus mutans* and *Lactobacillus* species) resident in dental plaque is responsible for decalcification of tooth enamel. These bacteria can produce organic acids from fermentable carbohydrates (dietary sugars).
- Other bacteria associated with dental caries include *S. sanguinis, S. sobrinus, S. salivarius* and *S. mitior.*
- *Actinomyces spp. (e.g., A. viscosus)* are associated with the development of root caries.
- Other contributing factors involved in the development of dental caries include hyposalivation (xerostomia) caused by systemic medications and disorders, and radiation.
- Early childhood caries is due to frequent nursing with fluids containing high concentration of sugars.

Clinical Features

- Clinically, dental caries can be classified as pit and fissure caries and smooth surface caries (Figure 6.1).
    - Initially, carious lesion (white spot lesion) is asymptomatic. As an early symptom, the affected individual may experience dentin hypersensitivity due to dentinal exposure.
    - Pit and fissure caries involves pits and fissures on the occlusal surfaces of molars and premolars, buccal surfaces of molars and palatal surfaces of maxillary incisors.
    - Smooth surface caries develops on the proximal surfaces of teeth and on the gingival third of the buccal surfaces of molars (cervical caries).

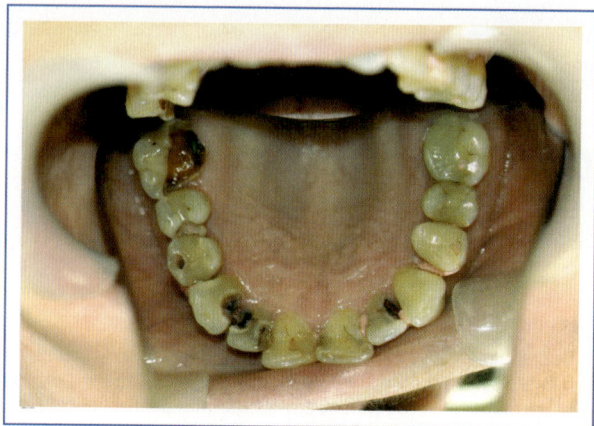

Figure 6.1   Dental caries of the maxillary teeth.
Reproduced with permission from: Dr. Matthew Hoyle, School of Dentistry & Health Sciences, Charles Sturt University.

- Early carious lesions present as opaque white area on the enamel. This mimics the opacity produced by enamel hypoplasia. In advanced cases, carious lesions appear as brown discoloured cavities.
- Radiation caries (cervical caries) occurs due to radiation therapy doses exceeding 4000 cGy to the salivary gland region.
- Nursing bottle caries, also called childhood caries, involves multiple teeth and is rampant.
- When caries advances and affects dental pulp, pain is a common symptom, due to pulpitis.

Diagnosis

- History and clinical examination using dental probe and bitewing or periapical radiographs of the teeth are adequate for detecting carious lesions.

Management

- In the early stages of dental caries, that is, before tooth cavitation, the following strategies are used:
  - ♦ Advise the patient to:
    - Brush at least twice a day with fluoride toothpaste and to floss immediately before brushing. Interdental cleaning aids are also useful in plaque-reduction exercise.
    - Avoid sucrose in sticky forms or as sweet snacks between meals.
    - Use antimicrobial agents, such as chlorhexidine gel.
    - Use remineralising agents, such as fluoride rinses (0.2–1 mg/mL). After rinsing the mouth, to spit out the wash and do not swallow it.

  – For white spot caries, topical application of remineralising agents is effective.
- Refer the patient to a dentist for further advice and treatment.

RAMPANT TOOTH DECAY (RAMPANT CARIES)

Definition/Description

- Rampant tooth decay (rampant caries) refers to an aggressive form of caries that involves many or all teeth in the dentition. This form of caries is generally resistant to traditional preventive measures and progresses rapidly.

Cause

- Multifactorial causes. These include frequent consumption of carbohydrates, hyposalivation resulting in xerostomia, ineffective dental care and poor oral hygiene. Xerostomia may be due to causes such as radiation, medication, use of illicit drugs and salivary gland disorders.

Clinical Features

- Caries affects multiple teeth (Figure 6.2).
- Mostly involves the facial surfaces of the anterior teeth and inter-proximal surfaces of the lower incisors.
- In preschool children, rampant caries involves pits and fissures, smooth surfaces and anterior teeth.

Diagnosis

- History and clinical examination.

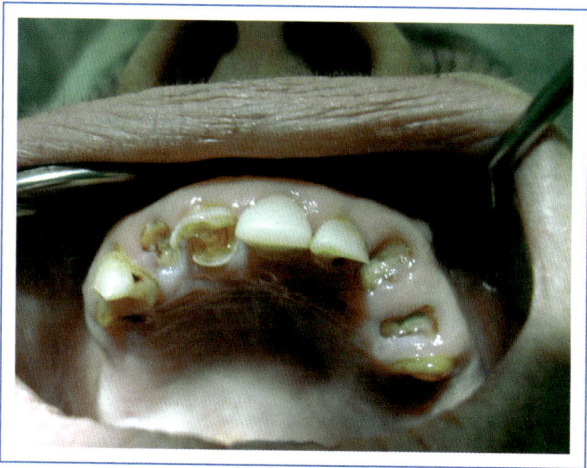

Figure 6.2   Rampant caries resulting in gross destruction of tooth substance.
Courtesy: Paul Abbott.

Management

- Management of dental caries needs both preventive and therapeutic approach.
- Diet modification.
- Use of fluoride-releasing agents and antibacterial mouth rinses (e.g., chlorhexidine).
- Identification, treatment and control of systemic diseases, if present.
- Refer the patient to a dentist for caries control, oral hygiene education and maintenance.

EARLY CHILDHOOD CARIES (BABY BOTTLE TOOTH DECAY)

Early childhood caries (baby bottle tooth decay) is found in children with deciduous teeth. Deciduous maxillary anterior teeth are commonly involved. Usually, these children are allowed to fall asleep with sweetened liquids in their feeding bottles. Feeding children with sweetened drinks multiple times during the day can also cause early childhood caries. There is no scientific evidence that confirms that breastmilk is associated with caries development.

SUGGESTED READINGS

Oral and Dental Expert Group. Dental caries. In: *Therapeutic Guidelines: Oral and Dental*. Version 2. Melbourne: Therapeutic Guidelines Limited; 2012. pp. 47–54.

Fejerskov O, Kidd E, editors. *Dental Caries: The Disease and Its Clinical Management*. 2nd ed. Oxford, U.K.: Blackwell Munskgaard; 2003.

Ribeiro NM, Ribeiro MA. Breastfeeding and early childhood caries: a critical review. *J Pediatr (Rio J)*. 2004;80(5 suppl):S199–210.

Chapter 7

Abnormal tooth wear

S. R. Prabhu

TOOTH ATTRITION

Definition/Description

- Tooth attrition refers to a process of physiological wearing of teeth as a result of a normal function, such as mastication.

Cause

- One of the common causes of tooth attrition is the excessive grinding of the teeth and/or excessive clenching of the jaw. This is a parafunctional habit called bruxism.

Clinical Features

- Primary and permanent dentitions may be involved in attrition. In individuals with attrition, occlusal surfaces are generally flattened and vertical height may be reduced (Figure 7.1). In certain types of malocclusion, buccal or lingual surfaces may be affected. Usually, this condition is asymptomatic.

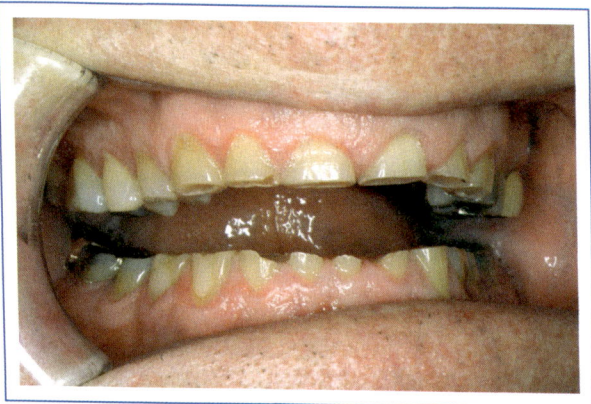

Figure 7.1 Generalised attrition leads to significant reduction in vertical height.
Courtesy: Nagamani Narayana.

Diagnosis

- History and clinical examination.

Management

- If parafunctional habits are found to be aetiologically associated, their management should be carried out.
- Refer the patient to a dentist for correction of malocclusion and/or for restorative treatment.

TOOTH ABRASION

Definition/Description

- Tooth abrasion refers to tooth substance loss due to mechanical forces derived from a foreign object such as toothbrush, toothpick, tooth floss and other agents.

Cause

- Common causes of abrasion include abrasive dentifrices, cigars, pipes, improper tooth-brushing techniques, excessive use of tooth floss or toothpick and holding needle or thread between upper and lower incisors.

Clinical Features

- Incisal or occlusal wear relates to the habit or use of abrasive agents. Cervical wear due to improper tooth-brushing techniques results in a V-shaped groove (abfraction injury) (Figure 7.2).

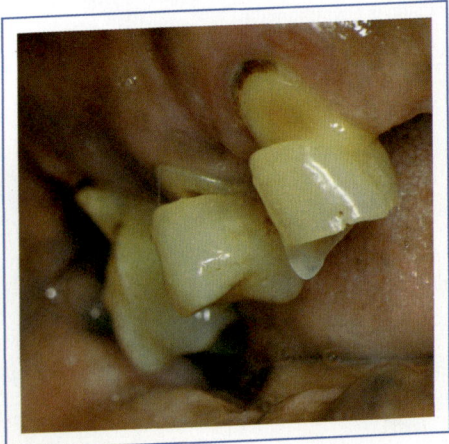

Figure 7.2 Abfraction injury. V-shaped tooth abrasion due to faulty tooth-brushing technique.
Reproduced with permission from: Titipong Prueksrisakul, Department of Oral Medicine, Faculty of Dentistry, Chulalongkorn University BKK, Thailand.

Diagnosis

- History and clinical examination.

Management

- Improvement of habits and elimination of the causative factors.
- Refer the patient to a dentist for restorative dental treatment.

TOOTH EROSION

Definition/Description

- Tooth erosion refers to tooth substance loss due to exposure of the tooth to a chemical such as acid from external sources.

Cause

- Causes of tooth erosion include occupational exposure to acids, acidic beverages, chronic regurgitation of gastric contents (as in gastroesophageal reflux disease) and bulimia (self-induced vomiting)-related vomiting.

Clinical Features

- In gastroesophageal reflux disease and bulimia-related disorders, erosions are located on the lingual surfaces of the anterior teeth (Figure 7.3).
- In beverage- or occupation-related erosion (e.g., in the battery and galvanising industry workers), the defects are located on the labial surfaces.

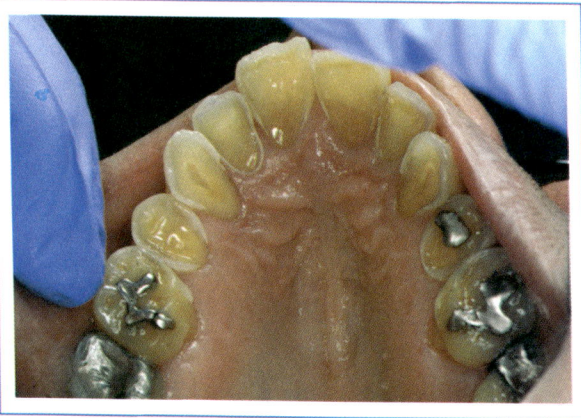

Figure 7.3 Erosion of palatal aspect of maxillary teeth; rule out bulimia and gastric reflux.
Courtesy: Nagamani Narayana.

- Primary dentition is more susceptible to erosion than permanent dentition.
- Smooth, shiny, round yellow surface depressions (on the palatal, incisal or occlusal surfaces) are characteristic features of dental erosions. Occasionally, these can be sensitive to hot or cold because of dentin exposure.

Diagnosis

- History and clinical appearance.

Management

- Identify and eliminate the causative factors.
- Refer the patient to a dentist for restorative treatment.

SUGGESTED READINGS

Kaidonis JA. Oral diagnosis and treatment planning: part 4. Non-carious tooth surface loss and assessment of risk. *Br Dent J*. 2012;213:155–61.

Rees JS, Jagger DC. Abfraction lesions: myth or reality? *J Esthet Restor Dent*. 2003;15:263–71.

Chapter 8

Developmentally missing teeth

S. R. Prabhu

HYPODONTIA, OLIGODONTIA AND ANODONTIA

Definition/Description

- The tooth is said to be developmentally or congenitally missing if it has not emerged in the oral cavity and is not detectable in the radiograph.
- All primary teeth erupt by the age of 3 years, and all permanent teeth except the third molars erupt between the ages of 12 years and 14 years.
- Congenitally missing primary teeth become evident in children between the ages of three years and four years, and congenitally missing permanent teeth (except third molars) become evident between the age of 12 years and 14 years. There are three terminologies used to denote congenitally missing teeth: hypodontia, oligodontia and anodontia.
  - ♦ **Hypodontia** refers to congenital absence of less than six permanent teeth, excluding the third molars.
  - ♦ **Oligodontia** refers to congenital lack of more than six teeth, excluding the third molars.
  - ♦ **Anodontia** refers to congenital lack of all teeth.

Cause

- Tooth agenesis is the cause of all three forms of congenital absence of teeth.
- Causes of congenitally missing teeth include environmental and genetic factors.
- Children treated for cancer with irradiation or chemotherapy at the time of tooth-developing ages are at a greater risk for agenesis of teeth.
- Viral infections during odontogenesis may also be associated with congenital lack of teeth.
- The use of thalidomide (an immunomodulatory drug) by pregnant women is known to cause congenitally missing teeth in their children.
- Of the genetic causes, mutations in MSX1 and PAX9 genes are found to be associated with oligodontia.
- Arrested tooth development leading to hypodontia is also associated with trauma in the dental region such as fractures and surgical procedures on the jaw bones.

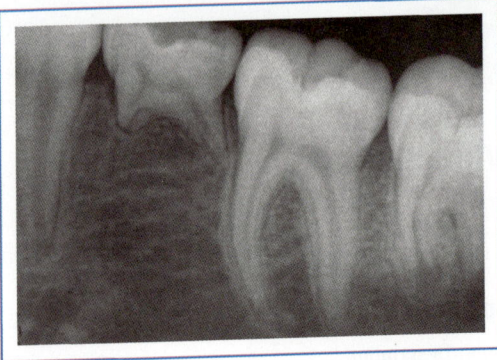

Figure 8.1 Hypodontia. Radiograph shows no sign of lower second premolar, which is congenitally missing. Also, note a retained deciduous molar.
Reproduced with permission from: Charles Dunlap. Formerly, Professor of Oral and Maxillofacial Pathology, UMKC, USA.

Clinical Features

- Congenitally missing teeth are not as common in primary dentition as in permanent dentition.
- Hypodontia and oligodontia are not rare, whereas anodontia is a rare condition.
- Most commonly missing teeth in hypodontia include third molars followed by mandibular second premolars (Figure 8.1), maxillary lateral incisors and maxillary second premolars.
- Hypodontia involving teeth other than those listed above is very rare.
- Most individuals with hypodontia lack only one or two permanent teeth.
- An ectodermal defect called hypohydrotic ectodermal dysplasia involves all ectodermal derivatives, including the teeth. Ectodermal dysplasia is characterised by sparse hair, eyelashes and brows, dystrophic nails and marked oligodontia (Figure 8.2 A and B).
  - Both primary and permanent dentitions may be involved.
  - Erupted teeth are cone-shaped.
  - Sweat glands are diminished, resulting in patient's inability to regulate body temperature.
- Isolated hypodontia is also known to occur in other syndromic forms such as oral-facial-digital syndrome type I, Down syndrome, syndromic craniosynostosis and orofacial clefting syndrome.

Diagnosis

- History, clinical examination and radiography of the jaws are essential diagnostic steps.
- History of loss of tooth or teeth due to extraction or trauma should be ruled out.

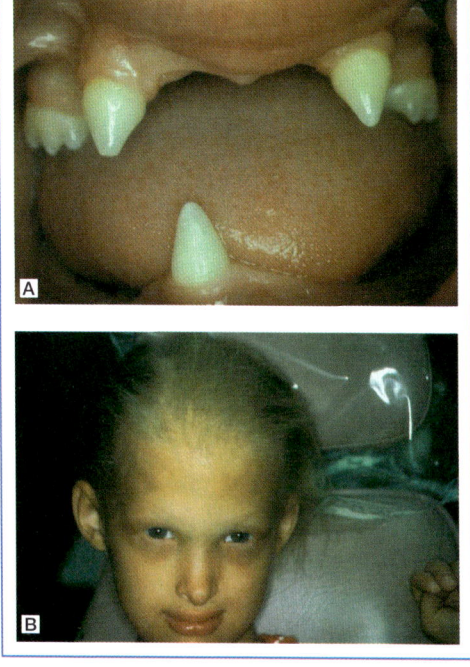

Figure 8.2 (A) Oligodontia in a patient with hypohydrotic ectodermal dysplasia and (B) typical facies of the condition.
Reproduced with permission from: Charles Dunlap. Formerly, Professor of Oral and Maxillofacial Pathology, UMKC, USA.

- Syndromic cases (e.g., ectodermal dysplasia) require a thorough clinical examination of the dental, oral and extraoral structures.
- Panoramic radiography of the jaws is essential in all syndromic and nonsyndromic cases.

Management

- Refer the patient to a dentist for restoration of aesthetic and functional aspects of the dentition.
- Syndromic patients need to be referred to relevant specialists.

SUGGESTED READINGS

Sciuba J, Regezi JA, Rogers RS. Tooth abnormalities. *PDQ Oral Disease: Diagnosis and Treatment*. Hamilton, Ontario, Canada: BC Decker Inc; 2002. pp. 304–22.

Dunlap C. *Abnormalities of Teeth*. MO: UMKC; 2004. Available from: https://dentistry.umkc.edu/Practicing_Communities/asset/AbnormalitiesofTeeth.pdf

Chapter 9

Extra number of teeth

S. R. Prabhu

SUPERNUMERARY TEETH (HYPERDONTIA)

Definition/Description

- Teeth that form in addition to the normal complement of teeth (20 primary and 32 permanent) are called supernumerary teeth.
- Supernumerary teeth commonly involve anterior maxilla. They can remain impacted and inverted.
- Multiple supernumerary teeth are often associated with syndromes such as Gardner syndrome, cleidocranial dysplasia (Figure 9.1), cleft lip and cleft palate
- Supernumerary teeth may cause prevention or delay of eruption of associated permanent teeth, crowding of teeth and root resorption of the adjacent teeth.

Cause

- Both genetic and environmental factors play a role in the causation of supernumerary teeth.
- Supernumerary teeth may develop from a second tooth bud arising from a dental lamina or from splitting the regular tooth bud of a normally forming tooth.

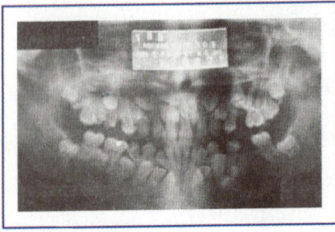

Figure 9.1 Supernumerary teeth in a patient with cleidocranial dysplasia.
Reproduced with permission from: Charles Dunlap. Formerly, Professor of Oral and Maxillofacial Pathology, UMKC, USA.

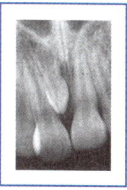

Figure 9.2 Radiographic image of a mesiodens. This is an extra incisor located in the midline between the two permanent central incisors. Reproduced with permission from: Charles Dunlap. Formerly, Professor of Oral and Maxillofacial Pathology, UMKC, USA.

Clinical Features

- Supernumerary teeth can be classified according to their shape and location in the dental arch. Following types of supernumerary teeth are known.
  - ◆ **Mesiodens:** Mesiodens is the most common supernumerary tooth located in the midline of the maxillary arch between the two central incisors (Figure 9.2). It is conical in shape and is smaller than any of the incisors in the maxillary arch.
  - ◆ **Paramolar:** It is a supernumerary tooth commonly located in the interproximal space buccal to the maxillary second and third molars.
  - ◆ **Distomolar:** It is the fourth permanent molar located distal to the third molar.
  - ◆ **Conical supernumerary tooth:** It is a small peg-shaped tooth with normal root.
  - ◆ **Tuberculate supernumerary tooth:** It is a multicusped, short barrel-shaped tooth with normal-appearing crown.
  - ◆ **Supplemental teeth:** These are one of the normal series of tooth. Extra teeth that belong to one of the normal series of tooth are called supplemental teeth (Figure 9.3).
  - ◆ **Odontome:** A hamartomatous malformation of dental tissues.

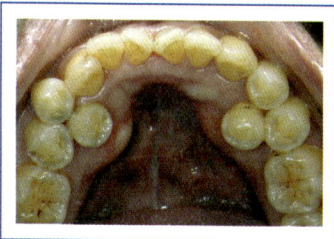

Figure 9.3 Supernumerary mandibular premolars located lingual to the first and second premolars. The size and shape of the supernumerary premolars are identical to the premolars in the dental arch. Reproduced with permission from: Getty Images Sales Australia Pty Ltd.

Diagnosis

- Clinical (number and shape) and radiographical examinations of the location of the suspected supernumerary tooth are essential to arrive at a definitive diagnosis.
- Syndromic association also needs to be checked if multiple supernumerary teeth are identified.

Management

- Asymptomatic supernumerary teeth do not require any treatment. Surgical extraction may be required if they pose any functional or aesthetic problems.
- Refer the patient to a dentist for evaluation.

SUGGESTED READINGS

Sciuba J, Regezi JA, Rogers RS. Tooth abnormalities. *PDQ Oral Disease: Diagnosis and Treatment*. Hamilton, Ontario, Canada: BC Decker Inc; 2002. pp. 304–22.

Dunlap C. *Abnormalities of Teeth*. Kansas, MO: UMKC; 2004. Available from: http://dentistry.umkc.edu/Practicing_Communities/asset/AbnormalitiesofTeeth.pdf

Chapter 10

Alterations in the size and shape of teeth

S. R. Prabhu

MACRODONTIA

Definition/Description

- A condition in which a tooth or teeth clinically and radiographically appear larger than normal for that particular type of tooth or teeth is called macrodontia. This condition is also called megadontia or megalodontia.

Cause

- Macrodontia is associated with disturbance in the tooth-forming tissues. When macrodontia is generalised (rare) and involves all teeth, a hormonal cause such as pituitary gigantism may be associated.

Clinical Features

- Majority of cases of macrodontia involve single tooth. Tooth size is larger than normal for the tooth in question. This should be confirmed clinically and radiographically.
- Radiograph shows single pulp chamber and root canal. Tooth is asymptomatic.
- Differential diagnosis should include conditions such as fusion (union of two adjacent teeth), dens invaginatus (also called dens-in-dente, meaning tooth within a tooth) and gemination (attempt by a single tooth bud to form two teeth). All these anomalies can exhibit tooth size larger than normal for the tooth in question.

Diagnosis

- Clinical and radiographic examination confirms the diagnosis. Tooth is large and is with one root canal.

Management

- Refer the patient to a dentist for evaluation.
- For asymptomatic patients with macrodontia, no treatment is required.

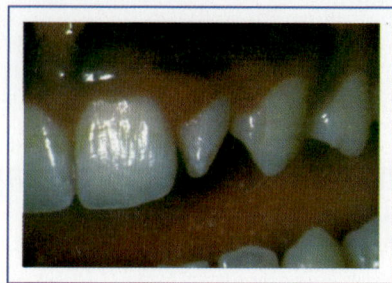

Figure 10.1 Microdontia (peg-shaped maxillary lateral incisor).
Reproduced with permission from: Charles Dunlap. Formerly, Professor of Oral and Maxillofacial Pathology, UMKC, USA.

MICRODONTIA

Definition/Description

- A condition in which a tooth or teeth clinically and radiographically appear smaller than normal for that particular type of tooth or teeth is called microdontia. Microdontia involving a single tooth is common.

Cause

- Developmental disturbances during morphodifferentiation of tooth development may cause alteration in the tooth size, including microdontia.

Clinical Features

- Generalised microdontia involving all teeth is rare. This may occur as a feature of conditions such as pituitary dwarfism.
- Often, microdontia is limited to a single tooth and may involve maxillary lateral incisors (peg-shaped laterals) (Figure 10.1) and third molars. Peg-shaped laterals may have a familial tendency.

Diagnosis

- History and clinical examination, including radiography.

Management

- Unless aesthetically unacceptable, treatment is not required.
- Refer the patient to a dentist for evaluation.

NOTCHED INCISORS

Definition/Description

- Notched incisors are characterised by a central notch in the incisal edge of an incisor.

Cause

- Notches can be derived from acquired causes, such as habits of holding a pencil, needle, thread or pipe between the teeth and biting seeds and nuts.
- Notched incisors of developmental origin can be seen in congenital syphilis. These are referred to as Hutchinson's incisors.

Clinical Features

- Notches are visible in different shapes, depending on the cause. Often the defect may cause sensitivity to cold.

Diagnosis

- History and clinical and radiographical findings.

Management

- Refer the patient to a dentist for evaluation.
- Restorative treatment may be necessary in some cases.

HUTCHINSON'S INCISORS

Definition/Description

- Hutchinson's teeth are centrally notched, widely spaced, peg (screwdriver teeth)-shaped upper permanent central incisors.

Cause

- Congenital syphilis.

Clinical Features

- The triad of Hutchinson's incisors (Figure 10.2), interstitial keratitis and sensorineural hearing loss are considered pathognomonic of congenital syphilis.

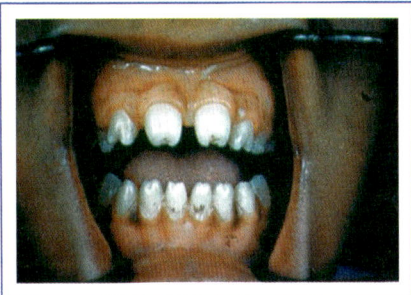

Figure 10.2 'Screwdriver'-shaped teeth (notched incisors) of congenital syphilis.
Reproduced with permission from: Charles Dunlap. Formerly, Professor of Oral and Maxillofacial Pathology, UMKC, USA.

Diagnosis

- History of congenital syphilis and clinical features aid the diagnosis of the condition

Management

- Refer the patient to a dentist for evaluation and restorative treatment.

MULBERRY MOLARS

Definition/Description

- Mulberry molars are permanent first molars with small occlusal surfaces and are characterised by the presence of several globular poorly formed cusps.

Cause

- Congenital syphilis.

Clinical Features

- Dental changes in congenital syphilis occur around the age of six years, as a result of which permanent central incisors and first molars are affected (Figure 10.3).
- First molars present several globular poorly formed cusps. These teeth show a narrower occlusal surface than its cervical third.

Diagnosis

- History and clinical grounds.

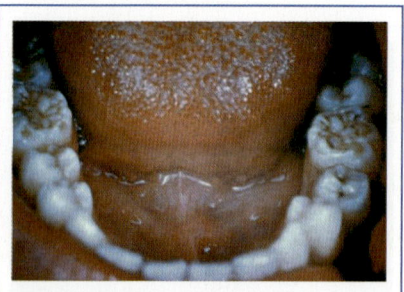

Figure 10.3 Mulberry molars of congenital syphilis. Note multiple poorly formed globular cusps of the right and left lower first permanent molars. Reproduced with permission from: Charles Dunlap. Formerly, Professor of Oral and Maxillofacial Pathology, UMKC, USA.

Management

- Refer the patient to a dentist for evaluation.

DILACERATION

- Severe bend in the long axis of the tooth located at the junction between the crown and the root is called dilaceration. This is caused by trauma before calcification and is detected on X-rays.
- Refer the patient to a dentist for evaluation. If extraction is required because of extensive decay, these teeth pose surgical difficulties.

TAURODONTISM

- Taurodontism (bull-like teeth) is characterised by abnormally long pulp chamber and short roots seen in molars. It is detected on X-rays.

GEMINATION AND FUSION OF TEETH

- Gemination of a tooth refers to an attempt by a single tooth germ to form two teeth (Figure 10.4 A and B). This process is also called twinning.
- Fusion refers to the fusion of two adjacent tooth germs to form a single tooth (Figure 10.4 C).

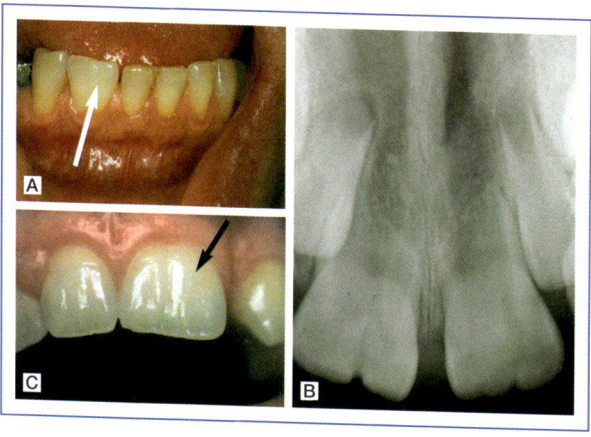

Figure 10.4 Gemination and fusion. (A–Arrow and B) All maxillary incisors are present in gemination. (C–Arrow) In fusion, note the missing left lateral incisor, which is fused with the central incisor.

Reproduced with permission from: Charles Dunlap. Formerly, Professor of Oral and Maxillofacial Pathology, UMKC, USA.

- Clinically, it is not easy to differentiate between the two conditions when the tooth looks large. Teeth need to be counted. In fusion, one tooth is missing.

SUGGESTED READINGS

Sciuba J, Regezi JA, Rogers RS. Tooth abnormalities. *PDQ Oral Disease: Diagnosis and Treatment*. Hamilton, Ontario, Canada: BC Decker Inc; 2002. pp. 304–22.

Dunlap C. *Abnormalities of Teeth*. Kansas, MO: UMKC; 2004. Available from: http://dentistry.umkc.edu/Practicing_Communities/asset/AbnormalitiesofTeeth.pdf

Chapter 11

Alterations in the structure of teeth

S. R. Prabhu

ENAMEL HYPOPLASIA

Definition/Description

- Enamel hypoplasia is characterised by deficient enamel formation, resulting in thin enamel surface. Underlying dentine is normal.

Cause

- Local causes of hypoplasia of permanent teeth include trauma derived from infection at the roots of the deciduous teeth. Turner's tooth is an example of the local factors that cause enamel hypoplasia.
- Systemic causes of hypoplasia of enamel include exanthematous fever or nutritional deficiencies during tooth development.

Clinical Features

- Clinically, surface of the enamel may be pitted or smooth. Hypoplastic milky white spots are common in this condition. Shape of the crown may be altered.

Diagnosis

- Clinical and radiographical findings.

Management

- Refer the patient to a dentist.
- Restorative treatment may be necessary in some cases.

TURNER'S TOOTH

Definition/Description

- Turner's tooth is characterised by hypoplasia of enamel and involves a single permanent tooth.

Cause

- Causes of Turner's tooth (Turner's hypoplasia) include traumatic injury to the deciduous teeth and periapical infection of the overlying deciduous teeth.

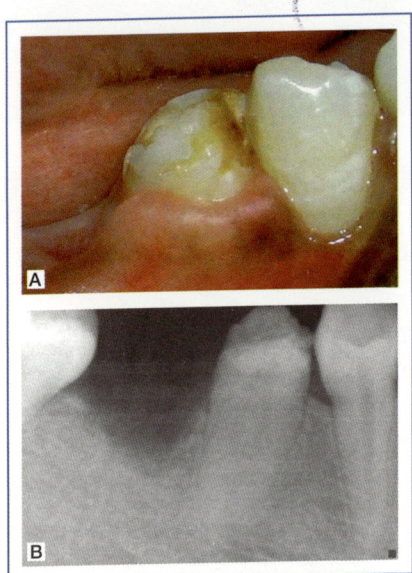

Figure 11.1 Turner's hypoplasia. Note (A) the yellowish-brown discolouration of the crown of the mandibular second premolar and (B) the radiographical image of the same tooth showing defective crown morphology.
Reproduced with permission from: Geeta Priya PR, John JB, Elango I. Turner's hypoplasia and non-vitality: a case report of sequelae in permanent tooth. *Contemp Clin Dent*. 2010;1:251–4.

Clinical Features

- Commonly involved teeth include premolars and maxillary central incisors. Surface of the involved permanent tooth may be pitted (Figure 11.1).

Diagnosis

- Clinical and radiographical findings.

Management

- Refer the patient to a dentist.
- Restorative treatment may be necessary.

AMELOGENESIS IMPERFECTA

Definition/Description

- Amelogenesis imperfecta (AI) represents a group of rare, inherited disorders characterised by abnormal enamel formation in the absence of systemic disorders.

- The condition is characterised by hypoplasia and/or hypominerali-sation of all or most of the primary and permanent teeth.

Cause

- It is an inherited disorder caused by X-linked or sporadic inheri-tance. Defective amelogenin (AMELX) genes on X and Y chromo-somes are mainly involved in its causation.

Clinical Features

Three types of AI include hypoplastic, hypomaturation and hypocalci-fied forms.

- In the hypoplastic form, the formation of enamel matrix is in-adequate. Enamel hardness is normal, but it is thin because of inadequate amount of enamel. The colour of enamel is normal (Figure 11.2 A).
- In the hypocalcified (hypomineralised) form, enamel is soft due to poor mineralisation, but the quantity of enamel is normal. The colour of the tooth is yellow to brown (Figure 11.2 B and C) and the tooth surface easily chips off. Caries susceptibility is low, but there is rapid rate of attrition.
- In the hypomaturation form, the crystal structure of the enamel is defective, which leads to mottled enamel with white to brown or yellow colour (Figure 11.2 D).

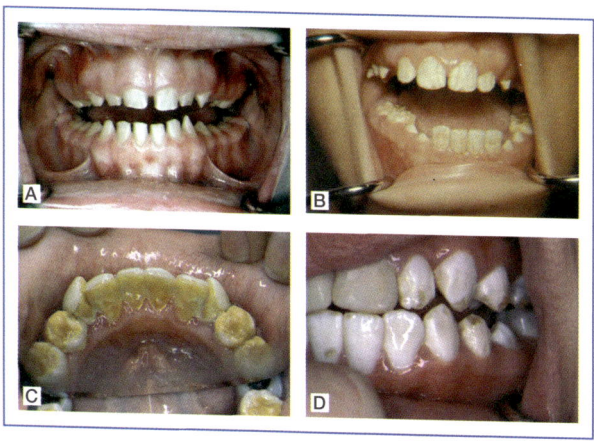

Figure 11.2 Amelogenesis imperfecta: (A) Hypoplastic type, (B and C) hypocalcified type and (D) hypomaturation type.
Reproduced with permission from: Charles Dunlap. Formerly, Professor of Oral and Maxillofacial Pathology, UMKC, USA.

Diagnosis

- History and clinical and radiographical features.

Management

- Genetic counselling is recommended.
- Refer the patient to a dentist for evaluation.
- Full crown restorations for aesthetics are carried out by dentists.

DENTINOGENESIS IMPERFECTA

Definition/Description

- Dentinogenesis imperfecta, also called hereditary opalescent dentin, represents a group of hereditary disorders characterised by abnormal dentine formation.
- This disorder may be seen alone or in association with the systemic hereditary disorder of the bone called osteogenesis imperfecta.

Cause

- Dentinogenesis imperfecta is a genetic disorder.
- Altered dentin matrix in dentinogenesis imperfecta is related to defective degradation of dentin phosphoprotein during the formation of dentin.

Clinical Features

- Both primary and permanent dentitions are affected in dentinogenesis imperfecta. However, primary dentition is more severely affected.
- Teeth exhibit grey to brownish opalescence (Figure 11.3 A and B). Enamel is normal but fractures easily due to underlying abnormal dentin.

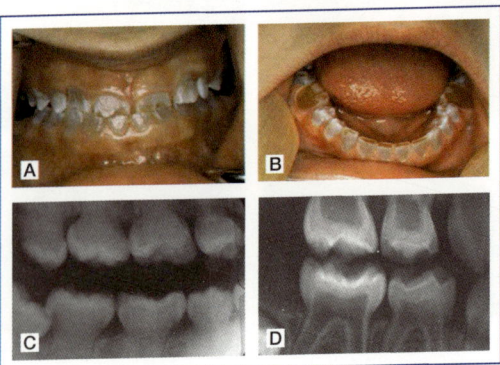

Figure 11.3   (A and B) Dentinogenesis imperfecta. (C and D) Radiographs of the premolars and molars show cervical constriction at the neck of the teeth. Reproduced with permission from: Charles Dunlap. Formerly, Professor of Oral and Maxillofacial Pathology, UMKC, USA.

- Exposed dentin undergoes severe tooth wear. This may cause the involvement of the dental pulp and dental abscess.
- Radiographical images show short roots, calcifications in the pulp and pronounced cervical constriction of the teeth (Figure 11.3 C and D) ('Tulip' profile).
- In patients with dentinogenesis imperfecta associated with osteogenesis imperfecta, the teeth exhibit blue-grey to yellow-brown colour, excessive breakdown of enamel and blue sclera.

Diagnosis

- History (in particular, family history) and clinical and radiographical examinations.

Management

- Genetic counselling is recommended.
- Refer the patient to a dentist for evaluation.
- Aesthetic restorations are required.

SUGGESTED READINGS

Sciuba J, Regezi JA, Rogers RS. Tooth abnormalities. *PDQ Oral Disease: Diagnosis and Treatment*. 2002. Hamilton, Ontario, Canada: BC Decker Inc; 2002. pp. 304–22.

Dunlap C. *Abnormalities of Teeth*. Kansas, MO: UMKC; 2004. Available from: http://dentistry.umkc.edu/Practicing_Communities/asset/AbnormalitiesofTeeth.pdf

Chapter 12

Delay and failure of tooth eruption

S. R. Prabhu

DEFINITION/DESCRIPTION

- A delay in the eruption of teeth refers to the condition where teeth fail to make their appearance in the mouth at the expected age.
- **Teething:** The process of sequential appearance of primary teeth emerging through the gums in infants and children is called teething. Teething is a normal process, and any systemic illness, particularly infections during the period of teething, is coincidental. Teething is totally harmless.
- **Tooth eruption:** The movement of the tooth from its site of development in the alveolar bone of the jaws to the occlusal plane in the oral cavity is called tooth eruption.
- The first teeth appear between the age of six months and nine months, and it may take two years to complete the eruption of all 20 primary teeth.
- Eruption of the primary teeth and their shedding, followed by the eruption of the permanent teeth, is a sequential event. In clinical practice, significant deviations in eruption time are frequently observed. Premature eruption and total failure of eruption are rare, whereas delayed eruption is common.
- The time of eruption of the deciduous and permanent teeth is shown in Chapter 1 (Examination of the mouth and the teeth).

CAUSE OF DELAY AND FAILURE OF ERUPTION

- Eruption of a single tooth may sometimes be prevented by local obstruction.
- In the permanent dentition, premature exfoliation of primary predecessor may cause a delay in the eruption of the permanent teeth due to closure of the available space.
- Other causes of delay or failure of eruption include malocclusion, loss of function and bony ankylosis of teeth.
- Some systemic syndromes are associated with delay or failure of tooth eruption. These include rickets, cleidocranial dysplasia, cherubism and gingival fibromatosis.
- It must be noted that gender differences in the timing of eruption do exist. Permanent teeth erupt earlier in girls than in boys.
- Trauma to the primary teeth and periapical cystic lesions of the nonvital primary incisors may cause delay in the eruption of the permanent successor.

- Arch-length deficiency can also cause a delay in the eruption of teeth. Severe malnourishment in children can lead to delayed eruption.
- Patients with hypothyroidism, hypopituitarism and hypoparathyroidism are known to exhibit delayed tooth eruption.
- In some syndromes such as Gardner's syndrome, cleidocranial dysplasia and Apert syndrome, delay in tooth eruption is common.
- Preterm babies (babies born before 37 weeks of gestation or those with birth weight less than 2500 g) commonly have delayed tooth eruption of both primary and permanent dentitions.

CLINICAL FEATURES

- When teeth do not make their appearance in the mouth at the expected age, a delay in eruption can be expected, and evaluation should be done to identify the causes.

DIAGNOSIS

- History (in particular, medical and family history), clinical examination and panoramic radiographs are essential.

MANAGEMENT

- Treatment considerations are based on the causes.
- Refer the patient to a dentist for evaluation.
- Some of the causes (e.g., removal of obstruction and creating space) can be corrected by the dentist.
- Patients with eruption delay of more than two years should be referred to a dentist or paediatric dentist for further investigation.

SUGGESTED READINGS

Sciuba J, Regezi JA, Rogers RS. Tooth abnormalities. *PDQ Oral Disease: Diagnosis and Treatment*. Hamilton, Ontario, Canada: BC Decker Inc; 2002. pp. 304–22.

Dunlap C. *Abnormalities of Teeth*. Kansas, MO: UMKC; 2004. Available from: http://dentistry.umkc.edu/Practicing_Communities/asset/AbnormalitiesofTeeth.pdf

Chapter 13

Tooth impactions

S. R. Prabhu

DEFINITION/DESCRIPTION

- In general, teeth that are completely or partially retained in the jaw bone beyond their normal date of eruption are regarded as impacted teeth. Mandibular third molars, followed by maxillary third molars and maxillary canines, are the commonly involved impacted teeth. In rare cases, second premolars and mandibular second molars may be impacted.

CAUSE

- Lack of space for tooth eruption due to inadequate arch length, crowding of teeth, dense overlying bone, excessive soft tissue in the path of eruption and genetic abnormality can cause impaction of teeth.
- Impacted canines are most likely due to an extended development period and the long, tortuous path of eruption before the teeth emerge into full occlusion.

CLINICAL FEATURES

- Impacted teeth may or may not present any symptoms. The number of teeth present in the dentition is less due to impaction.
- Symptomatic patients with mandibular third molar impaction may experience referred pain in the ears or paraesthesia of the lips.
- Some patients complain of food impaction beneath the soft tissue covering the partially impacted tooth. This is called pericoronitis and is commonly experienced in mandibular third molar impactions. This may lead to symptoms such as pain, swelling and inability to open the mouth.

DIAGNOSIS

- History and clinical and radiographical examinations are routinely carried out for the diagnosis of impactions.
- Radiographs provide information on the angulations of impactions. Impacted third molars, for example, can be seen as mesioangular, distoangular, horizontal or vertical impactions. Other features that can be detected on radiographs include the depth of impacted teeth, proportion of the crown to the root, the proximity of the impacted tooth to the inferior alveolar nerve (in lower third molar impactions) and also the presence of cysts and other pathologies associated with the impacted teeth.

MANAGEMENT

- Asymptomatic impacted teeth (in particular, third molars) generally do not require removal. Teeth presenting with symptoms require removal.
- Refer the patient to a dentist or an oral surgeon for evaluation.

SUGGESTED READINGS

Miloro M, Ghali GE, Larsen P, Waite P. *Peterson's Principles of Oral and Maxillofacial Surgery.* 2nd ed. Hamilton, Ontario, Canada: BC Decker; 2004.

Richardson G, Russell KA. A review of impacted permanent maxillary cuspids: diagnosis and prevention. *J Can Dent Assoc.* 2000;66: 497–501. Available from: https://www.cda-adc.ca/jcda/vol-66/issue-9/497.html

Chapter 14

Tooth discolourations

S. R. Prabhu

TOOTH DISCOLOURATION

Definition/Description

- Teeth often show normal range of variation in the colour and shade of enamel. When the enamel shows discolouration beyond the normal limit, the tooth is said to be discoloured.
- Tooth discolouration can occur due to internal or external factors.
- In internal discolouration, pigments of various types are incorporated into the dental hard tissues during tooth formation.
- External staining of the teeth occurs on the tooth surface. It occurs due to dietary factors or tobacco use.

INTRINSIC DISCOLOURATION

Definition/Description

- Intrinsic discolouration of the tooth can be defined as the discolouration that is incorporated into the structure of dental hard tissues.
- These stains cannot be removed by prophylactic measures or tooth brushing and can affect single tooth or the entire dentition, depending on the cause.

Cause

- Single tooth discolouration may be due to an injury to the tooth germ. For example, discolouration of a permanent incisor can occur due to an infection or trauma from a deciduous predecessor and discolouration of premolars can occur due to periapical infection of the primary molars.
- Nonvital teeth due to trauma or infection can also cause tooth discolouration.
- Other causes of tooth discolouration include the following:
    - ◆ Excessive intake of fluoride (fluorosis) during tooth formation.
    - ◆ Tetracycline staining as a result of tetracycline treatment for childhood infections or administration to pregnant women after 14 weeks of gestation.
    - ◆ Enamel hypoplasia due to exanthematous fevers or severe nutritional deficiencies during childhood.
    - ◆ Erythroblastosis foetalis due to Rhesus (Rh) incompatibility and inherited disorders such as amelogenesis imperfecta and dentinogenesis imperfecta.

Clinical Features

- Discolouration may be confined to a single tooth or the entire dentition.
- Colour may vary from yellow and brown to green, depending on the causes involved.
- In fluorosis, the discolouration varies from mild opacity to dark yellow-brown discolouration (Figure 14.1). The severe form of fluorosis with yellow-brown discolouration with pits and grooves on the surface of enamel is called mottling.
- In tetracycline staining, the pattern of discolouration changes from light yellow to localised dark grey, purple, blue or brown colour. The colour depends on the type of tetracycline used (Figure 14.2 A and B).
- Aureomycin® gives grey-brown colour, whereas Achromycin® gives yellow colour. When viewed under ultraviolet light, teeth show bright-yellow fluorescence.
- Greyish-brown discolouration of a single tooth (e.g., maxillary central incisor) is due to necrotic pulp derived from trauma, ischaemia or bacterial infection.
- Internal resorption of dentine can give rise to pink discolouration.

Diagnosis

- A detailed history is essential for determining the cause of intrinsic discolouration of teeth. This process includes the following:
    - ◆ Medical history, mother's obstetric history, history of neonatal illness and drugs taken.

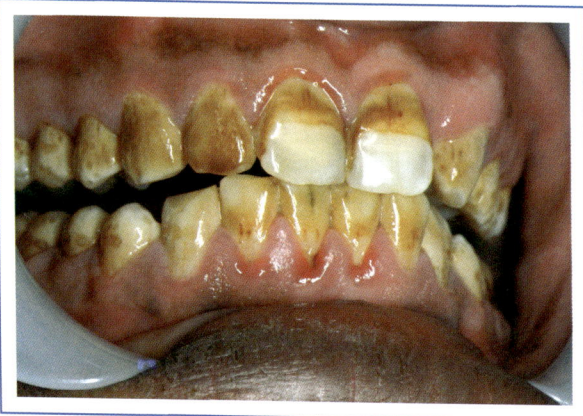

Figure 14.1   Generalised yellow-brown tooth discolouration due to fluorosis. Also, note gingival recession in relation to three lower incisors, possibly due to trauma from occlusion.
Courtesy: Nagamani Narayana.

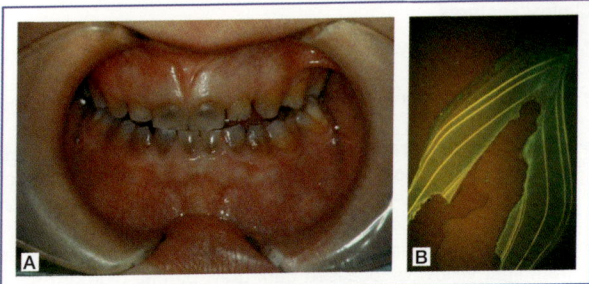

Figure 14.2 (A) Tetracycline staining of teeth and (B) section of the tooth viewed with fluorescent light shows yellow band of fluorescence in the dentin, suggesting an episode of treatment with tetracycline.
Reproduced with permission from: Charles Dunlap. Formerly, Professor of Oral and Maxillofacial Pathology, UMKC, USA.

- ◆ History of trauma, residence history related to drinking water and fluoridation areas and dental history.
- ◆ Social history with respect to smoking and intake of tea, coffee and red wine.
- Clinical examination includes a detailed oral and dental examination and intraoral X-ray of the full mouth.

Management

- Restorative treatment for aesthetic reasons may be required.
- Refer the patient to a dentist for evaluation.

EXTRINSIC DISCOLOURATION

Definition/Description

- Extrinsic discolouration of teeth is the discolouration in which stains are deposited on the surface of the teeth from external sources and they can be removed by oral prophylactic measures.

Cause

- Extrinsic stains of teeth are due to external sources. These include tobacco smoking or chewing; use of areca, betel, and drinks such as tea, coffee and red wine; use of chlorhexidine (mouth rinses), stannous fluoride, silver nitrate and coloured juices and fruits; presence of dental calculus; and arrested caries.
- Discolouration of teeth may range from yellow and brown to black, depending on the cause and its duration.

Diagnosis

- History and clinical examination.

Management

• Refer the patient to a dentist for evaluation and removal of stains.

SUGGESTED READING

Dunlap C. *Abnormalities of Teeth*. Kansas, MO: UMKC; 2004. Available from: http://dentistry.umkc.edu/Practicing_Communities/asset/AbnormalitiesofTeeth.pdf

Chapter 15

Abnormal mobility of the permanent teeth

S. R. Prabhu

DEFINITION/DESCRIPTION

- Normal physiological tooth mobility is approximately 0.25 mm.
- Mobility of the permanent tooth above the normal range of the tooth movement can be regarded as pathological. Pathological mobility is usually due to the loss of periodontal support.
- Close to the time of exfoliation, teeth become loose in the deciduous dentition. This is called physiological mobility.

CAUSE

- Permanent teeth exhibit increased mobility when alveolar bone resorption occurs due to local or systemic causes.
- Gingival diseases alone do not cause increased mobility of teeth unless periodontal tissues (periodontal ligament and alveolar bone) are affected.
- Common local and systemic causes of the increased mobility of teeth include the following:
  - Dental trauma resulting in root fracture.
  - Bruxism and traumatic occlusion, gingival recession with periodontal involvement, necrotising ulcerative periodontitis and chronic plaque-induced periodontitis.
  - Pathology of periapical tissues, such as periapical granuloma, cyst and abscess.
  - Bone tumours or gingival carcinomas that invade periodontal tissues.
  - Dentin dysplasia (rootless teeth).
  - Uncontrolled diabetes.
  - Pregnancy (due to the increased levels of progesterone and oestrogen).
  - Papillon-Lefevre syndrome, Chediak-Higashi syndrome, hypophosphatasia, Langerhans cell histiocytosis, neutropaenia and leukaemia.

DIAGNOSIS

- Abnormal tooth mobility in clinical practice can be diagnosed by tapping the tooth between two instrument handles and evaluating the movement of the tooth between the two extreme positions.

- It must be noted that on the basis of the underlying systemic and local factors, gingival swelling and bleeding may also accompany increased tooth mobility.
- Radiographical examination is an important aspect of the diagnosis of abnormal tooth mobility. Radiographs reveal alveolar bone loss and root resorption.
- If systemic causes are suspected, appropriate blood tests need to be done.

MANAGEMENT

- Refer the patient to a dentist for evaluation.
- Local causes should be identified and eliminated. If systemic causes are suspected, appropriate investigations need to be carried out and treatment should be offered.

SUGGESTED READING

Mittal S, Kataria P, Arya V, Taneja Arya L. Tooth mobility: a review. *Heal Talk*. 2012;5:40–2. Available from: http://oaji.net/articles/2014/1143-1412674504.pdf

Chapter 16

Malocclusion and crowding of teeth

S. R. Prabhu

DEFINITION/DESCRIPTION

- Occlusion refers to a manner in which the upper and lower teeth intercuspate between each other in all mandibular positions and movements.
- Malocclusion refers to incorrect occlusion, where teeth of upper and lower arches approach each other as the jaw closes.
- The crowding of teeth is characterised by teeth in the jaw that are too close to each other, thus resulting in overlapping.

CAUSE

- Oral habits such as thumb sucking, tongue thrusting, pacifier sucking (beyond the age of three years), prolonged use of feeding bottle, nail biting and biting on pen or pencil during active skeletal growth.
- Abnormal posture and deglutition disorders are also associated with malocclusion.
- Malocclusion can also be hereditary.
- Misalignment of jaw fractures after severe injury, birth defects such as cleft lip and cleft palate, impacted teeth and supernumerary teeth are other causes of malocclusion.

CLINICAL FEATURES

- Malocclusion is classified as class I, class II and class III malocclusions.
  - Class I malocclusion is the most common. It is characterised by normal bite; however, there is slight overlapping of the lower teeth by the upper teeth.
  - Class II malocclusion, also known as retrognathism, is a severe overlapping of the lower jaw and teeth by the upper jaw and teeth.
  - Class III malocclusion, also known as prognathism, is characterised by the protrusion of the lower jaw, which causes the lower jaw and lower teeth to overlap the upper jaw and teeth.
  - Symptoms of malocclusion include abnormal alignment of teeth, difficulty or discomfort in chewing or biting and mouth breathing.
- Other common terminologies used in clinical practice are as follows:
  - Overjet: The distance between the upper and lower incisors in the horizontal plane.
  - Overbite: The overlap of the incisors in the vertical plane.

- Deep or complete overbite: The contact of the lower incisors with the upper incisors or the palatal mucosa.
- Anterior open bite: A space that is seen between the upper and lower incisor edges when the teeth are in occlusion. This is viewed from the front.
- Crossbite: A deviation from the normal buccolingual relationship. This may be anterior, posterior and/or unilateral or bilateral.

DIAGNOSIS

- Malocclusion and crowding of teeth are easily diagnosed during routine oral examination.
- Diagnostic radiographs assist the clinician to confirm the diagnosis.

MANAGEMENT

- Refer the patient to a dentist for evaluation.
- Orthodontic treatment is recommended.

SUGGESTED READING

Hassan R, Rahima AK. Occlusion, malocclusion and method of measurements: an overview. *Archives of Orofacial Sciences*. 2007;2:3–9.

Chapter 17

Orofacial infections of dental origin

S. R. Prabhu and H. Al Bayaty

DENTAL ABSCESS (DENTOALVEOLAR ABSCESS, PERIAPICAL ABSCESS OR TOOTH ABSCESS)

Definition/Description

- Dental abscess is the localised collection of pus associated with an infected tooth. On the basis of its duration, this may occur in the acute or chronic forms.
- When abscess develops due to periapical infection, it is called periapical abscess. This is the most common form of dental abscess.
- If the abscess is due to periodontal infection, it is called periodontal abscess.

Cause

- Bacterial infection of the dental pulp (due to caries, failed root canal treatment or trauma) or of the periodontal tissues is the major cause of dental abscess.

Clinical Features

- Tooth involved in the formation of abscess is tender to touch. Abscess may be confined to the periapical or the gingival tissues and may not cause any noticeable extraoral swelling.
- When periapical abscess perforates the bone and causes infection of the surrounding tissues, facial swelling develops (Figure 17.1). Symptoms include mild to severe localised pain that is continuous, throbbing, sharp or shooting. Skin over the swelling is tender on palpation.
- Cervical lymphadenopathy with tender nodes is common.

Diagnosis

- History, clinical examination and radiography.
- Sometimes, microbiology, including antibiotic sensitivity tests, may be required.

Management

- Antibiotics and drainage (untreated cases may develop osteomyelitis, cellulitis or Ludwig's angina.)
- Refer the patient to a dentist or oral surgeon for the management of the involved tooth, which, in majority of patients, requires extraction.

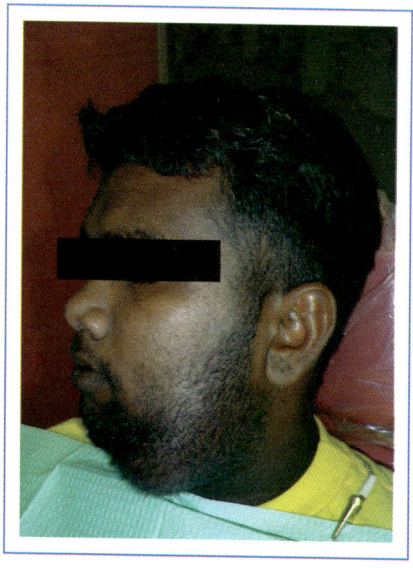

Figure 17.1 Dental abscess due to infection of the left first lower molar. *Courtesy*: Haytham Al Bayaty.

OSTEOMYELITIS OF THE JAW BONES

Definition/Description

- Osteomyelitis refers to the inflammation of the bone marrow.

Cause

- Osteomyelitis of the jaw bones is mainly due to odontogenic infections derived from the dental tissues.
- Other causes include infection of the fracture sites or of the surgery sites.
- Osteomyelitis is predominantly caused by haemolytic streptococcal infection and anaerobic bacteria such as *Peptostreptococci, Fusobacteria and Prevotella*. These bacteria are common in odontogenic infections.
- Underlying predisposing factors may include alcoholism, malnutrition, diabetes, leukaemia, anaemia, therapeutically irradiated bone, osteopetrosis, Paget's disease, and florid osseous dysplasia.

Clinical Features

- On the basis of the duration and severity of the inflammation, osteomyelitis can occur in two forms: acute and chronic.
- The third type called suppurative osteomyelitis is characterised by the infection of all three components of bone: periosteum, cortex and the marrow.

- Depending on the type of osteomyelitis, symptoms include deep-seated throbbing pain; extraoral swelling (which is tense, tender and red); trismus; dysphagia; cervical lymph node enlargement; paraesthesia in the area of distribution of mental nerve (for mandibular involvement); fever; malaise; a decayed and infected tooth; loose tooth; pus (at a later stage) and fetid odour. Mandible is involved in majority of cases.
- In chronic osteomyelitis, fragments of necrotic bone are separated from the vital bone (sequestra). If large segments of necrotic bone exist, they may be surrounded by granulation tissue and a new bone called involucrum.
- In chronic osteomyelitis, the swelling may be firm and mildly painful or tender. Sinus tracks opening to the external surface of the skin may be present.

Diagnosis

- History and clinical examination. Radiographs, computed tomographic scans and magnetic resonance imaging are used in the diagnostic protocol.
- Radiographical changes in the bone do not appear until 10 to 12 days from the start of the infection. Sequestra may be seen at a later stage.
- Subperiosteal bone formation may give rise to buccal swelling and may be visible on lateral radiographs. 'Moth-eaten' radiographical appearance characterised by radiopacity of the sequestra and the radiolucency of the pus is a sign of chronic and suppurative osteomyelitis.
- Radiographs are also useful in detecting the original site of infection, such as a decayed tooth or fracture site.

Management

Refer the patient to an oral surgeon. The following treatment protocol is recommended in a hospital setting:

- Acute osteomyelitis: Place drains, carefully remove the necrotic bone, obtain aspirate for microbiological examination and empirically provide antibiotic cover until the antibiotic sensitivity report is received.
- Chronic osteomyelitis: Drain the sinus tract, debride and obtain tissue for culture and consider sensitivity-directed antibiotic therapy. Also, consider hyperbaric oxygen and positron emission tomographic scans as follow up procedures.

OROFACIAL AND CERVICOFACIAL CELLULITIS, INCLUDING LUDWIG'S ANGINA

Definition/Description

- Orofacial cellulitis refers to the spread of infection to the soft tissue spaces of the orofacial region. In this condition, inflammatory exudate forms the vehicle for the spread of infection.

- Ludwig's angina is characterised by a rapidly progressive cellulitis of the soft tissues of the neck and the floor of the mouth. Infection is bilateral.

Cause

- Anaerobic bacteria are mainly involved. In majority of cases, the infection originates from the apical sites of the mandibular molars.
- Dental infections from the infected lower second and third molars account for the majority of cases of Ludwig's angina. Roots of these teeth lie at the level of the mylohyoid muscle, and periapical infection of this anatomical region can spread to the submandibular space.
- Mixed infections (i.e., infections with both aerobes and anaerobes) associated with cellulitis and Ludwig's angina include infections with α-haemolytic streptococci, staphylococci and bacteroides groups.
- HIV-infected patients, diabetes patients, transplant recipients and alcoholics are at risk of infection from a variety of atypical organisms.
- Less common causes of Ludwig's angina include mandibular fracture, neck trauma, tongue piercing, sialadenitis, neoplasms and peritonsillar abscess.

Clinical Features

- On the basis of the fascial spaces involved, cervicofacial cellulitis can occur in three forms: sublingual, submandibular and parapharyngeal (Figure 17.2).

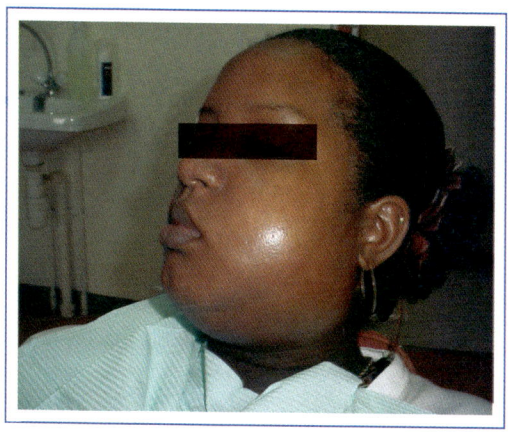

Figure 17.2 Cellulitis involving the left submandibular space due to acute infection of the left first lower molar.
Courtesy: Haytham Al Bayaty.

- When sublingual and submandibular spaces are bilaterally and simultaneously involved, the condition is called Ludwig's angina.
- Ludwig's angina is potentially a life-threatening condition, which causes airway obstruction due to progressive swelling of the soft tissues and elevation and posterior displacement of the tongue.
- In Ludwig's angina, patients report with dental pain or a history of recent dental procedures, neck pain and swelling, fever, dysphonia, dysphagia and dysarthria.
- Less than one-third of adults will present with respiratory distress with dyspnoea, tachypnoea or stridor.
- On physical examination in Ludwig's angina, more than 95% of patients have bilateral submandibular swelling and an elevated or protruding tongue.
- The submandibular swelling is often characterised as brawny (or 'woody') and tense, with overlying erythema. Suprahyoid swelling ('bull's neck') is tender and nonfluctuant.
- Cervical lymphadenopathy may be absent in patients with Ludwig's angina because the infection spreads to the structures of the anterior neck via connective tissue, muscle and fascial planes rather than by the lymphatic system.
- In advanced infection, cavernous sinus thrombosis and brain abscess may occur.

Diagnosis

- Diagnosis of cellulitis and Ludwig's angina is done on clinical grounds.
- Panoramic radiographs show dental source of infection.
- Computed tomographic scans show the extent of soft tissue swelling, the presence of gas, fluid collection and airway compromise. Magnetic resonance imaging is also a useful diagnostic technique.

Management

Immediate referral to a hospital setting is essential. The treatment protocol is as under:

- Cervicofacial cellulitis: Establishment of drainage and use of injectable systemic antibiotics, antipyretics and analgesics.
- Ludwig's angina: Protection of the airway is of foremost importance during the initial management. Hospitalisation of the patient is essential.
- Consultation with an anaesthetist and maxillofacial or ENT surgeon and transfer of the patient to the operating theatre should be considered immediately.
- Tracheotomy remains the gold standard for securing the airway. Once the airway is secured, aggressive intravenous administration of antibiotic agent should begin. High doses of penicillin and metronidazole, clindamycin, amoxicillin-clavulanate are used for these patients.
- Surgical drainage is indicated when suppuration is seen. Removal of the infected teeth is also essential.

SUGGESTED READINGS

Horswell BB. Diagnosis and treatment of infections. In: Laskin DM, editor. *Clinician's Handbook of Oral and Maxillofacial Surgery*. Hanover Park, IL: Quintessence Publishing Co; 2010. pp. 258–77.

Bruce Donoff R. Odontogenic infection. In: Bruce Donoff R, editor. *Manual of Oral and Maxillofacial Surgery*. St. Louis, MO: Mosby; 1997. pp. 207–21.

Cawson RA, Odell EW. Major infections of the mouth, jaws and perioral tissues. *Cawson's Essentials of Oral Pathology and Oral Medicine*. 8th ed. London, U.K.: Churchill Livingstone; 2008. pp. 99–114.

Chapter 18

Temporomandibular joint disorders

S. R. Prabhu

DEFINITION/DESCRIPTION

- Temporomandibular joint disorder (TMJD) is a collective term used to indicate a disorder or dysfunction within the muscles of mastication and/or the temporomandibular joint (TMJ), with the possibility of other associated structures being involved. TMJDs are a major source of orofacial pain in the general population.

CAUSE

- No specific cause is identified for TMJDs. However, predisposing, precipitating and perpetuating factors have been found to be associated with this disorder.
  - ◆ **Predisposing factors** include occlusal malrelations, jaw or face trauma, bruxism, clenching, whiplash, iatrogenic causes, new restorations, third molar extractions, oral intubation for surgery, poor general health, orthopaedic imbalances and mental distress.
  - ◆ **Precipitating and/or perpetual factors** include skeletal deformity, poor posture, nutritional deficiencies, metabolic disturbances, depression and anxiety, middle ear infection, rheumatoid arthritis, sinusitis, chewing gum and sleep disturbances.

CLINICAL FEATURES

- Pain in the TMJ is a common complaint.
- Increase in pain occurs with jaw movement (e.g., chewing and yawning).
- Other symptoms include periauricular pain, ear pain, facial pain, limited and deviated jaw opening, jaw 'locking', joint sounds and recurrent headaches.

DIAGNOSIS

- Detailed history: Pain history, medical history and dental history.
- Measurement of level of pain on a pain scale of 0 to 3 (0 = no pain, 1 = slight pain or discomfort, 2 = moderate pain and 3 = severe pain).
- Clinical examination of the joints and muscles of mastication.
- Palpation: Lateral aspects of the TMJ, with mouth closed and open. Pain in the joint indicates capsulitis, sinovitis or osteoarthritis.
- Palpation of the muscles of mastication: Bilateral palpation for comparison for rigidity, pain and size.

- Mouth opening by using a metal ruler: normal 40 mm; range: 35 to 45 mm, depending on the size of the mouth.
- Measurement of mandibular deviation (left or right) or 'S'-shaped opening, if any.
- Intraoral examination for dental occlusion and palpation of lateral and medial pterygoid muscles.
- Palpation and/or auscultation of the sounds of the TMJ: clicks, pops or crepitus.
- Imaging: Orthopantamography and transcranial radiographs for TMJDs and magnetic resonance imaging for soft tissue derangements.

MANAGEMENT

Refer the patient to a dentist for evaluation and treatment. Treatment protocol includes the following:

- Nonsurgical therapy
  - ◆ Moist heat and cold spray
  - ◆ Local anaesthetic injections in muscle trigger zones
  - ◆ Passive and active exercises
  - ◆ Medications: muscle relaxants and analgesics
  - ◆ Splints
  - ◆ Acupuncture
  - ◆ Physiotherapy
  - ◆ Transcutaneous electrical neural stimulation
  - ◆ Dental therapy

SUGGESTED READING

Nassif J. Temporomandibular disorder. In: Prabhu SR, editor. *Textbook of Oral Medicine*. New Delhi, India: Oxford University Press; 2004. pp. 71–90.

Part III

Presenting complaints related to the gums, oral mucosa and oral environment

Chapter 19

Gingival and oral soft tissue lumps and swellings

S. R. Prabhu and D. F. Wilson

GINGIVAL LUMPS AND SWELLINGS

Fibrous Epulis

Definition/Description

- The term 'epulis' means a localised growth on the gingiva. Fibrous epulis refers to a fibrous growth on the gingival or alveolar mucosa.

Cause

- The cause of fibrous epulis is hyperplasia of the oral mucosal fibrous tissue, which results from the tissue's response to mild and chronic local irritation or trauma. Sometimes, fibrous epulis is referred to as peripheral fibroma of the gingiva.

Clinical Features

- Fibrous epulis is commonly located on the gingiva between two teeth. The lesion is usually seen as a pink-white firm nodule, sessile or pedunculated (Figure 19.1).
- Fibrous epulis is asymptomatic in most cases and has a history of slow growth.

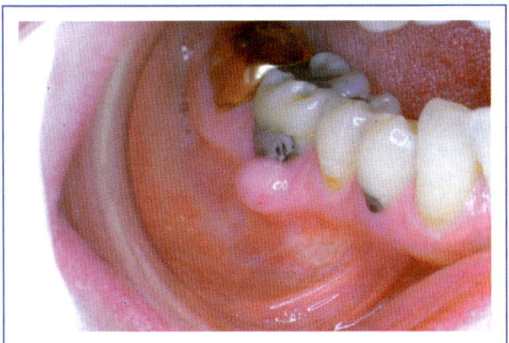

Figure 19.1 Fibrous epulis.
Courtesy: David Wilson.

Diagnosis

- History and clinical examination.
- Histological examination is recommended for confirmation.

Management

- Refer the patient to an oral surgeon for conservative surgical excision.

Pyogenic Granuloma

Definition/Description

- Pyogenic granuloma is a highly vascular, localised inflammatory lesion. The term 'pyogenic' is a misnomer, since this lesion does not produce pus. When a pyogenic granuloma occurs in pregnant women, the condition is called pregnancy epulis or pregnancy tumour.

Cause

- Pyogenic granuloma is an exuberant tissue response to local irritation or trauma.
- In pregnancy, the lesion may also be related to the effects of female hormones.

Clinical Features

- Pyogenic granuloma occurs commonly but not exclusively in women.
- Facial surfaces of gingival tissues are commonly involved.
- The lesion is painless, mildly painful or tender.
- The surface is smooth or lobulated, and red or purple in colour (Figure 19.2).
- It may show ulceration, and in some cases, the lesion is pedunculated.
- There may be a history of rapid growth.

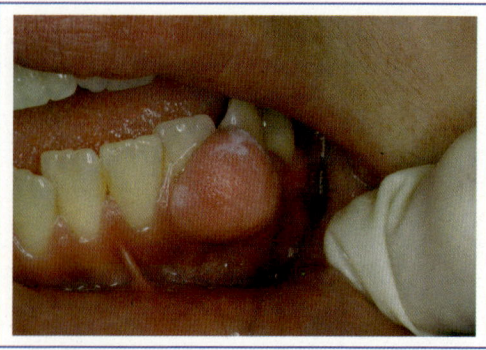

Figure 19.2 Pyogenic granuloma.
Courtesy: Nagamani Narayana.

Diagnosis

- History and clinical examination are helpful in the diagnosis. Histological evaluation is confirmatory.

Management

- Refer the patient to a dentist or an oral surgeon.
- Conservative surgical excision with a wide margin is the treatment of choice.
- Scaling of adjacent teeth is required to eliminate the sources of irritation or infection.
- Recurrences are common.

Peripheral Giant Cell Granuloma (Giant Cell Epulis)

Definition/Description

- Peripheral giant cell granuloma (PGCG), also called giant cell epulis, is a reactive lesion on the gingiva and is characterised by the histological presence of vascular, cell-rich fibrous connective tissue containing multinucleated giant cells.

Cause

- Lesions occur as a result of a reactive response to irritation or trauma.

Clinical Features

- Gingiva or alveolar ridges are commonly involved, with a predilection for the maxilla.
- Peripheral giant cell granuloma is a bluish-purple nodule and may be sessile or pedunculated (Figure 19.3).
- It may show signs of surface ulceration.

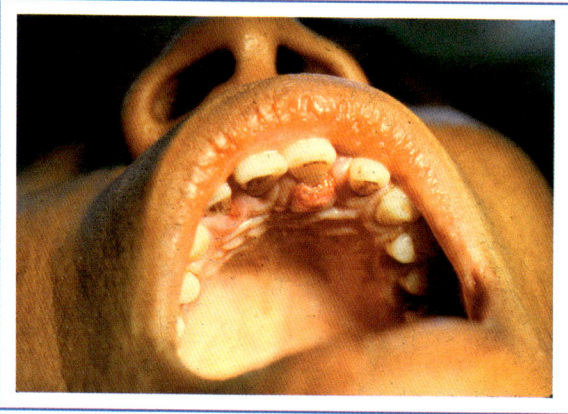

Figure 19.3 Peripheral giant cell granuloma.
Courtesy: David Wilson.

Diagnosis

- Clinical examination alone may not be useful for the diagnosis of PGCG because other epulides can also present a similar clinical picture.
- Histological evaluation confirms the diagnosis.
- PGCG lesions are characterised by the histological presence of multinucleated giant cells, ovoid-spindle stromal cells, red blood cells, haemosiderin and occasionally reactive bone.

Management

- Refer the patient to a dentist or an oral surgeon.
- Conservative surgical excision with a margin is the treatment of choice.
- Adjacent teeth should be scaled, and patients should be followed up because 10% of PGCGs show recurrence.

Peripheral Ossifying Fibroma (Ossifying Fibroid Epulis or Calcifying Fibroblastic Granuloma)

Definition/Description

- Peripheral ossifying fibroma (POF), also known as ossifying fibroid epulis, refers to a gingival lesion that is characterised by the histological presence of fibroblastic proliferation and bone or cementum-like mineralised structures.
- Fibroblasts are derived from the periosteum or periodontal ligament.

Cause

- POF is due to a reactive response to low-grade irritation.

Clinical Features

- Lesions are found on the gingiva, with a predilection for the maxilla, particularly in the incisor-canine region.
- The lesion is a pink or red nodule and is either sessile or pedunculated (Figure 19.4), with a history of slow growth.

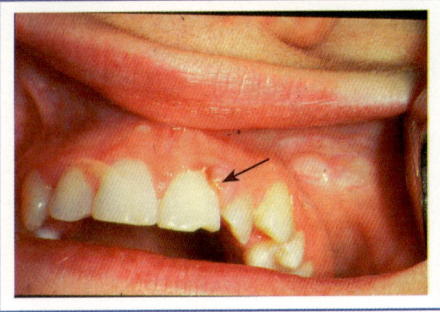

Figure 19.4 Peripheral ossifying fibroma (arrow).
Courtesy: David Wilson.

Diagnosis

- History, clinical examination and histological findings.
- Clinically, this lesion mimics other epulides.
- Biopsy for histological confirmation is necessary.

Management

- Refer the patient to a dentist or an oral surgeon.
- Conservative surgical excision is the treatment of choice.
- Adjacent teeth should be scaled, and patients should be followed up because as 16% of POFs show recurrence.

Denture Granuloma (Epulis Fissuratum, Denture Epulis or Denture Hyperplasia)

Definition/Description

- Denture granuloma, also called epulis fissuratum, is a hyperplastic lesion that may be located on an edentulous ridge or adjacent sulcus in a denture wearer.

Cause

- Denture granuloma is caused by chronic irritation derived from an ill-fitting or overextended denture flange.

Clinical Features

- This is a pink hyperplastic lesion usually creased by a trough, which is produced by the denture flange (Figure 19.5).
- The lesion is firm, persistent and painless. It may be ulcerated.

Diagnosis

- History, clinical appearance and microscopical examination confirm the diagnosis.

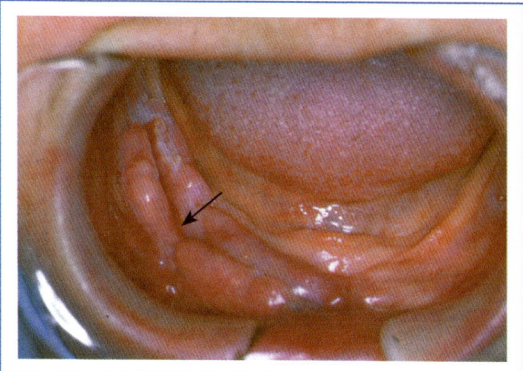

Figure 19.5 Epulis fissuratum (arrow).
Courtesy: David Wilson.

Management

- Refer the patient to a dentist or an oral surgeon.
- Treatment includes surgical removal of the hyperplastic tissue and denture relining or construction of new dentures.

Inflammatory Gingivitis

Definition/Description

- Inflammatory gingival enlargement results from bacterial-plaque-associated chronic inflammation of the gingival mucosa.
- The condition is similar to pregnancy gingivitis and pubertal gingivitis but occurs in patients without these histories.

Cause

- Bacterial plaque.

Clinical Features

- Generalised gingival enlargement, with the disappearance of stippling, is common.
- Gums are shiny due to inflammatory oedema.
- Halitosis and gingival bleeding on brushing of teeth are common features.
- This condition responds to mechanical debridement of the teeth and gums.

Diagnosis

- History and clinical examination.

Management

- Refer the patient to a dentist for oral prophylaxis.

Gingival Abscess

Definition/Description

- Gingival abscess is a localised inflammatory condition of the gingiva and is characterised by purulent exudates, without attachment loss.

Cause

- Localised infection secondary to injury to the gingival tissues from toothbrush bristle, fish bone, foreign body impaction (dental floss, toothpick, etc.) or other external agents.

Clinical Features

- Pain in the gum for one to two days, accompanied by a red localised swelling confined to the marginal gingival tissues.

Diagnosis

- History of the chief complaint and clinical examination of the abscess offer useful clues to clinical diagnosis.

Management

- Refer the patient to a dentist. This may be considered a dental emergency.
- Drainage of the gingival abscess is required. The use of antibiotics may be necessary, depending on the severity of the infection.

Drug-induced Gingival Hyperplasia

Definition/Description

- Drug-induced gingival hyperplasia refers to generalised gingival enlargement associated with the use of systemic medication.

Cause

- This condition is characterised by an abnormal response of the gingival tissue to the use of certain systemic medications.
- It has strong associations with phenytoin (an anticonvulsive agent), cyclosporine (an immunosuppressant) and nifedipine (calcium channel blocker for hypertension).
- The incidence of gingival hyperplasia is 50%, 25% and 25% in phenytoin users, cyclosporine users and nifedipine users, respectively.
- The anterior gingival facial surface is commonly involved. The degree of enlargement depends upon patient's level of oral hygiene.

Clinical Features

- Gingival hyperplasia typically begins one to three months after starting the treatment.
- The gingiva is pink and firm. If inflamed, the gingiva is red and oedematous and may completely cover the crowns of the teeth (Figure 19.6).

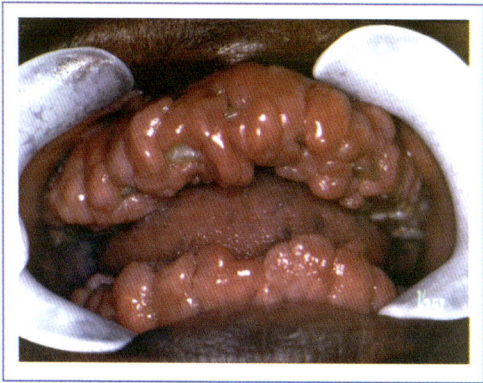

Figure 19.6 Drug (cyclosporine)-induced gingival hyperplasia. *Courtesy*: David Wilson.

Diagnosis

• History and clinical examination.

Management

• Change of medicine without compromising patient's general health may be required.
• Refer the patient to a dentist or an oral surgeon for prophylaxis, gingivectomy and periodic reevaluation.

Leukaemic Gingival Enlargement

Definition/Description

• Leukaemic gingival enlargement refers to generalised enlargement of the gingivae, predominantly in acute myelogenous leukaemia.

Cause

• Leukaemic infiltrate of the gingival tissues.

Clinical Features

• Gingival enlargement is generally boggy and nontender.
• Ulceration of the gingiva and adjacent oral mucosa due to neutro-paenia is frequently present.
• Constitutional symptoms include fatigue and fever. Infection and bleeding are also common in these patients.

Diagnosis

• A complete blood count should be performed; typically, elevated white blood cell count is present.
• Other investigations include peripheral blood smear and bone marrow aspiration.

Management

• The patients with leukaemic gingival enlargement respond when they receive chemotherapy for leukaemia.

Hereditary Gingival Fibromatosis (Familial Gingival Hyperplasia)

Definition/Description

• Hereditary gingival fibromatosis is an inherited disorder characterised by diffuse fibrous enlargement of the gingival tissues.

Cause

• Genetic aetiology.
• Increased synthesis of collagen and a decreased degradation or alteration of fibroblast proliferation.

Clinical Features

• Both men and women are affected.
• Gingival enlargement presents normal colour and is firm.
• Buccal and lingual aspects of the gums are involved and often cover the entire dentition (Figure 19.7).
• Gingival enlargement starts as permanent teeth erupt.

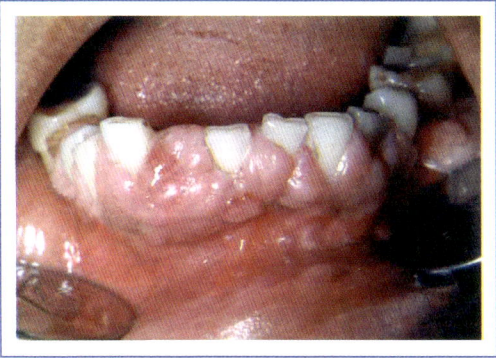

Figure 19.7 Familial gingival hyperplasia.
Reproduced with permission from: Ramadas K, Lucas E, Thomas G, et al. *A Digital Manual for the Early Diagnosis of Oral Neoplasia*. IARC, Lyon, 2008. Available from: http://screening.iarc.fr/atlasoral.php?lang=1

Diagnosis

• History, clinical examination and histological evaluation.

Management

• Refer the patient to a dentist or a periodontist for management. Serial surgical removal of the hyperplastic tissue is required for aesthetical and functional reasons.
• Oral prophylaxis and oral home care are essential aspects of the management. Recurrence is common.

ORAL SOFT TISSUE LUMPS AND SWELLINGS

Fibroepithelial Polyp (Traumatic Fibroma or Irritation Fibroma)

Definition/Description

• The fibroepithelial polyp, also known as traumatic fibroma or irritation fibroma, is a sessile fibrous nodule usually seen on the buccal mucosa. Less common sites include the labial mucosa, tongue and gingiva. A gingival fibroepithelial lesion is called a fibrous epulis.

Cause

• Reactive hyperplasia of the oral mucosal fibrous connective tissue due to chronic irritation or trauma.

Clinical Features

• The fibroepithelial polyp is a solitary, well-circumscribed, firm, painless and pink nodule attached to the underlying mucosa with a broad base. The overlying mucosa may be normal or occasionally ulcerated due to trauma (Figure 19.8).

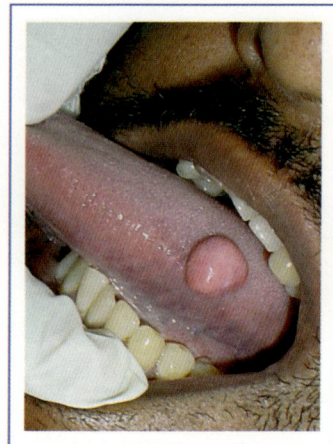

Figure 19.8 Fibroepithelial polyp (irritation fibroma) of the lateral border of the tongue.
Courtesy: Haytham Al Bayaty.

Diagnosis

- A history of trauma or the presence of the lesion on a trauma-prone site and clinical examination. Histopathological evaluation of the lesion obtained from excision biopsy is confirmatory.

Management

- Refer the patient to an oral surgeon for surgical removal of the lesion. If adequate excision is carried out, recurrence is unlikely.

Lipoma

Definition/Description

- A lipoma is a slow-growing benign neoplasm of mature adipose tissue.

Cause

- Exact cause is not known. May represent a proliferative response of lipocytes to local trauma.

Clinical Features

- A lipoma is a sessile, circumscribed lesion with a soft to firm consistency.
- This lesion is painless and usually seen as a yellow, circumscribed lesion, whereas deeper lesion is usually pink in colour (Figure 19.9). Preferred intraoral sites of occurrence include the buccal mucosa, ventral surface of the tongue and floor of the mouth.

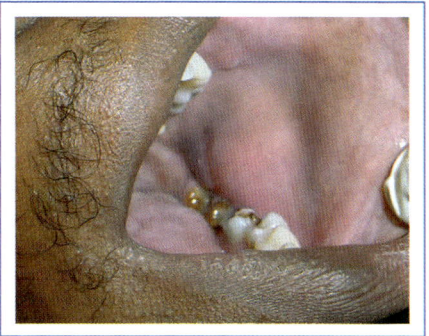

Figure 19.9   Lipoma of the buccal mucosa.
Courtesy: Haytham Al Bayaty.

Diagnosis

• History, clinical examination and histopathological evaluation of the
lesion obtained by excision biopsy.

Management

• Refer the patient to an oral surgeon for surgical excision.
Recurrences are unlikely.

Neurofibroma

Definition/Description

• Neurofibromas are benign neoplasms of the Schwann cells and
perineural fibroblasts.
• Solitary neurofibroma of the oral tissues is rare. Intraoral neurofibromas often appear as a part of multiple neurofibromatosis (von
Recklinghausen's disease).

Cause

• The cause of the solitary neurofibroma is not known. Multiple neurofibromatosis is inherited as an autosomal dominant trait in about
50% of cases.

Clinical Features

• Solitary neurofibroma is a circumscribed, painless, pink, firm nodule
with a broad base. Common intraoral sites include the tongue and
the buccal mucosa.
• Neurofibromatosis lesions are multiple and occur on the skin
accompanied by skin pigmentation referred to as *cafe-au-lait*
macules.

Diagnosis

• History and clinical examination. Histopathological evaluation of
the lesion is confirmatory.

Management

- Refer the patient to an oral surgeon for surgical removal. Fifteen percent of the patients with multiple neurofibromatosis develop neurofibrosarcomas.

Traumatic Neuroma

Definition/Description

- Traumatic neuroma, also known as amputation neuroma, is a lesion that results from trauma to a nerve, usually during a surgical procedure.

Cause

- In the majority of cases, traumatic injury to a nerve bundle secondary to tooth extraction is the cause. Most cases involve the mental nerve.

Clinical Features

- A circumscribed, pink, firm nodule with a broad base. Common intraoral sites include mucosa over the mental foramen and dorsal surface of the tongue.
- Lesions can be painful when pressure is applied.

Diagnosis

- History of trauma and clinical examination. Histopathological examination of the lesion is confirmatory.

Management

- Refer the patient to an oral surgeon for surgical removal of the lesion.

Mucocoele and Ranula

Definition/Description

- 'Mucocoele' is a clinical term used to describe a single or multiple blister-like painless, soft, smooth spherical fluctuating swelling caused by pooling of saliva from a severed or obstructed minor salivary gland duct.
- Mucocoeles are grouped as extravasation and retention types.
- Ranula is a large dome-shaped mucocoele of the extravasation type, located in the floor of the mouth. When ranula dissects through the mylohyoid muscle, it presents as a swelling in the neck (cervical ranula).

Cause

- Mucocoeles of the extravasation type are caused by mechanical trauma to the excretory duct of the gland, leading to rupture and consequent pooling of mucin into the connective tissue stroma. These are common on the lower lips and buccal mucosa.
- Mucocoeles of the retention type are retained in the duct and/or acini as a result of duct obstruction by sialolith or strictures. These are usually found on floor of the mouth, hard palate and upper lip.

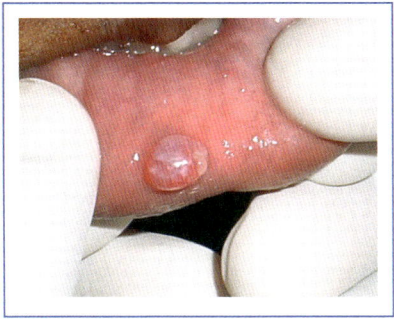

Figure 19.10   Mucocoele of the lower lip.
Courtesy: Nagamani Narayana.

Clinical Features

- Mucocoele is painless, smooth and dome-shaped (Figure 19.10).
- On rupturing, mucocoele may be slightly painful because of the inflammation. Ruptured mucocoele heals within a few days.
- Most mucocoeles are fluid-filled fluctuant vesicles or blisters in the superficial mucosa. When located deep within the connective tissue, they are fluctuant and nodular in consistency. Spontaneous rupture of the superficial mucocoeles may occur. These are recurrent.
- Mucocoeles are common in the second decade of life.
- Lower lip is the most commonly affected site.
- Colour of mucocoele may be pink or blue.
- Ranula is a large dome-shaped mucocoele of the extravasation type, located in the floor of the mouth (Figure 19.11). It often results in the elevation of the tongue.

Diagnosis

- History and clinical examination.

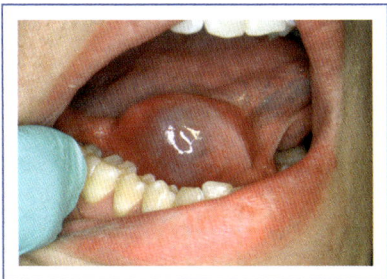

Figure 19.11   A ranula in the floor of the mouth.
Courtesy: Nagamani Narayana.

- Shape, size, location and fluctuant nature of the lesion offer important clues for the diagnosis.
- Histological examination is confirmatory.

Management

- Refer the patient to an oral and maxillofacial surgeon for complete excision of the lesions.
- Cryosurgery, carbon dioxide lasers and electrocautery are often used.

Pleomorphic Adenoma of Minor Salivary Glands

Definition/Description

- Pleomorphic adenomas are benign tumours of the salivary glands. They are composed of both epithelial and myoepithelial components. These lesions are sometimes called 'mixed' tumours.

Cause

- Benign neoplastic change involving the epithelial and myoepithelial components of the minor salivary glands.

Clinical Features

- The majority of pleomorphic adenomas are located in the superficial lobe of the parotid gland.
- When found in the minor salivary glands, the hard palate is the most frequently involved site, followed by the upper lip (Figure 19.12). The lower lip is generally spared.
- Pleomorphic adenomas are painless, slow-growing tumours and are of firm consistency.
- Pleomorphic adenomas are located on the palate away from the midline.
- Pleomorphic adenomas do not invade palatal bone.

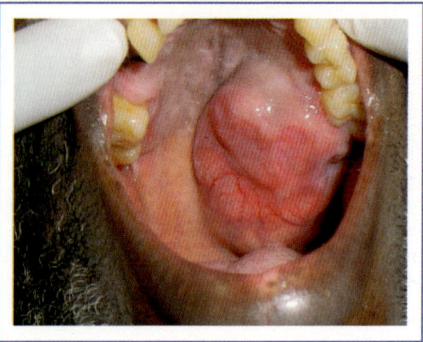

Figure 19.12   Pleomorphic adenoma of the palate.
Courtesy: Haytham Al Bayaty.

Diagnosis

- History and clinical examination.
- Computed tomographic scan is helpful in determining the extent of the tumour.
- Histopathological evaluation is confirmatory.

Management

- Refer the patient to an oral and maxillofacial surgeon for biopsy and surgical removal of the neoplasm. Recurrence is likely if the tumour is not completely removed.

Adenoid Cystic Carcinoma and Mucoepidermoid Carcinoma of the Minor Salivary Glands

Definition/Description

- Adenoid cystic carcinoma is an epithelial malignancy composed of epithelial and myoepithelial salivary gland cells.
- Mucoepidermoid carcinoma is a malignant neoplasm of glandular tissues, arising especially from the salivary gland ducts. The tumour contains mucinous and epidermoid squamous cells.
- Based on their histological features and clinical behaviour, mucoepidermoid carcinomas are classified as being low-grade, intermediate-grade and high-grade mucoepidermoid carcinomas.

Cause

- Causes of salivary gland malignant tumours are unknown. A number of risk factors have been implicated. These include exposure to radiation, viruses, carcinogenic chemicals and genetic predisposition.

Clinical Features

- Both adenoid cystic carcinoma and mucoepidermoid carcinomas occur in major and minor salivary glands.
- Adenoid cystic carcinoma is the most common oral minor salivary gland malignancy, whereas mucoepidermoid tumour is common in major salivary glands. About 15% to 20% of mucoepidermoid carcinomas are found in the oral cavity, mostly in the palate.
- Adenoid cystic carcinoma grows slowly (despite its malignant nature). It may show mucosal ulceration on the palate in about 50% to 60% of cases.
- On the tongue, adenoid cystic carcinoma may appear as an asymptomatic or painful lump and, sometimes, with unilateral tongue paresis due to invasion of nerve by the tumour.
- A low-grade mucoepidermoid carcinoma of the palate may or may not show surface ulceration at presentation. A high-grade mucoepidermoid carcinoma of the palate may be infiltrative, ulcerated and destructive of the palate mimicking squamous cell carcinoma.

Diagnosis

- History, clinical examination, CT scan, MRI (to assess spread and bone invasion) and microscopic evaluation of the lesion obtained from incision biopsy.

Management

- Refer the patient to an oral and maxillofacial surgeon.
- Low-grade mucoepidermoid carcinoma can be treated by surgical removal, whereas intermediate- and high-grade mucoepidermoid carcinomas and adenoid cystic carcinomas require surgical removal (hemi-maxillectomy for palatal tumours), followed by radiotherapy.

Orofacial Granulomatosis

Definition/Description

- Orofacial granulomatosis is the term used to describe noncaseating granulomas in the orofacial soft tissues.

Cause

- The cause of orofacial granulomatosis is unknown; however, it may represent an abnormal immune response in patients with predisposing genetic factors.

Clinical Features

- Lips become protuberant and present fissuring, which may occur in the midline of the lips (median cheilitis) or at the angles of the mouth (angular cheilitis).
- Swelling may also involve the cheeks, thus producing a cobblestoned appearance. It may cause enlargement of the gums or tongue as well.
- Painful mouth ulcers may resemble recurrent aphthous ulcers.
- The tongue may demonstrate fissuring.

Diagnosis

- History, clinical and histopathological examination.
- Presence of other conditions such as Crohn's disease and Wegener's granulomatosis should be ruled out.

Management

- Corticosteroids (intralesional) and systemic corticosteroids are useful.
- Refer the patient to an oral and maxillofacial surgeon.
- Surgical correction of the lips may be required for some patients.

SUGGESTED READINGS

Scully C. Lumps and swellings. In: Scully C, editor. *Oral and Maxillofacial Medicine*. 2nd ed. Edinburgh: Churchill Livingstone; 2008. pp. 93–6.

Cawson RA, Odell EW. Gingivitis and periodontitis. In: Cawson RA, Odell EW, editors. *Cawson's Essentials of Oral Pathology and Oral Medicine*. 8th ed. Edinburgh: Churchill Livingstone; 2008. pp. 77–96.

Laskaris G. Gingival enlargement. In: Laskaris G, editor. *Pocket Atlas of Oral Diseases*. 2nd ed. New York: Thieme; 2006. pp. 223–50.

Savage NW, Daly CG. Gingival enlargements and localized gingival overgrowths. *Aust Dent J*. 2010;55(91 suppl):55–60.

Demirer S, Özdemir H, Şencan M, Marakoglu I. Gingival hyperplasia as an early diagnostic oral manifestation in acute monocytic leukaemia: a case report. *Eur J Dentv*. 2007;1:111–4. Available from: http://www.ncbi.nlm.nih.gov/pmc/articles/PMC2609944/

Chapter 20

Gingival, oral and postextraction bleeding

S. R. Prabhu

GENERAL CONSIDERATIONS

A clinically significant bleeding episode is the one with the following features:

- Continues beyond 12 hours.
- Causes the patient to call or return to the medical or dental practitioner or medical emergency care.
- Results in the development of haematoma or ecchymosis within the soft tissues.
- Requires blood product support.

A Detailed History

A detailed history should consist of the following:

- Any previous unusual bleeding episode after surgery or trauma, spontaneous bleeding and easy or frequent bruising.
- Family history with bleeding disorders.
- Drug history, including the use of anticoagulation medicines.
- Use of recreational drugs, such as heroin.
- Alcohol abuse and possible liver damage.
- Viral hepatitis and associated liver damage.

General and Oral Examination

This step may indicate bleeding tendencies. One should look for the following symptoms:

- Gingival inflammation and bleeding tendencies.
- Purpura on the skin and/or oral mucosa.
- Haematomas and swollen joints due to haemarthrosis.

Laboratory Tests of Relevance

Laboratory tests are not to be used routinely. However, when indicated, the following tests should be considered:

- Bleeding time
- Activated partial thromboplastin time
- International normalised ratio
- Platelet count

GINGIVAL BLEEDING

- Healthy gingiva does not show bleeding tendencies.
- Gingival bleeding is a common complaint in persons with chronic gingivitis.

Causes of Gingival Bleeding

- Gingival bleeding due to gingivitis is common. Other causes include mechanical trauma such as brushing, use of toothpicks and food impaction or biting into solid foods.
- In some systemic conditions, spontaneous bleeding occurs even in the absence of gingival inflammation or mechanical trauma.
- Systemic conditions include idiopathic thrombocytopaenic purpura, vitamin K deficiency, vitamin C deficiency, haemophilia and leukaemia.
- Gingival bleeding may also occur in persons on anticoagulant medicines, such as dicoumarol and heparin.
- In pregnancy, there is an increased tendency of gingival bleeding.

Clinical Features

- Bleeding may be acute or chronic.
- In gingivitis, gums are inflamed, swollen and bleed easily. This condition is associated with poor oral hygiene and dental plaque (bacterial biofilm).
- Lacerations of the gingiva (even in the absence of inflammation) by toothbrush bristles during aggressive brushing of teeth are commonly reported.
- In patients with acute necrotising ulcerative gingivitis, slight provocation of the gingival tissue can result in spontaneous bleeding.
- Gingival bleeding in leukaemia is usually associated with gingival enlargement.

Diagnosis

- History and oral and general examination.
- Laboratory tests, where relevant.
- A search for systemic causes is necessary.

Management

- When the local cause (gingivitis or periodontitis) of gingival bleeding is suspected, refer the patient to a dentist for the management of gingival and periodontal inflammations.
- Patients with acute necrotising ulcerative gingivitis should also be referred to a dentist. These patients require irrigation and debridement of the necrotic area and tooth surfaces, instruction on oral hygiene, oral rinses and appropriate antibiotics.
- If systemic factors are the causes of gingival bleeding, patient must be treated accordingly.
- Referral of the patient to a haematologist is necessary if blood disorders are suspected as the causes of bleeding.

ORAL BLEEDING

Oral bleeding may present as haematoma, ecchymosis, petechiae or purpura.

Haematoma and Ecchymosis

Definition/Description

- Haematoma and ecchymosis refer to extravasation of blood into the soft tissues.

Cause

- Trauma is the main cause of haematoma and ecchymosis.

Clinical Features

- Submucosal lesions of haematoma or ecchymosis may be of red, brown or black colour.
- Fresh lesions are red in colour. Lesions may be raised.
- Usually, haematomas resolve in two weeks.
- Lesions of haematoma/ecchymosis are larger than pinpoint spots (petechiae) and do not blanch with pressure.

Diagnosis

- History of trauma and clinical examination.
- Where trauma is ruled out, blood dyscrasia, anticoagulant therapy or liver disease should be suspected.
- For ecchymosis of suspected systemic causes, relevant blood tests for coagulation factors, partial prothrombin time and bleeding and clotting time should be carried out.

Management

- Generally, no treatment is required for superficial haematoma or ecchymosis due to trauma. Follow-up may be necessary.
- For bleeding and clotting disorders, the patient should be referred to a specialist for treatment.

Petechiae

Definition/Description

- Petechiae are characterised by pinpoint haemorrhages in the mucosa or submucosa. The lesions of petechiae measure less than 3 mm.

Cause

- Petechiae may result from trauma, streptococcal pharyngitis, viral infections (such as infectious mononucleosis and measles), rickettsial infections, thrombocytopaenia, leukaemia, vasculitis and disseminated intravascular coagulation.

Clinical Features

- Oral petechiae are pinpoint red lesions.
- Usually, petechiae are located on the soft palate and buccal mucosa.
- Petechiae do not blanch under pressure.

Diagnosis

- History and examination.
- If thrombocytopaenia and leukaemia are suspected, complete blood count, differential count, platelet count, bone marrow aspiration and bleeding and clotting time are carried out.

Management

- Petechiae due to trauma and viral aetiology do not require treatment. In these cases, observation is adequate.
- For petechiae due to thrombocytopaenia, leukaemia and other systemic disorders, treatment of the underlying disorder by specialists is required.

Purpura

Definition/Description

- Purpura refers to the bleeding underneath the skin or mucosa. The lesions of purpura measure 3 to 10 mm (the lesions of ecchymoses are greater than 1 cm).
- Purpura is essentially the result of platelet disorders.
- In conditions characterised by purpura, the bleeding time is prolonged but the clotting functions are normal (with the exception of von Willebrand disease, in which both the bleeding time and the clotting functions are abnormal).
- Spontaneous bleeding can occur when the platelet count is less than 50,000/μL.

Cause

- Idiopathic thrombocytopaenic purpura
- Acute leukemias
- Drug-associated purpura
- HIV/AIDS-associated purpura

Clinical Features

- The palate is the typical intraoral site for purpura. Blood blisters and excessive gingival bleeding are other features of purpura.
- Systemic manifestations of the underlying disorder (e.g., thrombocytopaenia) may also be present.

Diagnosis

- History, clinical examination and complete blood count.

Management

- For purpura due to thrombocytopaenia, leukaemia and other systemic disorders, treatment of the underlying disorder by specialists is required.
- Referral to a haematologist is necessary.

POSTEXTRACTION BLEEDING

- In most instances of postextraction bleeding, there is no cause for concern, because tooth sockets ooze slightly for 24 hours after the extraction.

- Usually, two to three hours after extraction, reactionary haemorrhage occurs due to wearing off of vasoconstrictor effect of the local anaesthetic.
- If haemorrhage occurs at any time within the first week after extraction, the cause of bleeding in most cases is the infection of the socket.
- Management of patients with bleeding disorders should begin with a careful family, medical and drug history.
- Significant postextraction bleeding due to anticoagulant medication is rare.
- In most cases, changing or stopping a patient's anticoagulant medicines is not necessary because such a move may put the patient at an increased risk of morbidity or mortality.
- Almost all patients taking anticoagulant therapy can have dental extractions.

Initial Management of Postextraction Bleeding

- Ask the patient about family history of bleeding, anticoagulant therapy and previous experience with unusual bleeding.
- Clear any packing and clot from the bleeding site.
- Identify the bleeding source: soft tissue or the tooth socket(s).
  ◆ Bleeding from the soft tissue: Application of digital pressure or asking the patient to bite on a rolled-up gauze swab moistened with saline or water.
  ◆ Bleeding from the socket or bone: Bleeding continues after digital pressure or biting on a wet gauze swab. If local measures as listed above fail, the patient should be referred to a dentist or an emergency department of the hospital as soon as possible.

Management Options of Postextraction Bleeding

- Administration of local anaesthetic with a vasoconstrictor is useful.
- Bleeding from the soft tissue can be stopped by placing a horizontal mattress suture across the socket.
- Bleeding from the socket or bone can be stopped by using a haemostatic cellulose pack.

Normal clot lysis occurs within 7 to 10 days postoperatively. If bleeding occurs during this period, infection of the socket may be the cause. The infection must be treated.

Coagulopathy as the cause of postextraction bleeding is rare. Therefore, laboratory clotting studies need not be carried out routinely, unless there is a suspicion that they might be abnormal.

Systemic Agents Used for the Management of Postsurgical Bleeding Due to Coagulopathies

Systemic agents used for the management of patients with bleeding disorders (congenital or acquired) include the following:

- Platelet transfusion for thrombocytopaenic purpura.
- Fresh, frozen plasma for undiagnosed bleeding disorder.
- Cryoprecipitate for haemophilia A, von Willebrand disease and fibrinogen deficiency.

- Factor VIII concentrate for haemophilia A and von Willebrand disease.
- Factor IX concentrate for haemophilia B.
- Desmopressin for active bleeding in patients with von Willebrand disease, liver failure and kidney failure with uraemia.
- Epsilon-aminocaproic acid or tranexamic acid for any bleeding disorder as an adjunct to support the formation of blood clot.

SUGGESTED READINGS

Lockhart PB, Gibson J, Pond SH, Leitch J. Dental management considerations for the patient with an acquired coagulopathy. Part 1. Coagulopathies from systemic disease. *Br Dent J*. 2003; 195:439–45.

Gupta A, Epstein JB, Cabay RJ. Bleeding disorders of importance in dental care and related patient management. *J Can Dent Assoc*. 2007;73:77–83.

Chapter 21

Mucosal white lesions

S. R. Prabhu and D. H. Felix

MATERIA ALBA

Definition/Description

- The term 'materia alba' refers to the accumulation or aggregation of microorganisms, desquamated epithelial cells, white blood cells and a mixture of salivary proteins loosely adherent to the surface of dental plaque, teeth, gingivae or dental appliances.

Cause

- Poor maintenance of oral hygiene, which leads to microbial growth.

Clinical Features

- Clearly visible, yellow or greyish-white, soft, sticky deposit on the gingival third of the teeth, dental calculus, gingivae and restorations.
- Halitosis may be present.

Diagnosis

- History and clinical examination.

Management

- Materia alba can be flushed away by using a water spray.
- Referral of the patient to a dentist for oral prophylaxis measures, patient education and home oral care.

LINEA ALBA

Definition/Description

- It is a linear raised white line extending from the angle of the mouth to the posterior part of the buccal mucosa along the occlusal plane. Linea alba is usually seen bilaterally.

Cause

- Friction from occlusion.
- Often results from habitual cheek, lip or tongue chewing.

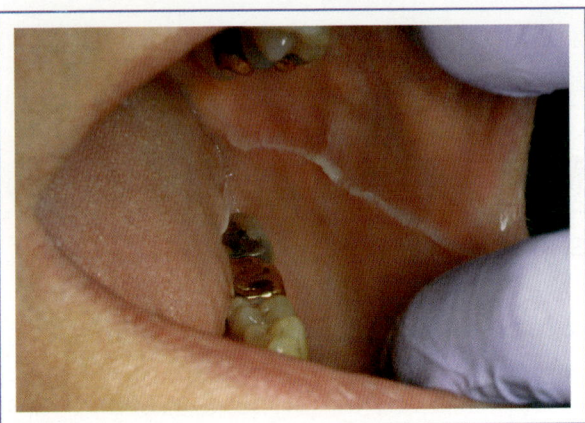

Figure 21.1 Linea alba on the cheek mucosa at the level of occlusion. *Courtesy*: Nagamani Narayana.

Clinical Features

- Asymptomatic white line on the buccal mucosa at the occlusal plane (Figure 21.1) in individuals with full complement of dentition.
- Present bilaterally in most individuals.

Diagnosis

- Clinical examination.

Management

- No treatment is required. Patient reassurance is recommended.

GEOGRAPHIC TONGUE (MIGRATORY GLOSSITIS)

Definition/Description

- Geographic tongue is characterised by irregular map-like structures usually seen on the dorsal surface of tongue.

Cause

- Largely unknown.
- Haematinic deficiencies, the use of spicy foods and the consumption of alcohol may cause symptoms.

Clinical Features

- Map-like structures are usually asymptomatic. Occasionally, mild burning sensation is reported.
- Lesions keep on migrating from one area to the other on the dorsal surface of the tongue (hence called migratory glossitis).
- The lesions are bordered by whitish lines (Figure 21.2).

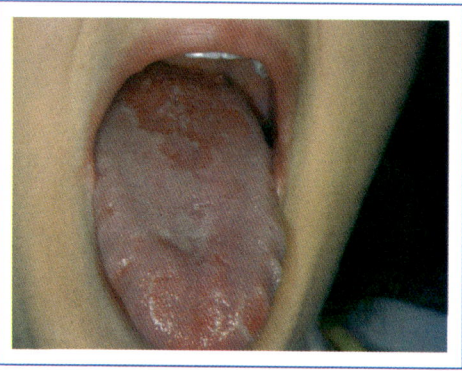

Figure 21.2 Geographic tongue with white borders.
Courtesy: Nagamani Narayana.

Diagnosis

- Clinical examination.

Management

- No treatment is required. Patient reassurance is recommended.

FURRED AND WHITE HAIRY TONGUE

Definition/Description

- Furred tongue is a white coating on the tongue of patients with poor oral hygiene or febrile diseases. It is common in edentulous adults who are on a soft diet.
- White hairy tongue is a disorder due to the accumulation of keratin on the filiform papillae.

Cause

- Predisposing factors of furred tongue include poor oral hygiene, febrile illness, fasting and xerostomia. Accumulation of epithelial, microbial and food debris can also result in furred tongue.
- There is no known single cause of white hairy tongue. Factors associated with hairy tongue include poor oral hygiene, chronic use of mouthwashes containing oxidising agents, excessive smoking, bacterial and candidal infections and prolonged use of antibiotics.

Clinical Features

- White coating on the dorsal surface of the tongue is a common feature of furred tongue (Figure 21.3).
- Halitosis and alteration in taste sensation may be present.
- In white hairy tongue, white hair-like structures on the dorsum of the tongue are seen.

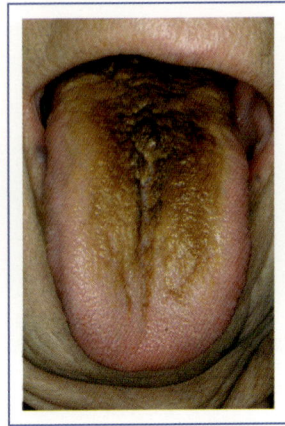

Figure 21.3 Furred tongue shows a white coating, which can be removed with gentle scraping. When hair-like projections are seen on the dorsum of the tongue, the condition is called hairy tongue. Hair-like structures cannot be scraped off easily. In both instances, colour may occasionally appear brown or black due to the heavy use of coffee or tobacco.
Courtesy: Nagamani Narayana.

- These structures may show brown or black colour due to tobacco stains.
- Patients may complain of altered taste and gagging.

Diagnosis

- History and clinical examination.
- In furred tongue, coating can be rubbed off with a gauze, whereas in white hairy tongue, hair-like structures cannot be rubbed off.

Management

- Management of furred tongue include the following:
  - ♦ Identification and elimination of the cause.
  - ♦ Patient education.
  - ♦ Maintenance of oral hygiene.
- Management of white hairy tongue include the following:
  - ♦ Elimination of causes or predisposing factors.
  - ♦ Restoration of oral hygiene improves the condition.
  - ♦ Application of trichloroacetic acid is effective.

THERMAL BURN

Definition/Description

- Thermal burn is one of the common lesions on the central palate. It is associated with eating hot pizza or pie with cheese.

Cause

- Pizza burn may result in superficial necrosis of the epithelium from the heat-holding cheese.
- Reverse smoking or accidental injury resulting from cautery used to treat oral conditions may also lead to thermal burns.
- These burns may also result when dentists accidentally apply hot dental forceps, dental wax or impression materials to the oral soft tissues.

Clinical Features

- The condition is painful and appears red.
- Because of the exposure to intense heat, the tissue may result in desquamation, leaving exposed red erosive surfaces.

Diagnosis

- History and clinical examination.

Management

- Generally, no treatment is required.
- Damaged tissue heals within a week. In some cases, symptomatic treatment may be required.

CHEMICAL BURN

Definition/Description

- Chemical burn is the burn that occurs as a result of exposure of the oral mucosa to chemicals.

Cause

- Chemical burn of the oral mucosa can occur due to self-medication with agents such as aspirin placed in the vestibule adjacent to a painful tooth. This results in the formation of a white pseudomembrane.
- When some agents used in dental procedures such as silver nitrate, pure eugenol, sodium hypochlorite and formocresol accidentally come in contact with the oral mucous membrane, they result in chemical burns.
- Laboratory workers are occasionally exposed to chemicals. This exposure results in chemical burns of the oral mucosa.

Clinical Features

- Clinically, the affected mucosa is covered with a white membrane due to necrosis (Figure 21.4).
- The necrotic epithelium can easily be removed, leaving a red, bleeding surface. The lesions are painful and tender.

Diagnosis

- History and clinical examination.

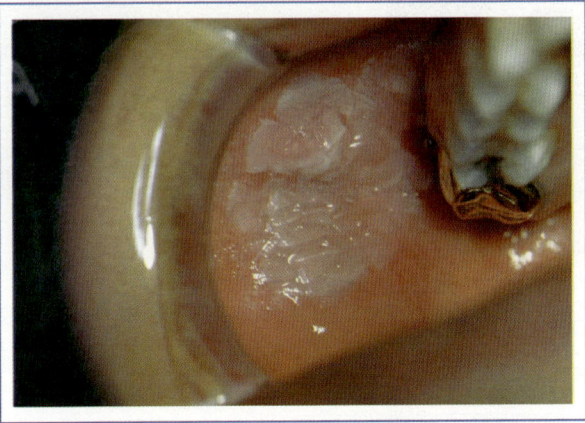

Figure 21.4 White chemical burn of the cheek mucosa, caused by topical local anaesthetic spray.
Courtesy: Nagamani Narayana.

Management

- Symptomatic treatment.
- Avoidance of causative agents.

RADIATION-INDUCED MUCOSITIS

Definition/Description

- Radiation-induced mucositis is an inflammation of the oral mucosa caused by radiation exposure of the head and neck region for the treatment of cancer.

Cause

- Radiation treatment of head and neck cancer.

Clinical Features

- Erythema of the oral mucosa in the early stages of radiotherapy, followed by white sloughing of epithelium, which leaves erosive/ulcerative areas.
- Xerostomia, burning and loss of taste are other features of radiation-induced mucositis.

Diagnosis

- History and clinical examination.

Management

- Symptomatic treatment is required. Vitamin B complex and low doses of corticosteroids are beneficial.

FRICTIONAL KERATOSIS

Definition/Description

- Frictional keratosis is characterised by the formation of keratotic lesion caused by friction mainly derived from teeth.

Cause

- Cusps of teeth rubbing against cheek mucosa or tongue (Figure 21.5 A and B) can result in keratotic lesions due to chronic friction.
- Patients with missing teeth may develop keratosis on the alveolar ridges.

Clinical Features

- Frictional keratosis presents as a white lesion with irregular borders. Patient may or may not be aware of its existence.

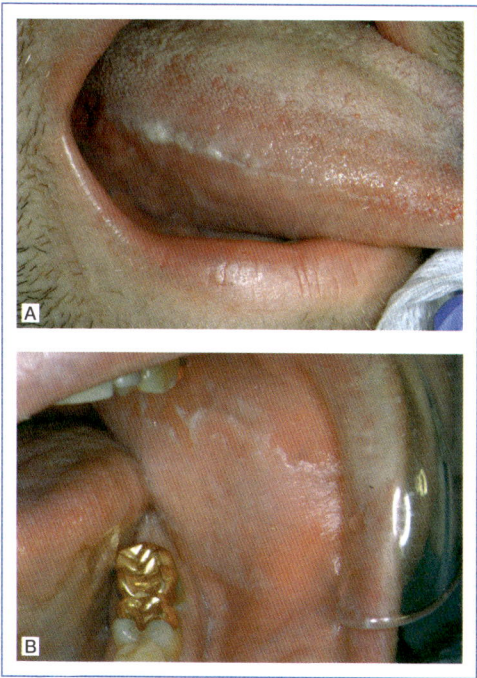

Figure 21.5 White keratotic lesions due to friction caused by chronic chewing habit (A) on the lateral border of the tongue and (B) on buccal mucosa.
Courtesy: Nagamani Narayana.

- When symptomatic, patient may complain of rough surface texture.
- Pain is not a consistent feature, unless the lesion is ulcerated.

Diagnosis

- History and clinical examination.

Management

- Identify the cause and eliminate it.
- Refer the patient to a dentist.

TOBACCO-INDUCED KERATOSIS

Definition/Description

- Tobacco-induced keratosis is an oral white lesion induced by the action of tobacco. When associated with smoking, the lesion is usually called smoker's keratosis.

Cause

- Causes of smoker's keratosis include the use of cigarette, pipe and cigar, and reverse smoking.
- Tobacco chewing or snuff-dipping also causes keratosis.

Clinical Features

- In cigarette smokers, mild keratosis may be seen on the lip or labial commissures.
- In pipe and cigar smokers, palatal lesions are characterised by red inflamed orifices of minor salivary glands against the white background (Figure 21.6 A). These lesions are also called smoker's keratoses, smoker's palate, stomatitis nicotina or nicotinic stomatitis.
- In reverse smokers, palatal changes are much more pronounced (Figure 21.6 B).
- In people with the habit of snuff-dipping, keratotic lesion of the gingival or labial/buccal mucosa can occur together with gingival recession. This is called snuff dipper's keratosis (Figure 21.6 C).

Diagnosis

- History and clinical examination.
- Biopsy is necessary for the lesions that are suspected to carry malignant potential.

Management

- Elimination of tobacco use.

ACTINIC KERATOSIS (SOLAR KERATOSIS)

Definition/Description

- Actinic keratosis, also known as solar keratosis, is characterised by a white lesion on the lower lip, caused due to chronic and excessive exposure to solar radiation.

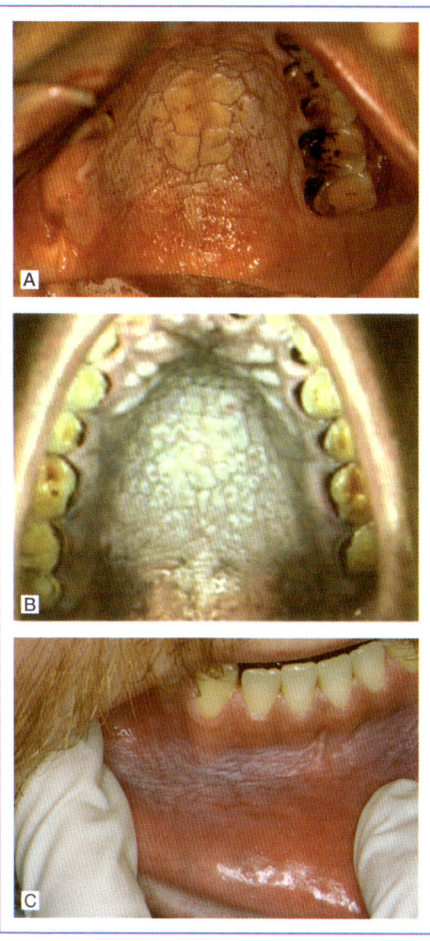

Figure 21.6 (A) Nicotinic stomatitis (smoker's palate). (B) Nicotinic stomatitis (smoker's palate) in a reverse smoker. (C) Snuff-dipper's keratosis of the lower labial mucosa.
Courtesy: (A) David Wilson. (B) S. R. Prabhu. (C) Nagamani Narayana.

Cause

- Chronic solar ultraviolet radiation.

Clinical Features

- In outdoor workers (in particular, farmers and fishermen), vermilion portion of the lower lip is commonly affected.

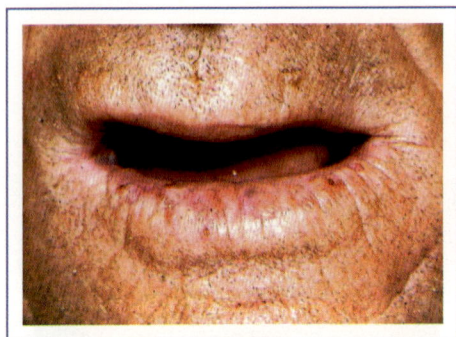

Figure 21.7 Actinic keratosis of the lower lip with crusty lesions.
Courtesy: David Wilson.

- Pale opaque keratotic lesion with intervening red atrophic areas are suggestive of actinic keratosis.
- In later stages, actinic keratosis may be accompanied by scaly, crusted lesions (Figure 21.7). These lesions carry malignant potential.

Diagnosis

- History of outdoor living and clinical examination of the lip lesion.
- Biopsy of the clinically suspicious lesions is necessary.

Management

- Further exposure to chronic solar radiation should be avoided.
- Sunscreens should be used in order to block damage from ultraviolet radiations.
- Surgical removal of keratotic lesion by laser is recommended.
- Topical application of 5-fluorouracil to the lesion is effective.

SUBLINGUAL KERATOSIS

Definition/Description

- Sublingual keratosis is a white patch located in the sublingual region. This lesion cannot be rubbed off with a gauze.

Cause

- The cause is unknown. Smoking and alcohol may be found to be associated with sublingual keratosis in some patients.

Clinical Features

- The lesion is white and has wrinkled surface, which extends from the anterior floor of the mouth onto the ventral surface of the tongue.

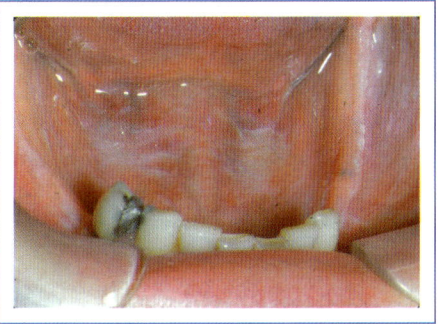

Figure 21.8 Sublingual keratosis. Note the wrinkled 'ebbing tide' appearance of the keratotic white lesion.
Courtesy: David Wilson.

- The lesion is irregular but shows a well-defined outline. See 'ebbing tide' appearance in (Figure 21.8).
- Sublingual keratosis is considered potentially malignant. Malignant transformation of these lesions may be as high as 24%.

Diagnosis

- Clinical examination and biopsy for histological evaluation.

Management

- Referral to a specialist is indicated for the surgical removal of the lesion. Follow-up is required.

FORDYCE SPOTS (FORDYCE GRANULES)

Definition/Description

- Fordyce spots or granules are asymptomatic yellowish-white granular lesions seen on the buccal mucosa and lips.

Cause

- Ectopic collection of sebaceous glands in the cheek mucosa and lips.

Clinical Features

- Fordyce granules are granular and appear whitish to yellow in colour (Figure 21.9). These should not to be mistaken for mucosal disease.
- Asymptomatic in the majority of individuals.
- Lesions cannot be rubbed off with a gauze.

Diagnosis

- Clinical examination.

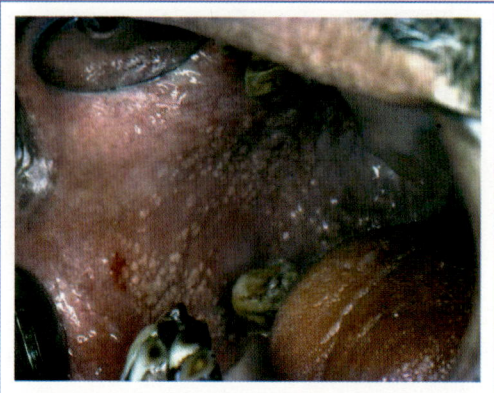

Figure 21.9 Fordyce granules on the buccal mucosa.
Reproduced with permission from: Ramadas K, Lucas E, Thomas G, et al.
A Digital Manual for the Early Diagnosis of Oral Neoplasia. IARC, Lyon,
2008. Available from: http://screening.iarc.fr/atlasoral.php?lang=1

Management

- No treatment is required.
- For patients who are concerned about the presence of granular whitish spots in the mouth, patient assurance is recommended.

LEUKOEDEMA

Definition/Description

- Leukoedema is characterised by a grey-white, diffuse milky opalescent film on the cheek mucosa, which blanches when stretched.
- Leukoedema is bilateral and is common in smokers and people of African or Asian descent.

Cause

- Genetic predisposition may be associated with this condition.

Clinical Features

- Milky, opalescent mucosa (Figure 21.10).
- The clinical appearance of leukoedema is due to the collection of intercellular water.

Diagnosis

- Clinical examination.

Management

- This condition can be regarded as a normal variation and does not require any treatment.

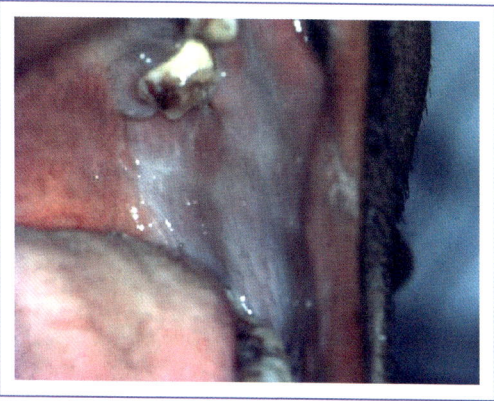

Figure 21.10 Leukoedema of the buccal mucosa in a smoker.
Reproduced with permission from: Ramadas K, Lucas E, Thomas G, et al.
A Digital Manual for the Early Diagnosis of Oral Neoplasia. IARC, Lyon,
2008. Available from: http://screening.iarc.fr/atlasoral.php?lang=1

WHITE SPONGE NAEVUS

Definition/Description

- White sponge naevus, also known as white folded gingivostomatitis or Cannon's disease, is a hereditary disorder
characterised by diffuse white keratotic patches involving oral
mucosa.

Cause

- An autosomal hereditary disorder due to keratin gene mutations.

Clinical Features

- Clinically seen as an asymptomatic folded (spongy) and thickened white mucosa, which becomes prominent in the second
decade.
- Buccal mucosa is commonly involved. White patch cannot be
rubbed off with a gauze.
- Family history is positive.
- White sponge naevus does not carry any malignant potential.

Diagnosis

- Family history and clinical appearance.

Management

- No treatment is required. Patient reassurance is recommended.

ORAL PSEUDOMEMBRANOUS CANDIDIASIS

Definition/Description

- Pseudomembranous candidiasis (candidosis), also known as thrush, is characterised by white flecks or curd-like white to yellow coloured lesions seen on the oral mucosal surfaces, usually in patients with underlying predisposing factors.

Cause

- Pseudomembranous candidiasis is caused by *Candida* species, in particular *C. albicans*.
- Predisposing factors for candidal infection include prolonged use of antibiotics or corticosteroids, xerostomia (due to different causes), endocrine defects, immune defects (e.g., AIDS), immunosuppressive treatment, leukaemia, lymphomas, cancers and diabetes.

Clinical Features

- Pseudomembranous candidiasis presents as creamy plaques (Figure 21.11) that can be easily wiped off with a gauze, leaving a red base.
- Lesions commonly appear in the posterior part of the maxillary buccal vestibule and on the soft palate.

Diagnosis

- History of the underlying predisposing factors is positive in majority of patients.
- Clinical examination (white patches are easily rubbed off with gentle scraping).
- Gram stain is useful in identifying hyphae of *Candida*.

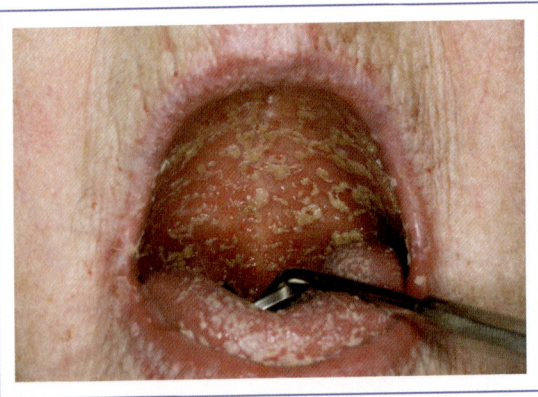

Figure 21.11 Pseudomembranous candidiasis presenting as white- and cream-coloured curd-like deposits on the oral mucosa. The patient was on costicosteroid inhalers and complained of dry mouth.
Courtesy: Nagamani Narayana.

Management

- Topical antifungal agents are useful. If topical application does not yield desired result, systemic use of antifungal agents may be required.
- Underlying predisposing factors need to be managed.

CHRONIC HYPERPLASTIC CANDIDIASIS (CANDIDAL LEUKOPLAKIA)

Definition/Description

- Chronic hyperplastic candidiasis, also known as candidal leukoplakia, refers to a *Candida*-associated white lesion that is fixed to the underlying structures.

Cause

- *Candida* species is associated with keratotic lesion. However, its aetiological role is not clear.

Clinical Features

- Candidal leukoplakia is a white keratotic lesion (Figure 21.12) that is adherent to the underlying mucosa.
- Labial commissures and dorsum of tongue are commonly involved.
- Majority of patients are smokers.
- White lesion cannot be scraped off.
- This lesion is considered a potentially malignant disorder.

Diagnosis

- Clinical examination of the lesion provides some diagnostic help.
- Biopsy is confirmatory.
- Histopathology reveals the presence of candidal hyphae in the superficial layers of the hyperplastic epithelium.

Management

- Long-term antifungal agents are useful.
- Periodic follow-up is recommended.

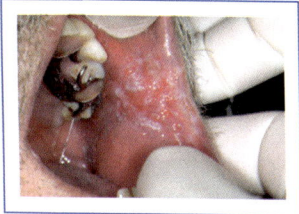

Figure 21.12 Chronic hyperplastic candidiasis of the labial commissure.
Courtesy: Haytham Al Bayaty.

ORAL HAIRY LEUKOPLAKIA

Definition/Description

- It is a white keratotic lesion located mainly on the lateral surfaces of the tongue of persons whose immune system is severely compromised.

Cause

- Epstein-Barr virus infection is the cause of oral hairy leukoplakia in an immunocompromised patient.

Clinical Features

- Asymptomatic white lesion with 'hair-like' and corrugated appearance, located on the lateral surfaces of the tongue (Figure 21.13).
- The white lesion cannot be rubbed off by gentle scraping. Occasionally, other mucosal surfaces in the mouth may be involved.
- Hairy leukoplakia does not carry any malignant potential.

Diagnosis

- History of compromised immune status and clinical appearance with hair-like projections on the lateral borders of the tongue help in the diagnosis.
- Biopsy of the lesion and *in situ* hybridisation techniques to confirm the presence of Epstein-Barr virus.

Management

- The lesions are typically asymptomatic and no treatment is required.
- Underlying immune defect must also be addressed in these patients.

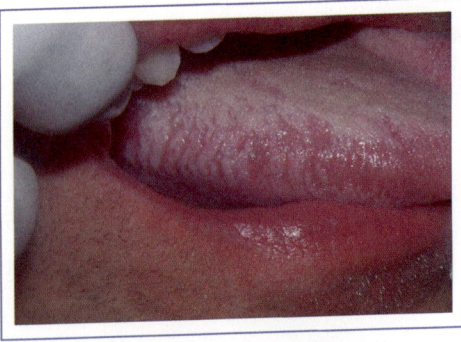

Figure 21.13   Hairy leukoplakia of the tongue in an HIV-infected patient. Reproduced with permission from: Dr. Steve Debbink, Dental Director, AIDS Resource Center of Wisconsin, and David Reznik. Available from: http://www.hivdent.org

ORAL PROLIFERATIVE VERRUCOUS LEUKOPLAKIA

Definition/Description

- Oral proliferative verrucous leukoplakia (OPVL) is a slowly progressive, aggressive and persistent form of oral leukoplakia. This condition is refractory to treatment and has a high risk of recurrence and malignant transformation.

Cause

- OPVL is associated with tobacco use.
- Some evidence points to the aetiologic role of human papillomavirus (HPV) types 16 and 18.

Clinical Features

- This condition an initially flat keratotic white lesion that progresses into a hyperkeratotic verrucous (warty) lesion with a friable surface (Figure 21.14).
- It is seen in the middle-aged and elderly individuals.
- It carries malignant potential and may transform into verrucous carcinoma or squamous cell carcinoma.

Diagnosis

- History, clinical examination and microscopical examination of the lesion.

Management

- Refer the patient to an oral surgeon for surgical excision. Follow-up is necessary.

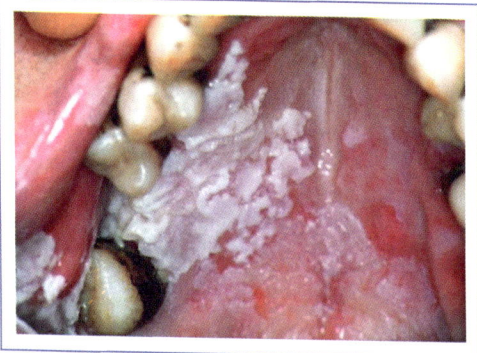

Figure 21.14   Proliferative verrucous leukoplakia. Note the extensive thick white plaques on the palate.

Reproduced with permission from: Ramadas K, Lucas E, Thomas G, et al. *A Digital Manual for the Early Diagnosis of Oral Neoplasia*. IARC, Lyon, 2008. Available from: http://screening.iarc.fr/atlasoral.php?lang=1

ORAL SUBMUCOUS FIBROSIS

Definition/Description

- Oral submucous fibrosis is a condition characterised by progressive closure of the mouth due to fibrosis of the oral submucosa.

Cause

- This disorder is common among those who habitually chew betel nut.
- There is a genetic predisposition in favour of people of Asian (in particular, Indian) origin.

Clinical Features

- Fibrous bands occur on lips, cheek mucosa and soft palate.
- Oral mucosa appears pale (marble-like), and patients complain of progressive inability to open the mouth (Figure 21.15).
- This condition is regarded as a potentially malignant disorder.

Diagnosis

- History of betel nut chewing.
- Clinical examination reveals marble-like pale mucosa and palpable vertical fibrous bands on buccal mucosa, lips and soft palate.
- Biopsy confirms the presence of fibrosis.

Management

- Intralesional injections of corticosteroids offer symptomatic relief.
- Surgical intervention of fibrous bands may be required based on the extent of the disorder.
- Permanent cure is not available.

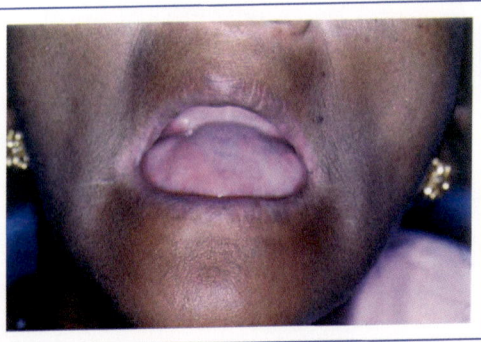

Figure 21.15 Oral submucous fibrosis. Blanching and extensive depapillation of the tongue are seen. Mouth opening is restricted.
Reproduced with permission from: Ramadas K, Lucas E, Thomas G, et al. *A Digital Manual for the Early Diagnosis of Oral Neoplasia*. IARC, Lyon, 2008. Available from: http://screening.iarc.fr/atlasoral.php?lang=1

ORAL LEUKOPLAKIA

Definition/Description

- Leukoplakia is a clinical entity that is defined as 'a white patch firmly attached to the underlying tissues, which cannot be classified as any other known disease entity'.
- Leukoplakia is considered a potentially malignant disorder.

Cause

- Exact cause is unknown.
- Predisposing factors include tobacco and alcohol consumption.
- In a small number of cases, *Candida* and HPV infections may be associated.

Clinical Features

- Three clinical forms of leukoplakia are recognised: homogeneous, speckled (heterogeneous) and verrucous (nodular) forms.
  - **Homogenous leukoplakia** is characterised by smooth white patches adhered to the underlying tissues (Figure 21.16 A). It is the most common variety of leukoplakia and shows minimal, if any, evidence of malignant potential.
  - **Speckled leukoplakia** is a mixture of white and red patched, for which reason it is also called erythroleukoplakia (Figure 21.16 B).

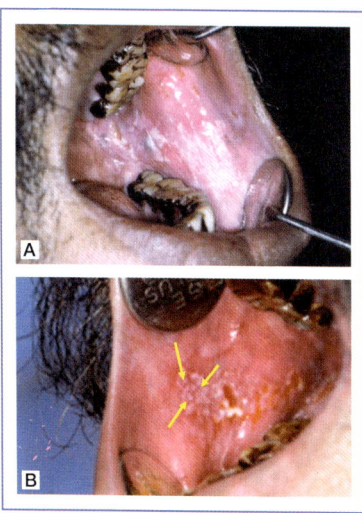

Figure 21.16 (A) Homogeneous and (B) nonhomogeneous/nodular (speckled) forms of oral leukoplakia.

Reproduced with permission from: Ramadas K, Lucas E, Thomas G, et al. *A Digital Manual for the Early Diagnosis of Oral Neoplasia*. IARC, Lyon, 2008. Available from: http://screening.iarc.fr/atlasoral.php?lang=1

♦ **Proliferative verrucous leukoplakia** is a raised warty white lesion (Figure 21.14).

- Both speckled and proliferative verrucous varieties of leukoplakia carry malignant potential.
- Leukoplakia cannot be scraped off by rubbing with a gauze.

Diagnosis

- History, clinical examination and histological evaluation of the lesion.

Management

- Surgical or laser removal of the lesions are recommended.
- Retinoids may have beneficial effects during the treatment.
- Follow-up is essential.
- Tobacco and other predisposing factors need to be eliminated.

For more information on leukoplakia, refer to Chapter 38 (Oral potentially malignant disorders I: Leokoplakia and erythroplakia).

LICHEN PLANUS

Definition/Description

- Lichen planus (LP) is a common chronic mucocutaneous condition believed to be due to an immune-mediated injury.
- Oral LP is usually found as white lesions with a variety of clinical appearances: reticular form, plaque form, erosive form, atrophic form and bullous form. In this chapter, only reticular and plaque forms of oral LP have been discussed because they present as white lesions.

Cause

- Exact cause of oral LP is not known. An inflammatory immune-mediated defect has been noted to be associated with the pathogenesis of this condition.
- Stress and anxiety have been found to occur in many LP patients.

Clinical Features

- Oral LP lesions are common in middle-aged persons (in particular, women).
- Lace-like pattern is a feature of the reticular form of LP (Figure 21.17 A and B).
- Papular LP is characterised by white papules.
- Plaque-like LP simulates leukoplakia and is characterised by thick raised white patch with radiating streaks.
- Occasionally, annular or circular pattern of LP may occur.
- Erosive and atrophic forms of LP are red lesions.
- Lesions are generally bilateral and asymptomatic.
- Oral lesions may occur concurrently with skin lesions.
- Skin lesions on the flexor surfaces of the limbs may be itchy, white or rough.
- Approximately 1% to 1.5% of oral LP (in particular, erosive form) are known to carry malignant potential over a 10-year period.

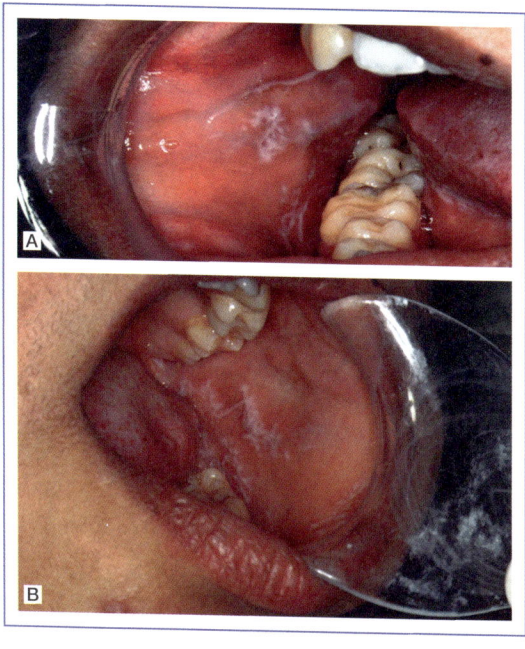

Figure 21.17   (A and B) Reticular type of oral lichen planus presenting lace-like white lesions.
Courtesy: Nagamani Narayana.

Diagnosis

- A thorough history regarding drug use should be obtained to rule out lichenoid reaction.
- Clinical appearance of the lesions offers useful clues for the diagnosis of LP.
- Biopsy is necessary if lesions show change in size or there are signs of ulceration.

Management

- Treatment of asymptomatic LP is not necessary.
- Topical corticosteroids are useful; however, there is no permanent cure.
- Systemic corticosteroids may be necessary in some cases. A periodic follow-up is also essential.
- If LP lesions are closely associated with amalgam restorations, removal of amalgam is advisable.
- If drugs are implicated (lichenoid reaction), patient's physician may be consulted to decide whether change of therapy is needed.

Detailed information on LP is presented in Chapter 39 (Oral potentially malignant disorders II: Oral lichen planus, oral lichenoid lesions, oral graft-versus-host disease and oral submucous fibrosis).

ORAL LICHENOID REACTIONS

Definition/Description

- The term 'oral lichenoid reactions' (OLRs) refers to lesions that are histologically and clinically similar to oral LP and the causative factor for these lesions can be identified.

Cause

- Drugs, direct contact with dental amalgam and other restorative materials, and graft-versus-host disease.
- Drugs associated with OLRs include antihypertensive drugs, antimalarials, antimicrobials, nonsteroidal anti-inflammatory drugs, hypoglycaemic drugs and angiotensin-converting-enzyme inhibitors.
- Dental restorative agents associated with OLRs include silver amalgam, gold, cobalt, palladium and epoxy resins.

Clinical Features

- Clinical features of OLRs are indistinguishable from oral LP lesions.
- However, OLR lesions are neither symmetrical nor bilateral like the oral LP lesions.
- When dental restorative materials are involved, OLRs are found in contact with the materials used. [See Chapter 39 (Oral potentially malignant disorders II: Oral lichen planus, oral lichenoid lesions, oral graft-versus-host disease and oral submucous fibrosis) for further details.]

Diagnosis

- History and clinical examination of the lesions.
- Cause is generally identifiable.

Management

- Identification of the triggering factor and elimination of exposure to the triggering factor is the first step of management.
- In case of systemic-drug-induced OLR patients, the risk and benefit of suspending the medicine must evaluated. In these cases, patient's physician should be contacted.

For more information on oral LP and lichenoid lesions, refer to Chapter 39 (Oral potentially malignant disorders II: Oral lichen planus, oral lichenoid lesions, oral graft-versus-host disease and oral submucous fibrosis).

LUPUS ERYTHEMATOSUS

Definition/Description

- Lupus erythematosus is an autoimmune disease that manifests as systemic lupus erythematosus (SLE) and discoid LE.
- In both forms of the disorder, oral mucosa may be involved in up to 20% of cases.

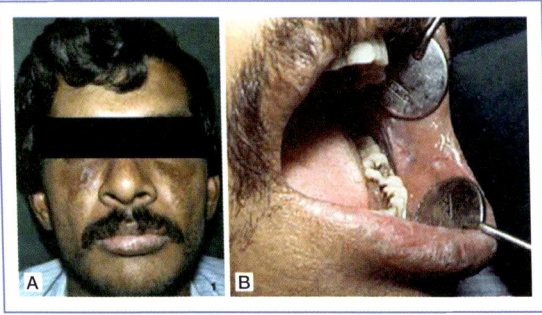

Figure 21.18 Patient with discoid lupus erythematosus with butterfly-shaped rash on the malar area. Also, note the lichen-planus-like lesion on the buccal mucosa.
Reproduced with permission from: Ramadas K, Lucas E, Thomas G, et al. *A Digital Manual for the Early Diagnosis of Oral Neoplasia*. IARC, Lyon, 2008. Available from: http://screening.iarc.fr/atlasoral.php?lang=1

Cause

- It is an autoimmune disorder.

Clinical Features

- Cutaneous scaly red lesions involving the bridge of the nose are characteristic ('butterfly' pattern) of SLE.
- Oral lesions are similar to those of oral LP.
- A central atrophic area surrounded by fine white striae radiating from the margin of the lesion is a feature of oral involvement of LE (Figure 21.18).

Diagnosis

- History and evaluation of antibodies.
- Anti-DNA antibodies are detected in SLE but not in discoid LE.

Management

- Corticosteroids are beneficial in both forms of LE.

ORAL SQUAMOUS CELL CARCINOMA

Definition/Description

- Oral squamous cell carcinoma (OSCC) refers to a malignant neoplasm arising from squamous cells of the oral epithelium.
- It has a wide range of clinical features. In approximately 5% to 8% of cases of early OSCC, the neoplasm presents as a white patch. This chapter discusses only the OSCC presenting as a white patch.

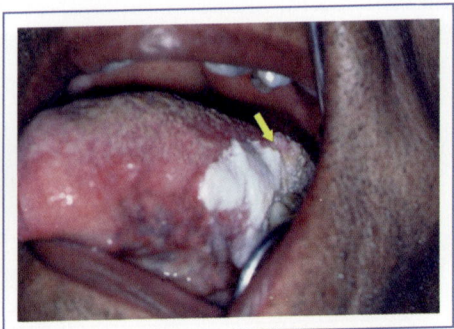

Figure 21.19 Malignant transformation (arrow) in a patient with homogeneous leukoplakia on the left lateral border of the tongue.
Reproduced with permission from: Ramadas K, Lucas E, Thomas G, et al. *A Digital Manual for the Early Diagnosis of Oral Neoplasia*. IARC, Lyon, 2008. Available from: http://screening.iarc.fr/atlasoral.php?lang=1

Cause

- In majority of cases, long-term use of tobacco and alcohol have been implicated as aetiological factors.
- A small percentage of OSCC is associated with HPV types 16 and 18 infection. These patients often have no alcohol or tobacco association.
- Factors such as chronic irritation from sharp cusps of teeth, extensive use of spices, poor oral hygiene, tertiary syphilis, chronic candidal infection of the oral mucosa and actinic radiation have also been attributed as contributing factors for the development of OSCC.

Clinical Features

- OSCC in its early stages may appear as a white patch, thus fulfilling the criteria of leukoplakia (Figure 21.19).
- Common locations include buccal mucosa, including the labial commissures, lateral borders of the tongue, floor of the mouth, palate and vermillion of the lower lip.
- Initially, the white patch is asymptomatic. The lesion may show ulceration and become symptomatic at a later stage.
- Cervical lymph node metastasis occurs as the lesion advances.

Diagnosis

- History, clinical examination and histological evaluation of the lesion.

Management

- Refer the patient to a specialist.
- Treatment modalities include surgery, radiotherapy and chemotherapy.

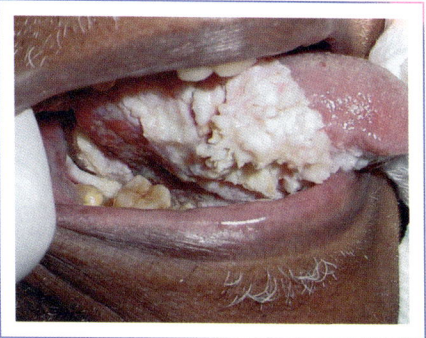

Figure 21.20 Oral verrucous carcinoma.
Courtesy: Haytham Al Bayaty.

Detailed information on OSCC is presented in Chapter 40 (Oral carcinoma and other malignant lesions of the mouth and jaws).

ORAL VERRUCOUS CARCINOMA

Definition/Description

- Oral verrucous carcinoma is a variant of squamous cell carcinoma. It is slow growing and exophytic in nature and has a white verrucous or papillomatous surface. It seldom metastasizes.

Cause

- Tobacco use (in particular, snuff-dipping), alcohol consumption and, occasionally, ill-fitting dentures.

Clinical Features

- Common in men aged more than 60 years.
- Gingiva, alveolar mucosa and buccal mucosa are the favoured sites.
- Exophytic and slow growing, with white pebbly surface (Figure 21.20).
- Invasive growth in most cases and rarely infiltrative.
- Usually does not metastasize to regional lymph nodes or to distant parts of the body.

Diagnosis

- History (of snuff-dipping or chewing and alcohol abuse) and clinical examination.
- Biopsy is confirmatory.

Management

- Refer the patient to a specialist.
- Surgery and laser therapy are effective.

SUGGESTED READINGS

Felix DH, Luker J, Scully C. Oral medicine. White lesions. *Dent Update*. 2013;40:146–8, 150–2, 154.

Scully C, Porter S. Orofacial disease: update for the dental clinical team: 3. White lesions. *Dent Update*. 1999;26:123–9.

Prabhu SR. White lesions of the oral mucosa. In: Prabhu SR, editor. *Textbook of Oral Medicine*. New Delhi, India: Oxford University Press; 2004. pp. 91–106.

Cawson RA, Odell EW. Benign chronic white mucosal lesions. *Cawson's Essentials of Oral Pathology and Oral Medicine*. Edinburgh, Scotland: Churchill Livingstone; 2008. pp. 252–9.

Birnbaum W, Dunne SM. White patches. In: Birnbaum W, Dunne SM, editors. *Oral Diagnosis: The Clinician's Guide*. Oxford, U.K.: Wright. pp. 210–25.

Chapter 22

Mucosal blisters, erosions and ulcers

S. R. Prabhu and D. H. Felix

PEMPHIGUS VULGARIS

Definition/Description

- Pemphigus vulgaris is an autoimmune disorder characterised by bullous lesions involving the skin and mucous membranes.

Cause

- Pemphigus vulgaris is an autoimmune disorder.
- Antibodies against epithelial intercellular attachments cause acantholysis, leading to blister formation.

Clinical Features

- There are different types of pemphigus. These include pemphigus vulgaris, pemphigus vegetans and paraneoplastic pemphigus.
- Pemphigus vulgaris is the most common type, which involves the oral mucosa.
- Bullous lesions on skin and oral mucosa are common.
- Middle-aged and elderly women are commonly predisposed to pemphigus. Genetic background is associated with the disorder.
- Gentle digital sliding pressure on the uninvolved adjacent skin causes stripping of the epithelium. This is called the Nikolsky sign.
- Oral bullous lesions are short-lived. Once ruptured, lesions leave erosions and ulcers (Figure 22.1).
- Soft palate, buccal mucosae, lips and gingivae are the common sites of oral involvement.

Diagnosis

- History, clinical examination, positive Nikolsky sign and immunostaining of the biopsy specimen and detection of antibodies in serum are required to diagnose the condition.

Management

- Systemic corticosteroids and immunosuppressant therapy are used to control the condition.

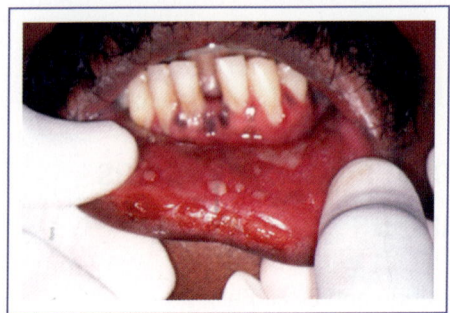

Figure 22.1 Pemphigus vulgaris lesions involving the labial mucosa.
Reproduced with permission from: Ramadas K, Lucas E, Thomas G, et al.
A Digital Manual for the Early Diagnosis of Oral Neoplasia. IARC, Lyon,
2008. Available from: http://screening.iarc.fr/atlasoral.php?lang=1

MUCOUS MEMBRANE PEMPHIGOID

Definition/Description

- Mucous membrane pemphigoid is an autoimmune disease characterised by the formation of blisters at the basement membrane zone
  of the mucous membranes.

Cause

- An autoimmune disorder in which autoantibodies are directed
  against epithelial basement membrane of the oral mucosa.

Clinical Features

- Usually, women in their fifth or sixth decade are affected.
- Gingivae and palate are the preferred sites of involvement.
- Blisters rupture, leaving ulcers with yellowish slough on their sur-
  faces (Figure 22.2 A and B).
- Other areas involved include conjunctiva, larynx and genital
  mucosa.
- Conjunctival involvement may lead to scarring.
- Skin involvement is rare.
- On the gingivae, mucous membrane pemphigoid may be seen as
  desquamative gingivitis (Figure 22.2 A).

Diagnosis

- History and clinical examination offer some clues, but confirmation is by histological and immunofluorescence examinations of the
  biopsy specimen.

Management

- Topical application of corticosteroids or tacrolimus yields good
  results.

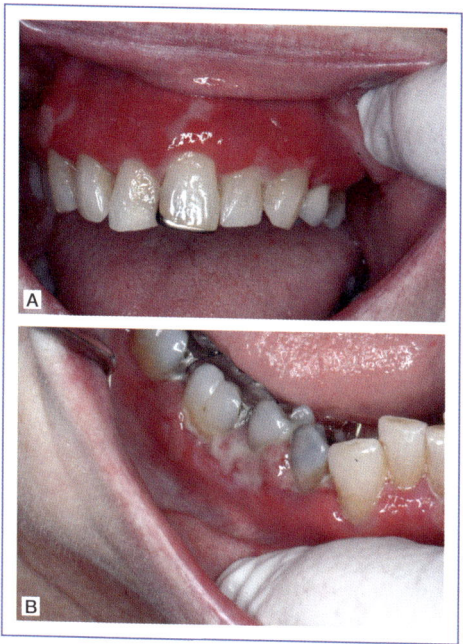

Figure 22.2 (A and B) Mucous membrane pemphigoid with vesiculobullous lesions seen on the gingivae.
Courtesy: Nagamani Narayana.

DERMATITIS HERPETIFORMIS

Definition/Description

- Dermatitis herpetiformis is a chronic blistering skin condition characterised by multiple blisters filled with fluid.
- Blisters clinically mimic those of herpes virus infection, hence the name dermatitis herpetiformis. This disorder is associated with coeliac disease.

Cause

- Dermatitis herpetiformis is an autoimmune disorder.

Clinical Features

- Dermatitis herpetiformis is primarily a skin disorder. Skin lesions appear as vesicular rash and have intense itchy sensation.
- Oral vesicles occur on palatal mucosa.

Diagnosis

- History, clinical examination and immunofluorescence of the biopsy specimen.

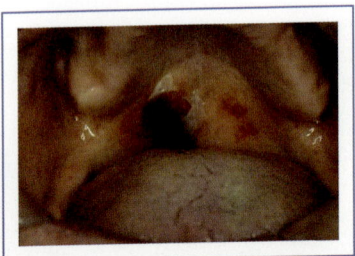

Figure 22.3 Blood blister on the soft palate in angina bullosa haemorrhagica. *Courtesy*: David H. Felix.

Management

- Dapsone and sulphonamides are effective.

ANGINA BULLOSA HAEMORRHAGICA

Definition/Description

- Angina bullosa haemorrhagica is a common disorder characterised by the formation of blood blisters most commonly on the soft palate.

Cause

- Unknown.

Clinical Features

- A large blood-filled blister on the soft palate, which may burst, leaving an empty epithelial sac (Figure 22.3).
- Condition is more common in people who use inhalers for asthma. The condition resolves within a week.

Diagnosis

- History and clinical examination.

Management

- This is a self-limiting lesion. Patient reassurance is recommended.

ERYTHEMA MULTIFORME

Definition/Description

- Erythema multiforme refers to a mucocutaneous disorder of unknown cause, possibly mediated by deposition of immune complexes in the superficial microvasculature of the skin and oral mucous membrane.

Cause

- Unknown. Possibly, an immunological disorder.
- This usually follows a viral infection or systemic drug exposure.

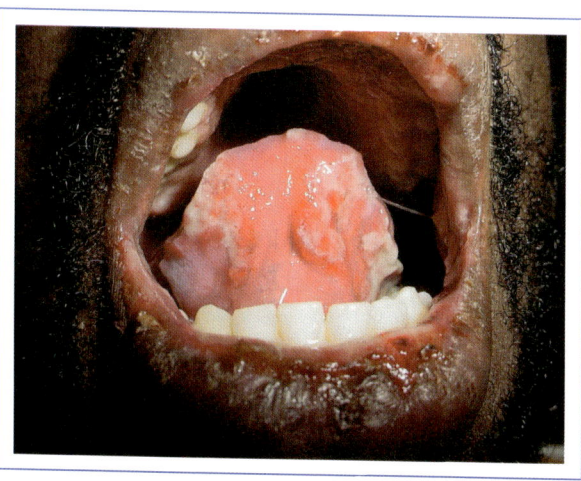

Figure 22.4 Erythema multiforme. Note erosive lesions on the ventral surface of the tongue and crusting of the lower lip.
Courtesy: Haytham Al Bayaty.

Clinical Features

- Oral mucosal involvement exhibits generalised erythema.
- Sometimes, it is accompanied by erosions or bullous lesions.
- Crusting of the lips is characteristic (Figure 22.4).
- Severe form of erythema multiforme is called Stevens-Johnson syndrome, in which oral, conjunctival and genital mucosae are involved.

Diagnosis

- History and clinical examination.
- Biopsy is confirmatory.

Management

- Discontinuation of systemic medicine and low doses of systemic corticosteroids are useful.
- Topical application of local anaesthetic agents or use of an anti-histaminic elixir rinse is useful to control the pain.

LICHEN PLANUS

Definition/Description

- Lichen planus (LP) is a chronic inflammatory disease of the skin and/or mucous membrane that has an immunological origin.
- Clinically, it may present in five different forms: reticular, papular, plaque-like, atrophic and bullous or erosive. In this chapter, only the erosive form is discussed.

Cause

- Causes of LP are poorly understood.
- Stress, anxiety and depression have been implicated as predisposing factors.
- Immunological and genetic factors may also play a role in its causation.

Clinical Features

- LP frequently occurs bilaterally in a symmetrical pattern.
- It is common on the buccal mucosa, gingiva and the dorsum of the tongue.
- Erythematous centre with radiating lines at the periphery is a common presenting feature (Figure 22.5 A and B).
- In bullous or erosive form, burning of the mucosa is a common complaint.
- It is indistinguishable from oral lichenoid reactions caused due to medicines (e.g., antihypertensive drugs).
- A small percentage of erosive LP lesions carries malignant potential.
- Occasionally, erosive forms of LP may be preceded by bullous lesions.

Diagnosis

- History, clinical examination and histopathological evaluation of the lesion.

Management

- Symptomatic treatment for pain.
- Topical application of corticosteroids (triamcinolone acetonide 0.1% cream).
- If topical applications are not responsive, intralesional injections or systemic administration of corticosteroids yield good results.

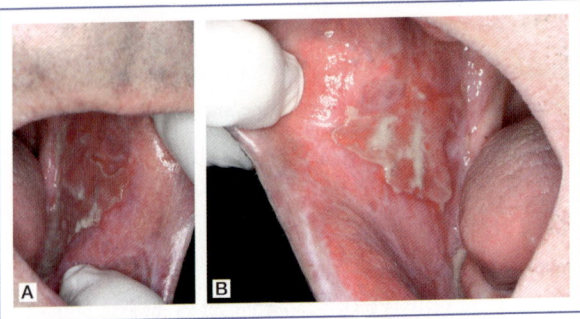

Figure 22.5 Erosive lichen planus of the (A) left and (B) right buccal mucosa in the same patient. Lichen planus lesions usually occur bilaterally. *Courtesy*: Nagamani Narayana.

- For severe cases, azathioprine may be helpful. However, the potential side-effects need to be considered.

   Detailed discussion on oral LP is presented in Chapter 39 (Oral potentially malignant disorders II: Oral lichen planus, oral lichenoid lesions, oral graft-versus-host disease and oral submucous fibrosis).

PRIMARY HERPES SIMPLEX VIRUS INFECTION (PRIMARY HERPETIC GINGIVOSTOMATITIS)

Definition/Description

- Primary herpes simplex virus (HSV) infection results in primary herpetic gingivostomatitis. This is a relatively common infection of the oral tissues, usually caused by HSV type 1.

Cause

- Infection with HSV type 1.

Clinical Features

- Usually, children are affected.
- Multiple vesicles occur on the gingival and other mucosal surfaces, which rupture, leaving shallow painful ulcers (Figure 22.6).
- Gingivae are swollen and oedematous.
- Systemic symptoms such as fever, malaise and anorexia may be present.
- Cervical lymph nodes are enlarged.

Diagnosis

- Diagnosis is based on history and clinical grounds.
- Diagnosis can be confirmed by polymerase chain reaction or viral culture. However, these investigations are not carried out in general practice.

Management

- Conservative treatment with symptomatic measures, including oral fluids, analgesics and antipyretics.

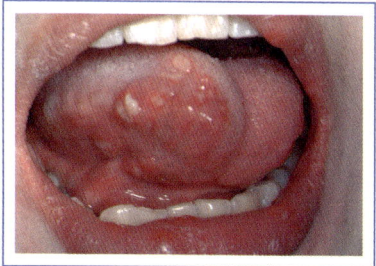

Figure 22.6   Ulceration due to herpes simplex virus infection. Reproduced with permission from: Patnarin Kanjanabuch.

- Antiviral therapy (acyclovir or famciclovir) may be indicated in immunosuppressed patients.

RECURRENT HERPES SIMPLEX VIRUS INFECTION (HERPES LABIALIS)

Definition/Description

- Reactivation of HSV causes recurrent infection. This is usually found on the lip at the mucocutaneous junction of the mouth. The condition is called herpes labialis and is commonly known as a 'cold sore'.

Cause

- Secondary or recurrent herpetic infection is caused by the reactivation of HSV (type 1 in most cases), which remains dormant in the sensory ganglia after the primary infection.
- Predisposing factors for reactivation of the dormant virus include sunlight or cold, psychological stress, menstruation, trauma, common cold and immunosuppression.

Clinical Features

- Recurrent herpetic infection has a prodromal phase. During this phase, itching and tingling sensation occurs a day before the appearance of multiple vesicles on the lip and sometimes on the side of the nose.
- Vesicles on the lips (Figure 22.7 A and B) rupture and heal without scarring.

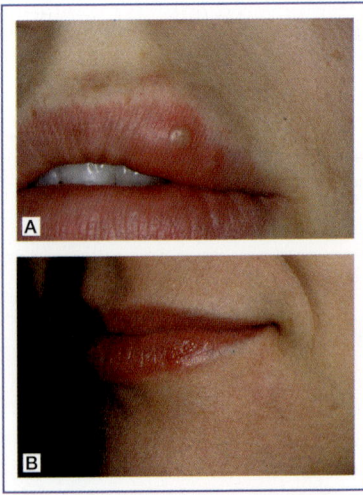

Figure 22.7 (A and B) Recurrent herpes simplex virus infection causing vesicles on the lips. This condition is also called herpes labialis. *Courtesy*: Nagamani Narayana.

- Intraoral involvement of recurrent herpetic infection is rare in immunocompetent individuals.
- The virus is present in the vesicles and saliva.

Diagnosis

- History and clinical examination.

Management

- Application of 5% aciclovir cream or 1% penciclovir during the prodromal phase is effective in reducing the clinical course of the condition.

HAND, FOOT AND MOUTH DISEASE

Definition/Description

- Hand, foot and mouth disease is a viral infection that presents with vesicular lesions on the hands, feet and the mouth.
- Hand, foot and mouth disease occurs in children, particularly in locations where the infection is epidemic.

Cause

- Causative virus is Coxsackie virus A16. Incubation period is 3 to 10 days.

Clinical Features

- Small blisters on the dorsal and lateral aspects of the fingers and toes and rashes on the hands and feet are consistent clinical features.
- Systemic symptoms include fever, malaise and lymphadenopathy. These symptoms are generally mild.
- Oral aphthous-like ulcers surrounded by erythema develop on the tongue and buccal mucosa.

Diagnosis

- History and clinical features.

Management

- Hand, foot and mouth disease is self-limiting and resolves within a week.
- Symptomatic treatment may be necessary.

HERPANGINA

Definition/Description

- Herpangina is a viral infection caused by Coxsackie virus.

Cause

- Causative virus is Coxsackie virus A2. Incubation period is two to seven days.

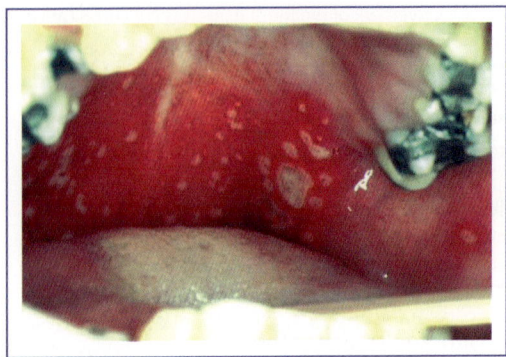

Figure 22.8 Herpangina: Multiple ulcers on the soft palate.
Courtesy: S. R. Prabhu.

Clinical Features

- Common in children.
- Systemic features include sore throat, fever, malaise and lymphadenopathy.
- Oral symptoms includes blisters, erosions and round ulcers, mainly seen on the soft palate (Figure 22.8).

Diagnosis

- History of illness and clinical appearance of lesions confined to soft palate and pharynx provide useful diagnostic clues.

Management

- Treatment is largely symptomatic.

CHICKENPOX

Definition/Description

- Chickenpox is a highly contagious primary infection caused by varicella-zoster virus. It is common in childhood.

Cause

- Primary infection with varicella-zoster virus.

Clinical Features

- Symptoms include fever, malaise, skin rash and vesicles on the trunk and the face.
- Painful oral vesicles and ulcers may occur in some patients. These are commonly seen on the palate.

Diagnosis

- History and clinical features.

Management

- Chickenpox is a self-limiting infection.
- Symptomatic treatment may be necessary.

HERPES ZOSTER (SHINGLES)

Definition/Description

- Herpes zoster, also known as shingles, is caused by the reactivation of varicella-zoster virus.

Cause

- Reactivation of the varicella-zoster (herpes zoster) virus in people who have had chickenpox in childhood.
- Varicella-zoster virus remains dormant in the sensory ganglia until reactivated.
- It is common in immunocompromised individuals.

Clinical Features

- Most commonly, it involves thoracic dermatomes. In 30% of cases, trigeminal involvement, usually the mandibular division, is seen.
- During the prodromal phase, the pain in the region is deeply seated and unilateral, often mimicking the pain of dental origin. This is followed by vesicles seen unilaterally along the distribution of the branches of the involved nerve.
- On the skin, these vesicles rupture and form crusts, whereas no crusting occurs intraorally. Shallow ulcers result due to the rupture of vesicles.
- If the maxillary division is involved (Figure 22.9), ulceration may also be found on the hard and soft palate.
- If the mandibular division is involved, the skin of the lower part of the face shows vesicles and ulceration.
- Corneal ulceration may result from ophthalmic division involvement.

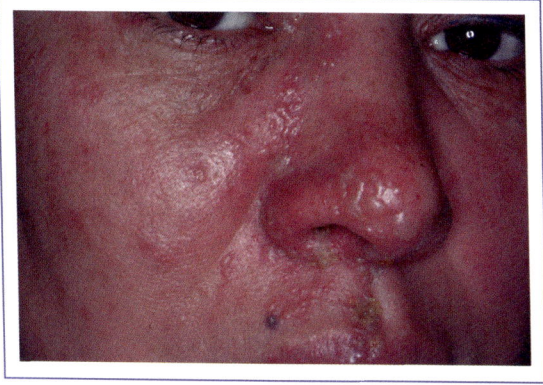

Figure 22.9   Shingles involving the maxillary division of the trigeminal nerve. *Courtesy*: Nagamani Narayana.

- Shingles is a painful condition.
- Systemic symptoms may include fever and malaise.
- Complication of herpes zoster may cause postherpetic neuralgia.

Diagnosis

- History and clinical features.

Management

- Antiviral agents: Aciclovir (800 mg, five times daily for seven days) is effective in reducing the severity of symptoms.
- Referral to an ophthalmologist is necessary if the ophthalmic division is affected.

ULCERS DUE TO CYTOMEGALOVIRUS INFECTIONS

Definition/Description

- Cytomegalovirus (CMV) belongs to the family of Herpesviridae (HHV-5).
- CMV infections mainly involve salivary glands.

Cause

- CMV infection.

Clinical Features

- Oral involvement is uncommon.
- In immunocompromised patients and those receiving immunosuppressive medicines, oral ulcers may be noted.
- Usually, a single ulcer is present. Tongue and buccal mucosa are the preferred sites.
- Ulcers mimic major aphthae.

Diagnosis

- Oral ulcers due to cytomeglovirus infections often mimic aphthous ulcers.
- Biopsy and histological examination of the lesions are useful; they show intranuclear and intracytoplasmic inclusion bodies.

Management

- CMV ulcers respond to ganciclovir.

ORAL ULCERS IN HUMAN IMMUNODEFICIENCY VIRUS INFECTION

- In human immunodeficiency virus (HIV) infection, more than 2% of patients develop oral ulcers. These ulcers are not exclusive to those with HIV infection or AIDS, but may also occur in immunocompetent individuals. Oral ulcers seen in HIV/AIDS patients are discussed in Chapter 37 (Oral lesions in HIV infection).

TRAUMATIC ULCERS

Definition/Description

- Traumatic ulcers are the ulcers that occur due to mechanical, thermal, chemical or radiation injury.

Cause

- Sharp cusps of teeth, periphery of denture or orthodontic appliances, accidental biting of the mucous membrane and self-inflicted or iatrogenic injury.

Clinical Features

- Patients remember the traumatic event.
- Acute ulcers are painful and chronic ulcers are mildly painful. Pain may be severe if they are secondarily infected.
- Ulcers are usually single and of irregular size and shape. Floor of the acute ulcer is yellow, and margins are not indurated.
- Traumatic ulcers heal within a few days upon elimination of the cause.
- Common sites include labial mucosa, buccal mucosa and lateral surface of the tongue (Figure 22.10).
- Chronic traumatic ulcers mimic malignant ulcers.
- Any oral ulcer that does not heal within two weeks after the removal of the cause should be biopsied to rule out malignancy.

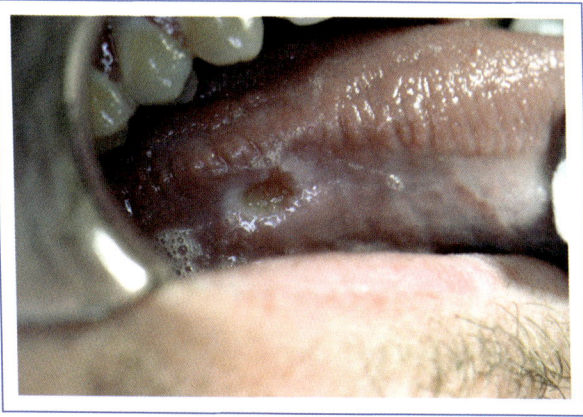

Figure 22.10   Chronic traumatic ulcer of the posteroventral surface of the tongue. This ulcer clinically mimics a malignant lesion. If the ulcer does not heal within two weeks after the elimination of trauma, a biopsy and histopathological evaluation of the ulcer are necessary to rule out malignancy. *Courtesy*: Nagamani Narayana.

Diagnosis

- History of the traumatic event, its duration and clinical presentation of the ulcer.
- Biopsy of the ulcer is necessary if the lesion fails to heal in two weeks after the removal of the cause.

Management

- Elimination of the cause and follow-up.
- Symptomatic treatment may be required, depending on the severity of symptoms.

RECURRENT APHTHOUS ULCERS

Definition/Description

- Recurrent aphthous ulcers (RAU), also known as recurrent aphthous stomatitis, is a common condition that affects nearly 20% of the population at some point in their lives.
- These recurrent ulcers present as three clinical types: minor, major and herpetiform.

Cause

- Exact aetiology is not known. However, cell-mediated immunological defect has been identified in patients with aphthous ulcers.
- Other contributing factors associated with RAU include nutritional deficiencies (most commonly iron deficiency; however, folic acid and vitamin B_{12} deficiencies may also be associated), genetic predisposition, smoking cessation, stress, trauma, hormonal imbalance and food allergies.
- Increased incidence of ulceration in patients with Crohn's disease and coeliac disease has also been observed.

Clinical Features

- RAUs are common. On the basis of their size, duration and type of healing, they present in one of the three clinical forms: minor, major or herpetiform.
- **Minor aphthous ulcers** are generally 3–10 mm in size, 1–10 in number, round or oval in shape and have a red halo (Figure 22.11). They generally heal within one to two weeks, without leaving a scar.
- Ulcers are painful. Minor aphthae are usually located on the lips, soft palate or buccal mucosa (nonkeratinised mucosa).
- **Major aphthous ulcers** are more than 1 cm in size (Figure 22.12), usually single and have an irregular border. They may take up to six weeks to heal and leave a scar.
- These lesions are deeper, painful and are usually located on the lips, soft palate or buccal mucosa (nonkeratinised mucosa).
- **Herpetiform aphthous ulcers** are less common. They present as pinpointed multiple ulcers (Figure 22.13) and have a clinical appearance similar to that of herpetic infection (hence the name).

- Ulcers are oval, shallow and yellow, which sometimes coalesce and form larger ulcers. They are also found on the gingiva. These ulcers may be associated with coeliac disease.

Diagnosis

- History and clinical presentation of ulcers.
- In patients with long-standing major recurrent aphthous ulcers, a biopsy of the ulcer is recommended to rule out malignancy.

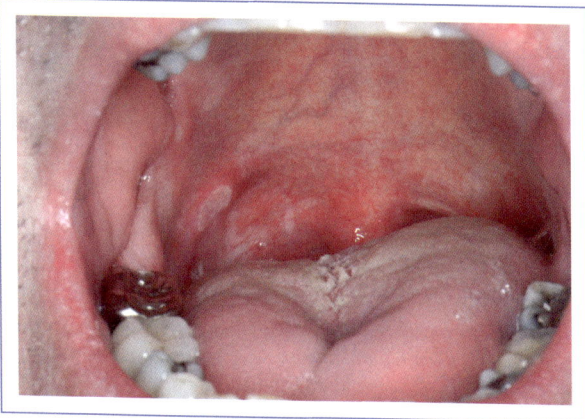

Figure 22.11   A minor recurrent aphthous ulcer on the soft palate.
Courtesy: Nagamani Narayana.

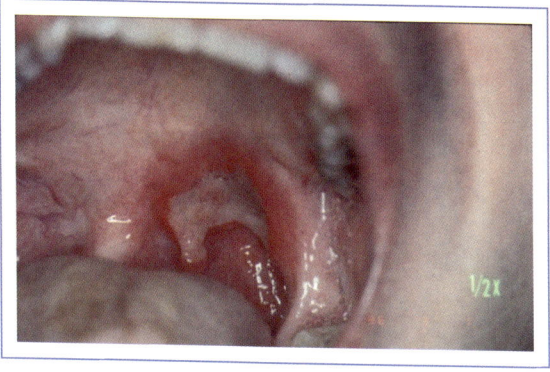

Figure 22.12   A major aphthous ulcer of the soft palate in an HIV-infected individual. Note the erythematous halo around the ulcer.
Reproduced with permission from: David Reznik. Available from: http://www.hivdent.org

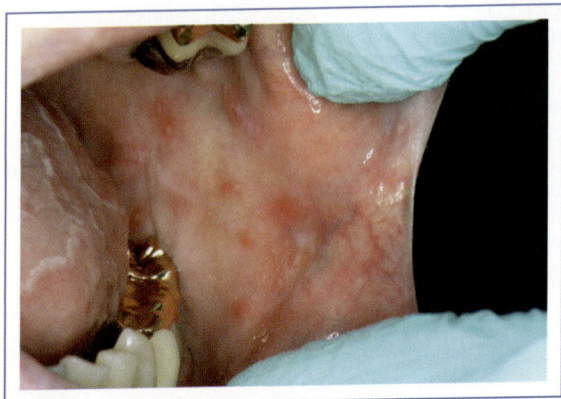

Figure 22.13 Herpetiform aphthous ulcers on the buccal mucosa.
Courtesy: Nagamani Narayana.

Management

- Underlying nutritional deficiency, if any, need to be excluded by carrying out full blood count, together with assays of ferritin, folic acid and vitamin B_{12}.
- Topical application of corticosteroids (e.g., beclomethasone 50 µg metered dose inhaler directed at the ulcer or soluble betamethasone 0.5 mg dissolved in water and used as a mouthwash) yields good results.
- If systemic diseases are associated with these lesions, appropriate treatment of the systemic disorder is required.

NECROTISING ULCERATIVE GINGIVITIS

Definition/Description

- Necrotising ulcerative gingivitis is a rapidly progressive ulcer that initially involves the interdental gingival papillae caused predominantly by anaerobic gram-negative organisms.

Cause

- Bacteria responsible for this condition predominantly include *Treponema vincentii*, *Fusobacterium fusiformis*, *Porphyromonas gingivalis*, *Leptotrichia buccalis* and *Prevotella intermedia*.

Clinical Features

- This condition is uncommon in otherwise healthy individuals.
- Predisposing factors include reduced general and local host resistance. Immunocompromised individuals, heavy smokers and drinkers and malnourished individuals are at a higher risk of developing this condition than healthy individuals.

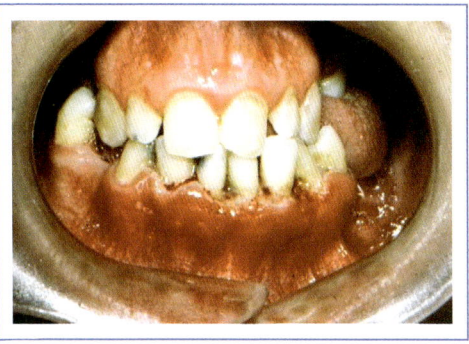

Figure 22.14   Necrotising ulcerative gingivitis in an HIV-positive patient. Note the destruction of interdental papillae.

Reproduced with permission from: David Reznik. Available from: http://www.hivdent.org

- Clinical features include necrotic ulcers of the interdental papillae (Figure 22.14). Ulcers exhibit a crater-like and punched-out appearance.
- Gingival bleeding, pain and halitosis are common.

Diagnosis

- History and clinical examination.
- Identification of gram-negative organisms in smears is confirmatory.

Management

- Treatment includes oral hygiene measures, oxygenating mouth rinses (hydrogen peroxide), antimicrobial therapy (e.g., metronidazole and amoxicillin) and symptomatic treatment of pain.
- Nutritional supplements are useful in building up the host resistance.

SYPHILITIC ULCER

Definition/Description

- Syphilis is a sexually transmitted disease. Oral lesions in syphilis are occasionally seen in primary, secondary and tertiary stages of the disease.

Cause

- Spirochaetes called *Treponema pallidum.*

Clinical Features

- **In primary syphilis,** an ulcerative lesion of the lip can occur at the site of entry of the spirochaete due to orogenital sexual contact. This ulcer is called chancre.
  - ♦ Chancre is a solitary painless ulcer that exhibits rolled borders and punched out appearance. This can be mistaken for carcinoma. Common sites include lips and tip of the tongue (Figure 22.15).

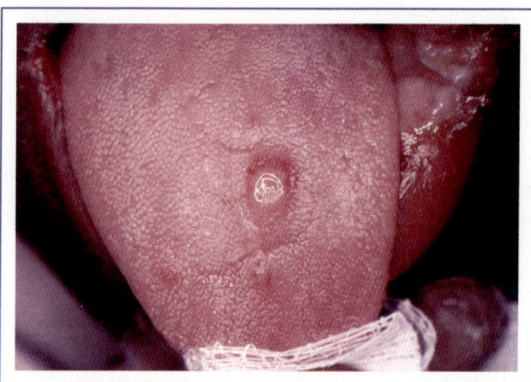

Figure 22.15 Primary syphilis: Chancre on the dorsum of the tongue. Reproduced with permission from: Centers for Disease Control and Prevention. Sexually Transmitted Diseases (STDs): Syphilis. Atlanta, GA: CDC. Available from: http://www.cdc.gov/std/syphilis/images.htm

- ◆ Cervical lymphadenopathy (rubbery consistency) is present. Ulcer may heal without treatment in about four weeks of its appearance.
- **In secondary syphilis,** mucocutaneous patches occur. Oral ulcers are flat and linear and are covered by a grey membrane. These are called snail-track ulcers.
  - ◆ On the skin, copper-coloured coin-like rashes appear in secondary syphilis.
  - ◆ Associated findings include fever, malaise, generalised lymphadenopathy and skin rashes. Serology is positive in this stage.
- **Tertiary syphilis** is very rare. In this stage of the disease, oral gummatous ulceration occurs, resulting in perforation of the tissue.
  - ◆ Gumma is usually seen on the palate. It is not infective.

Diagnosis

- Diagnosis includes detailed history, clinical examination of the ulcer and regional lymph nodes and tests for the presence of *T. pallidum* in the smear taken from chancre and ulcers.
- Samples are examined by dark-ground illumination method and nonspecific serologic tests (the Venereal Disease Research Laboratory test or VDRL test) and specific tests (such as *T. pallidum* haemagglutination test).

Management

- Ulcers of the primary and secondary stages respond to the systemic treatment of syphilis with antibiotics.
- Management of syphilis should be carried out by specialists.

Further details of syphilitic ulcer are presented in Chapter 31 (Oral mucosal infections).

TUBERCULOUS ULCER

Definition/Description

- Tuberculosis is a chronic infectious disease caused by acid-fast bacilli called *Mycobacterium tuberculosis*.
- Oral involvement of the disease is rare.

Cause

- Tuberculosis is caused by *M. tuberculosis.* Smoking, overcrowded conditions and poor living conditions are contributory factors.

Clinical Features

- Primary tuberculous ulcers of the oral tissues are rare.
- Occasionally, oral ulcers in a patient with untreated pulmonary tuberculosis occur as *Mycobacterium* gains entry into the oral tissues from the infected sputum.
- Dorsum of the tongue is a common site for tuberculous ulcers.
- Tuberculous ulcers typically show undermined borders and mucous-like material in the base of the ulcer. Often, these ulcers are mistaken for carcinoma.
- Cervical lymphadenopathy is a consistent feature.
- Systemic features include weight loss, night sweats, fever, cough and haemoptysis.

Diagnosis

- Detailed history and clinical examination of the ulcer and cervical lymph nodes.
- Diagnosis of the tuberculous ulcer can be confirmed by staining the tissue sample for acid-fast *Mycobacterium* (Ziehl-Neelsen stain).

Management

- When systemic treatment of pulmonary tuberculosis is given, oral ulcers heal.

    Detailed discussion of tuberculous ulcer is presented in Chapter 31 (Oral mucosal infections).

DRUG-INDUCED ORAL ULCERATIONS

Definition/Description

- Drug-induced oral ulcerations are adverse effects of the medications used for local or systemic conditions.

Cause

- Several kinds of drugs can cause oral ulceration. These include β-blockers, immunosuppressants, anticholinergic bronchodilators, platelet aggregation inhibitors, vasodilators, protease inhibitors, antibiotics, nonsteroidal anti-inflammatory drugs, antiretroviral agents, bisphosphonates (alendronate), potassium channel activators (nicorandil), systemic corticosteroid agents, antirheumatic drugs (methotrexate), antihypertensive agents and cytotoxic drugs (5-fluorouracil, methotrexate, bleomycin and cisplatin) used for the treatment of malignant lesions.

Clinical Features

- Widespread mucositis-associated ulceration is common in the patients receiving cytotoxic chemotherapy for cancer.
- Within a few days following the therapy, sloughing and ulcerations appear. Intense pain is a feature that often requires opioids.
- In other situations, fixed drug eruption may occur. In this condition, repeated development of treatment-resistant ulcers occurs.
- Single or multiple large oral ulcers are seen.
- Ulcers are not indurated.

Diagnosis

- Drug-induced oral ulcerations often pose diagnostic problems. Unless a detailed history is obtained and other non-drug-induced ulcers are ruled out, diagnosis of drug-induced lesions is difficult.
- Thorough clinical examination of the ulcers is also an important step in the diagnostic process.

Management

- Topical corticosteroids are not effective for most of these ulcers.
- A careful review of drug exposure must be done, and the medication suspected to cause the ulceration should be reduced in quantity or changed, in consultation with patient's physician.

Detailed discussion of drug-induced oral ulcerations is presented in Chapter 34 (Drug-induced oral adverse reactions, including medication-related osteonecrosis of the jaw).

MALIGNANT ULCERS

Definition/Description

- Malignant ulcers are chronic ulcers that fail to heal despite the removal of the possible factors that have caused the ulceration.

Cause

- Smoking, tobacco chewing, alcohol consumption, sunlight (for malignant ulcers of the lower lip) and, in a small number of cases, human papilloma virus.

Clinical Features

- In more than 95% of cases of oral malignancy (oral cancer), the neoplasm arises from the epithelial structures (squamous cell carcinoma).
- Oral ulceration is one of the several forms of squamous cell carcinomas. Other forms may appear as exophytic growths, white patches or red patches.
- Malignant ulcer is painless in the early stage and becomes painful in the advanced stage because of infiltration into the neural tissue or secondary infection.

- Eating and swallowing becomes difficult. Teeth become loose when the ulcer invades the gingival tissue and alveolar bone.
- Lateral borders of the tongue and buccal mucosa, floor of the mouth and alveolar ridges are the favoured sites.
- Malignant ulcer is round, crescentic or irregular in shape, with raised, rolled or everted edges (Figure 22.16 A and B).
- Base of the ulcer is indurated and fixed to the deeper tissues. Floor of the ulcer is granular and may bleed easily.
- Cervical lymph nodes are enlarged and nontender. Lymph nodes may become fixed to the adjacent tissues at the later stages of the disease.

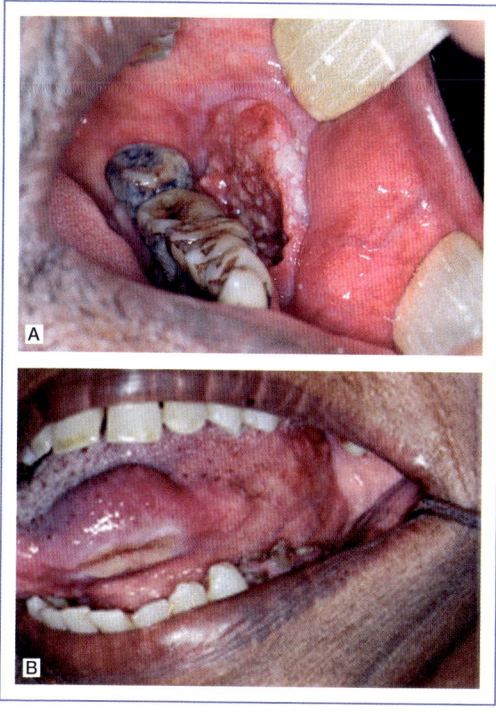

Figure 22.16 (A) Malignant ulcer (squamous cell carcinoma) of the buccal mucosa due to long-standing tobacco quid placement in the buccal vestibule. (B) Traumatic ulcer on the left lateral tongue margin, histologically confirmed with malignant features. Note the ulcerative lesion with rolled-out borders.

Reproduced with permission from: Ramadas K, Lucas E, Thomas G, et al. *A Digital Manual for the Early Diagnosis of Oral Neoplasia*. IARC, Lyon, 2008. Available from: http://screening.iarc.fr/atlasoral.php?lang=1

Diagnosis

- History, clinical examination of the ulcer and cervical lymph nodes and histopathological examination of the tissue obtained from the biopsy.
- Computed tomographic scans and magnetic resonance imaging are other useful tests.

Management

- Surgery, chemotherapy and radiation therapy are commonly used treatment methods. In the early stages of the disease, the prognosis is favourable.

SUGGESTED READINGS

Felix DH, Luker J, Scully C. Oral medicine: 1. Ulcers: aphthous and other common ulcers. *Dental Update*. 2012;39:513–9.

Felix DH, Luker J, Scully C. Oral medicine: 2. Ulcers: serious ulcers. *Dental Update*. 2012;39:594–8.

Leao JC, Gomez VB, Porter S. Ulcerative lesions of the mouth: an update for the general medical practitioner. *Clinics* [Internet]. 2007 [cited 2016 Jan 31];62:769–80. Available from: http://www.scielo.br/scielo.php?script=sci_arttext&pid=S1807-59322007000600018&lng=en

Porter SR, Leao JC. Review article: oral ulcers and its relevance to systemic disorders. *Aliment Pharmacol Ther*. 2005;21:295-306. doi: 10.1111/j.1365-2036.2005.02333.x.

Field EA, Allan RB. Oral ulceration-aetiopathogenesis, clinical diagnosis and management in the gastrointestinal clinic. *Aliment Pharmacol Ther*. 2003;18:949–62. doi: 10.1046/j.0269-2813.2003.01782.x.

Van Heerden WFP, Boy SC. Diagnosis and management of common non-viral ulcerations. *SA Fam Pract*. 2007;49:20–6.

Jinbu Y, Demitsu T. Oral ulcerations due to drug medications. *Jpn Dent Sci Rev*. 2014;50:40–6.

Lamey P-J, Lewis MAO. Oral ulceration. In: Lamey P-J, Lewis MAO, editors. *A Clinical Guide to Oral Medicine*. 2nd ed. London, U.K.: BDJ Books; 1997. pp. 7–12.

Laskaris G. Ulcerative lesions. In: Laskaris G, editor. *Pocket Atlas of Oral Diseases*. 2nd ed. New York: Thieme; 2006. pp. 137–96.

Prabhu SR. Ulcerative and erosive lesions of the oral mucosa. In: Prabhu SR, editor. *Textbook of Oral Medicine*. New Delhi, India: Oxford University Press; 2004. pp. 124–36.

Birnbaum W, Dunne SM. Ulcers. In: Birnbaum W, Dunne SM, editors. *Oral Diagnosis: The Clinician's Guide*. Oxford, U.K.: Wright; 2000. pp. 185–209.

Scully C. Common and important oral conditions. In: Scully C, editor. *Oral and Maxillofacial Medicine: The Basis of Diagnosis and Treatment*. 2nd ed. Edinburgh, Scotland: Churchill Livingstone; 2008. pp. 143–297.

Cawson RA, Odell EW. Diseases of the oral mucosa: non-infective stomatitis. In: Cawson RA, Odell EW, editors. *Cawson's Essentials of Oral Pathology and Oral Medicine*. 8th ed. Edinburgh, Scotland: Churchill Livingstone; 2008. pp. 220–45.

Qiao J, Fang H. Syphilitic chancre of the mouth. *CMAJ*. 2011;183:2015. doi: 10.1503/cmaj.110664.

Chapter 23

Mucosal red lesions

S. R. Prabhu

TRAUMATIC ERYTHEMA

Definition/Description

- When trauma is not severe enough to cause a breach in the mucosa, the resultant change is generally the one that clinically presents a red patch. This is called traumatic erythema.

Cause

- Traumatic erythema is due to inflammation or haemorrhage caused by trauma.
- Trauma is usually derived from mechanical sources or accidental biting of the oral tissues.

Clinical Features

- Clinically, the lesion is bright red because of the extravasation of blood, as in haematoma or ecchymosis.

Diagnosis

- History and clinical examination.

Management

- Elimination of the cause and symptomatic treatment are recommended.

ERYTHEMA DUE TO FELLATIO

Definition/Description

- Fellatio is the practice of oral sex. Repeated acts of oral sex may cause red lesion on the palatal mucosa.

Cause

- Trauma derived from fellatio.

Clinical Features

- Redness is usually found at the junction between hard palate and soft palate.
- Occasionally, petechiae or ecchymoses may be seen in these locations.

Diagnosis

- History and clinical examination.

Management

- No treatment is necessary. Patient needs to be informed of the cause of erythema.

CANDIDA-ASSOCIATED DENTURE STOMATITIS (CHRONIC ATROPHIC CANDIDIASIS)

Definition/Description

- Denture stomatitis (denture sore mouth) in early stages is a local-ised red area on the palate caused by chronic candidal infection in denture wearers.
- This condition should not be mistaken for allergic reaction to den-ture material. Detailed discussion on this condition is provided in Chapter 31 (Oral mucosal infections).

ERYTHEMATOUS CANDIDIASIS

Definition/Description

- Erythematous candidiasis is characterised by large red patches on the dorsum of the tongue and palate. A detailed discussion on this condition is provided in Chapter 31 (Oral mucosal infections).

ERYTHROPLAKIA

Definition/Description

- Erythroplakia is a red patch on the mucosa that cannot be classified as any other known clinical entity.
- This is a red counterpart of leukoplakia but has relatively higher malignant potential. A detailed discussion on erythroplakia is provided in Chapter 38 (Oral potentially malignant disorders I: Leukoplakia and erythroplakia).

HAEMATOMA, ECCHYMOSIS, PETECHIAE AND PURPURA

- Haematoma and ecchymosis refer to extravasation of blood into the tissues.
- Petechiae are characterised by pinpoint haemorrhages into the mucosa or submucosa. These are less than 3 mm in diameter.
- Purpura refers to red lesions of 3 to 10 mm diameter, caused due to bleeding under the skin or mucosa.

These lesions have been discussed in Chapter 20 (Gingival, oral and postexttraction bleeding).

HEREDITARY HAEMORRHAGIC TELANGIECTASIA

Definition/Description

- Hereditary haemorrhagic telangiectasia (HHT) is a genetic disorder characterised by the formation of abnormal blood vessel in the skin and mucous membranes. This condition is also called Osler-Weber-Rendu syndrome.

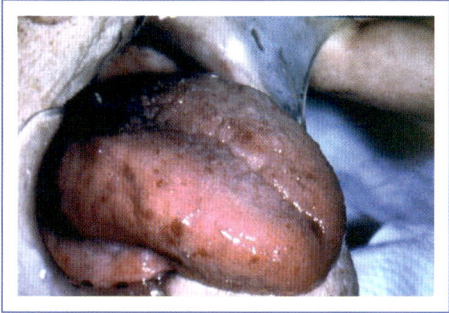

Figure 23.1 Hereditary haemorrhagic telangiectasia. Note red nodular lesions on the tongue.
Courtesy: S. R. Prabhu.

Cause

- HHT is a genetic disorder.

Clinical Features

- Multiple bright red papules or nodular lesions on lips, tongue and palate, which disappear on application of digital pressure (Figure 23.1).
- Mechanical trauma results in haemorrhage.
- Other features include nosebleeds and gastrointestinal haemorrhage.
- Skin lesions are usually located on the fingertips.
- Patient may be anaemic due to gastrointestinal bleeding.

Diagnosis

- Family history and clinical examination.
- Lesions blanch under pressure.

Management

- Observation of the condition is required.
- No treatment is necessary.

HAEMANGIOMA

Definition/Description

- Haemangioma is a developmental anomaly of the blood vessels.
- It can be grouped as congenital haemangioma and vascular malformations. The former is a hamartomatous lesion characterised by endothelial proliferation.
- Vascular malformations are generally due to abnormal morphogenesis of the arterial and venous structures.
- Both types develop during infancy and childhood. Haemangioma usually involutes as child grows, whereas vascular malformations persist and grow in size with the child growth.

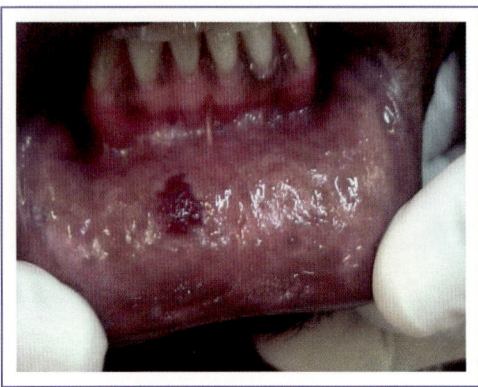

Figure 23.2 Haemangioma of the lower lip.
Courtesy: Haytham Al Bayaty.

Cause

- Haemangioma and vascular malformations are developmental defects of the blood vessels.

Clinical Features

- Haemangioma on the face or on the mucous membrane may present as flat or raised red lesions (Figure 23.2).
- Flat red lesions are usually due to capillary haemangioma, and the elevated lesions are caused by cavernous haemangioma and have large dilated sinuses filled with blood.
- When traumatised, lesions bleed heavily.
- Cutaneous (haemangioma-like) vascular malformation that involves facial and oral region following trigeminal nerve distribution is called encephalotrigeminal angiomatosis (Sturge-Weber syndrome).

Diagnosis

- History and clinical examination.
- Clinical test involves application of pressure (digital pressure or pressure using a glass slide) on the lesion, which results in the disappearance of the red lesion as long as the pressure is maintained. Once the pressure is released, the lesion returns. This test is called diascopy.

Management

- No treatment is required unless the lesions are traumatised, in which case patient should be referred to an oral surgeon for evaluation and appropriate treatment.
- Congenital haemangiomas usually involute over time.
- Sclerotherapy, cryosurgery, laser therapy and microembolisation followed by resection are some of the useful treatment methods.

DESQUAMATIVE GINGIVITIS

Definition/Description

- Desquamative gingivitis is not a specific disease, but it is a descriptive clinical term used for nonspecific gingival manifestations of underlying systemic or local conditions.

Cause

- Autoimmune mechanism may be involved in the causation of this disorder.
- Lichen planus, mucous membrane pemphigoid, linear immunoglobulin A disease, discoid lupus erythematosus (LE) and bullous pemphigoid are associated with desquamative gingivitis.

Clinical features

- Desquamative gingivitis is characterised by erythema with or without blisters or erosions on the marginal and attached gingivae (Figure 23.3).
- Lesions are painful and tender. The condition is common in middle-aged women.

Diagnosis

- History and clinical examination.
- Histological and immunological evaluations are also helpful.

Management

- Systemic corticosteroids or immunosuppressants are effective, based on the underlying disease.
- Oral hygiene should be maintained.

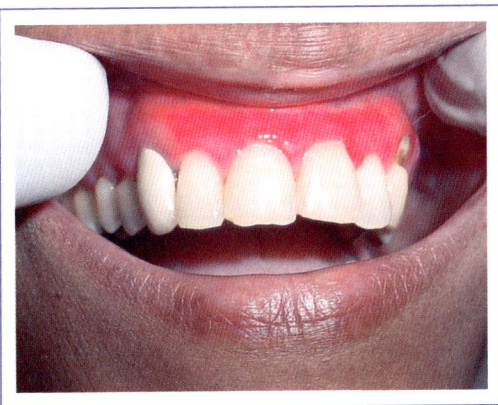

Figure 23.3 Diffuse erythema of the gingiva in desquamative gingivitis. *Courtesy*: Haytham Al Bayaty.

LINEAR GINGIVAL ERYTHEMA

Definition/Description

- Linear gingival erythema is characterised by linear erythema of the attached gingiva in HIV-positive patients. Detailed discussion on this condition has been provided in Chapter 31 (Oral mucosal infections) and Chapter 37 (Oral lesions in HIV infection).

CONTACT ALLERGIC STOMATITIS

Definition/Description

- Contact allergic stomatitis refers to an allergic reaction due to contact with certain allergens.

Cause

- Allergens include foods, restorative materials, toothpaste, lipstick and chewing gums.

Clinical Features

- In the acute form, erythema and oedema of the mucosa appear soon after contact with allergens.

Diagnosis

- History and clinical examination.
- Skin patch tests are useful in determining the antigenic agent.

Management

- Elimination and avoidance of suspected allergens.
- Topical or systemic corticosteroids and antihistamines are useful.

ERYTHEMA MULTIFORME

Definition/Description

- Erythema multiforme (EM) refers to a mucocutaneous disorder of unknown cause, possibly mediated by deposition of immune complexes in the superficial microvasculature of the skin and oral mucous membrane.
- This condition usually follows a viral infection or systemic drug exposure.

Cause

- Unknown. Possibly, an immunological disorder.

Clinical Features

- EM exhibits skin and oral mucosal lesions.
- Skin lesions are typically 'iris lesions'. Oral mucosal involvement exhibits generalised erythema. Sometimes, EM is accompanied by erosions or bullous lesions. Crusty lesions on the lips and erosive lesions on the tongue are often characteristic (Figure 23.4).
- Severe form of EM is called Stevens-Johnson syndrome, in which oral, conjunctival and genital mucosae are involved.

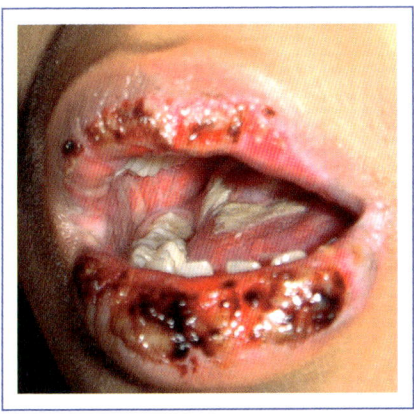

Figure 23.4 Erythema multiforme involving lips and intraoral tissues: Extensive erythematous lesions and crusty lesions are seen.

Reproduced with permission from: Joseph TI, Vargheese G, George D, Sathyan P. Drug induced oral erythema multiforme: a rare and less recognized variant of erythema multiforme. *J Oral Maxillofac Pathol*. 2012; 16:145–8. doi: 10.4103/0973-029X.92995.

Diagnosis

- History and clinical examination.
- Biopsy is required to confirm the diagnosis.

Management

- Discontinuation of medicine and low doses of systemic corticosteroids.
- Topical application of local anaesthetic agents or the use of antihistaminic elixir rinse is useful in controlling pain.

EROSIVE LICHEN PLANUS

Definition/Description

- Lichen planus is a mucocutaneous condition, which manifests in a variety of clinical forms. These include reticular, plaque, bullous and erosive forms. Oral involvement is sometimes seen as erosive lichen planus. A detailed discussion on this condition is provided in Chapter 39 (Oral potentially malignant disorders II: Oral lichen planus, oral lichenoid lesions, oral graft-versus-host disease and oral submucous fibriosis).

LUPUS ERYTHEMATOSUS

Definition/Description

- Lupus erythematosus (LE) is a multisystem autoimmune disorder. Two forms of LE exist: systemic LE and discoid LE.

Cause

- LE is an autoimmune disorder.

Clinical Features

- Oral lesions of LE are a combination of red and white lesions similar to those of lichen planus. 'Butterfly' lesions on the bridge of the nose are characteristic of skin involvement of the disorder.

Diagnosis

- History and evaluation of antibodies.
- Anti-DNA antibodies are detected in systemic LE but not in discoid LE.

Management

- Systemic use of corticosteroids is beneficial in both forms of LE.

MIGRATORY GLOSSITIS (GEOGRAPHIC TONGUE OR ERYTHEMA MIGRANS)

Definition/Description

- Migratory glossitis, also known as geographic tongue or erythema migrans, is generally not considered as specific disease entity.

Cause

- The cause is unknown, but hypersensitivity response to unknown agents has been implicated.

Clinical Features

- Dorsum of the tongue shows map-like depapillated smooth red areas with whitish-yellow borders (Figure 23.5) that migrate from one site to the other.

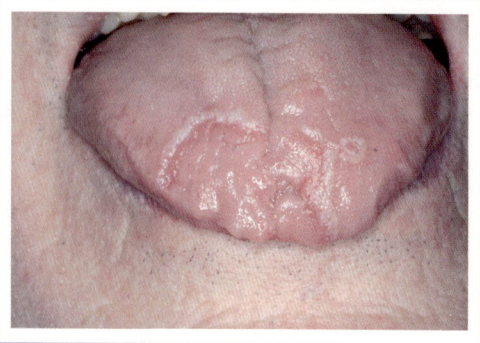

Figure 23.5 Migratory glossitis (geographic tongue). *Courtesy*: Nagamani Narayana.

- Sometimes, other mucosal areas may be affected, in which case the condition is called erythema migrans.
- Although asymptomatic, some patients may complain of burning sensation.
- Lesions may resolve within a few days but may appear at another mucosal site. Periods of exacerbation and remission are common.

Diagnosis

- Clinical examination.

Management

- No treatment is required.
- Reassuring the patient that the condition is a benign entity is necessary.

CENTRAL PAPILLARY ATROPHY (MEDIAN RHOMBOID GLOSSITIS)

Definition/Description

- Central papillary atrophy, which was previously known as median rhomboid glossitis, is characterised by a rhomboid area of papillary atrophy and erythema on the dorsal surface of the tongue anterior to the circumvallate papillae. Detailed discussion on this lesion is provided in Chapter 31 (Oral mucosal infections).

SUGGESTED READINGS

Rosebush MS, Anderson KM, Rawal YB. Normal oral cavity findings and variants of normal. In: Migliorati CA, Panagakos FS, editors. *Diagnosis and Management of Oral Lesions and Conditions: A Resource Handbook for the Clinician.* Rijeka, Croatia: InTech; 2014. pp. 1–12. doi: http://dx.doi.org/10.5772/57597.

Prabhu SR. Red lesions of the oral mucosa. In: Prabhu SR, editor. *Textbook of Oral Medicine.* New Delhi, India: Oxford University Press; 2004. pp. 117–23.

Laskaris G. Red lesions. In: Laskaris G, editor. *Pocket Atlas of Oral Diseases.* 2nd ed. Germany: Georg Thieme Verlag; 2006. pp. 43–78.

Chapter 24

Mucosal pigmented lesions

S. R. Prabhu

BLACK HAIRY TONGUE

Definition/Description

- Black and brown hairy tongue refers to a condition in which the filiform papillae elongate with black (or brown) discolouration, giving a black or brown hairy appearance.

Cause

- Causes or predisposing conditions of black hairy tongue include poor oral hygiene, smoking, radiation, xerostomia, the use of topical antibiotics (tetracyclines), antacids, chlorhexidine rinses, iron salts and excessive growth of fungal or bacterial organisms.

Clinical Features

- Hairy tongue occurs on the dorsum of the tongue, anterior to circumvallate papillae (Figure 24.1).
- The condition is asymptomatic. Some individuals may complain of dry mouth, bad taste, oral malodour or gagging sensation.

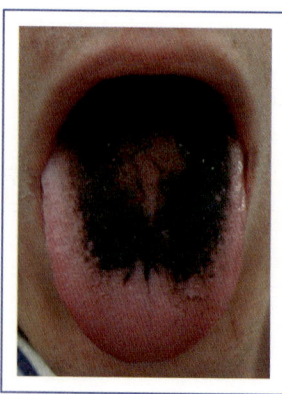

Figure 24.1 Black hairy tongue.
Reproduced with permission from: Wikimedia.org. Available from: http://upload.wikimedia.org/wikipedia/commons/1/16/Black_tongue.jpg

Diagnosis

- History and clinical examination.

Management

- Elimination of the predisposing conditions.
- Oral hygiene maintenance and tongue cleaning (by gentle scraping or brushing before sleep) are useful.
- Topical application of keratolytic agents such as podophyllins is also effective, but their intraoral use is generally not advisable due to their side-effects on repeated use.
- Reassurance is important.

RACIAL PIGMENTATION (PHYSIOLOGICAL PIGMENTATION)

Definition/Description

- Racial pigmentation (physiological pigmentation) of the oral mucosa is common in people of African, Asian or Mediterranean origin.

Cause

- Pigmentation is due to increased amount of melanocyte activity.

Clinical Features

- Gingival surface is the most favoured site. A dark-brown ribbon-like band is seen bilaterally on the attached gingiva [see Chapter 3 (Anatomical variants and normal structures often mistaken as pathological lesions), Figure 3.8].
- In some instances, dark-brown patches are seen on the buccal mucosa, hard palate, tongue or lips. These are asymptomatic.
- Racial pigmentation is not a potentially malignant lesion.

Diagnosis

- History of ethnic origin and clinical examination.

Management

- No treatment is required.
- If the patient is concerned (cancer-phobic), reassurance is necessary.

SMOKER'S MELANOSIS

Definition/Description

- Smoker's melanosis refers to smoking-related pigmentation of the oral mucosa in light-skinned people.

Cause

- Heavy smoking leads to smoker's melanosis.
- Increased production of melanocytes provides a biological defence against the adverse effects of tobacco smoke.

Clinical Features

- Anterior gingival surface is brown or black in colour.
- Buccal mucosa may also show brown or black colouration in heavy smokers.
- Women are more commonly affected, suggesting a possible synergistic action of female sex hormones and smoking. In three years after the cessation of smoking, pigmentation tends to disappear.

Diagnosis

- History and clinical examination.

Management

- Cessation of smoking.
- If pigmented areas show ulceration or surface elevation, biopsy is essential.

PEUTZ-JEGHERS SYNDROME

Definition/Description

- Peutz-Jeghers syndrome is a rare genetic disorder characterised by pigmented mucocutaneous macules and gastrointestinal polyposis.

Cause

- Genetic disorder caused due to mutation of the LKB1 gene on chromosome 19.

Clinical Features

- Multiple small melanotic spots are found on and around the lips (Figure 24.2). They are also found on the skin and other mucosal surfaces.
- These patients have an increased risk of malignancies of the small intestines, colon, stomach and breast.

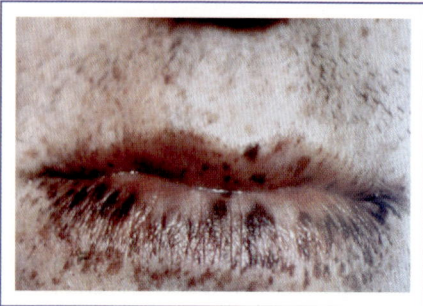

Figure 24.2 Perioral pigmentation in a patient with Peutz-Jeghers syndrome.
Courtesy: David Wilson.

Diagnosis

• History and clinical examination.

Management

• No treatment is required.
• Melanotic spots are not potentially malignant.

AMALGAM TATTOO

Definition/Description

• Amalgam tattoo is a focal blue-grey pigmentation, which is one of the common causes of intraoral pigmented lesions.

Cause

• Amalgam introduced in the soft tissues during dental procedures.

Clinical Features

• Localised blue-grey lesion on the gingival or alveolar mucosa (Figure 24.3) is the common appearance in majority of cases. Other oral mucosal areas may also be involved.
• Size of the pigmented lesions varies depending on the amount of amalgam embedded in the tissues.
• If amalgam particles are large, they may be detected on the periapical X-rays.
• There is no inflammatory response of the mucosa to amalgam.

Diagnosis

• History of amalgam restoration and traumatic extraction of the amalgam-filled tooth.
• Clinical examination of the pigmented lesion.

Management

• No treatment is required.
• Implanted amalgam is biologically inactive.

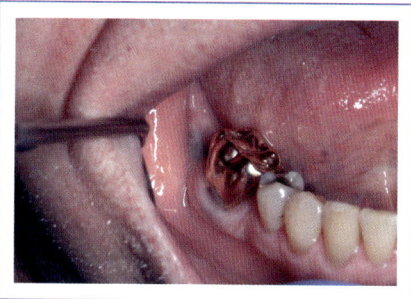

Figure 24.3   Amalgam tattoo seen on the alveolar ridge posterior to the first molar.
Courtesy: Nagamani Narayana.

DRUG-INDUCED MUCOSAL PIGMENTATION

Definition/Description

- A number of medicines cause oral pigmentation. Mucosal pigmentation is based on the type and duration of the drug used.

Cause

- Drugs that can cause mucosal pigmentation include antimalarials (chloroquine), antiretroviral drugs (zidovudine used for the treatment of HIV infection), antibiotics (tetracycline), oral contraceptives, antifungal drugs (ketoconazole), immunosuppressants (cyclophosphomide), bleomycin and 5-fluorouracil. Majority of these drugs may cause melanocyte stimulation.

Clinical Features

- The lesions are patchy and usually blue black or blue grey in colour.
- Hard palate, tongue and buccal mucosa are commonly involved.

Diagnosis

- History and clinical examination.
- Biopsy and histological evaluation are recommended.

Management

- No treatment is required for mucosal pigmentation.
- Change or reduction of the medicine may be required.

KAPOSI'S SARCOMA

Definition/Description

- Kaposi's sarcoma (KS) is a vascular malignancy seen predominantly in HIV/AIDS and severely immunosuppressed patients.

Cause

- Human herpesvirus 8 (HHV-8) is the causative agent in patients with immunodeficiency.

Clinical Features

- Hard palate, gingiva and tongue are the common sites of KS in the mouth. In the early stages, KS lesions present as brown to purple flat or slightly raised patches. Lesions are usually bilateral.
- In advanced stages, KS lesions are nodular and dark red or purple in colour (Figure 24.4). They may ulcerate and bleed easily.

Diagnosis

- History, clinical examination and histopathology.

Management

- Management of oral KS depends upon a variety of factors. These include local measures such as intralesional vinblastine injections or systemic administration of cytotoxic chemotherapy.

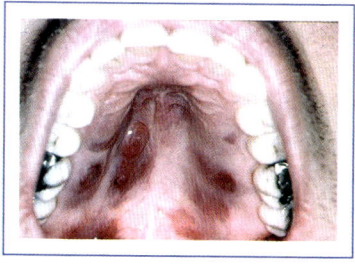

Figure 24.4   Kaposi's sarcoma of the palate, seen as purple-coloured maculopapular lesions in an AIDS patient.
Reproduced with permission from: David Reznik. Available from: www. HIVdent.org

MUCOSAL NAEVI (PIGMENTED NAEVI)

Definition/Description

• Mucosal naevi are rare developmental pigmented lesions found on the mucosa.

Cause

• Focal oral pigmentation because of the accumulation of naevus cells in the epithelial and/or connective tissue.

Clinical Features

• Mucosal naevus appears as a solitary flat dark-brown lesion (Figure 24.5). This is an example of junctional naevus.
• When the naevus is light brown in colour and dome-shaped, it is called intramucosal or compound naevus.

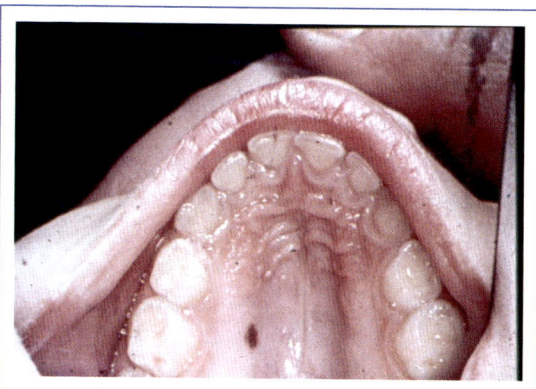

Figure 24.5   Pigmented naevus on the hard palate.
Courtesy: David Wilson.

- Intramucosal naevi are common. Buccal mucosa and hard palate are the favoured sites for oral naevi.

Diagnosis

- History and clinical appearance.
- Excision biopsy is recommended because occasionally, oral naevi may represent precursor lesions for oral melanomas.

Management

- Surgical removal of oral naevi is recommended.

MELANOTIC MACULE

Definition/Description

- Oral melanotic macule is a pigmented lesion commonly found on the lower lip. Other sites include gingiva, buccal mucosa and hard palate.

Cause

- Increased melanin production because of the increased number of melanocytes.

Clinical Features

- Melanotic macule is a brown-coloured lesion that is usually single and smaller than 1 cm, with clearly demarcated borders (Figure 24.6).
- Melanotic macule is common in women.

Diagnosis

- Clinical examination and histological evaluation.

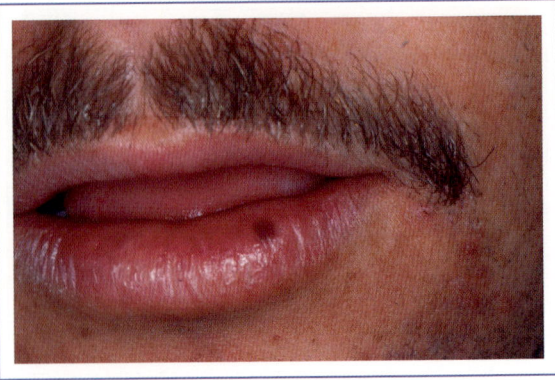

Figure 24.6 Melanotic macule of the lower lip.
Courtesy: David Wilson.

Management

- Melanotic macule is a benign lesion. Once the diagnosis is confirmed, no treatment may be necessary.

ORAL MALIGNANT MELANOMA

Definition/Description

- Oral malignant melanoma is a rare disease characterised by the proliferation of malignant melanocytes at the junction between the epithelium and connective tissues or within the connective tissue.

Cause

- Malignant proliferation of melanocytes.

Clinical Features

- Palate and gingiva are preferred intraoral sites for malignant melanoma.
- Melanoma may present as an asymptomatic brown or black patch with irregular borders. In some patients, melanoma may present as a rapidly growing black mass with ulceration, pain, bone destruction and bleeding (Figure 24.7).
- Some melanomas may not show discolouration. These are called amelanotic melanomas.
- Regional lymph node metastasis is a common feature.

Diagnosis

- History, clinical examination and histological evaluation.

Management

- Treatment should be offered as soon as the diagnosis is confirmed by histology.

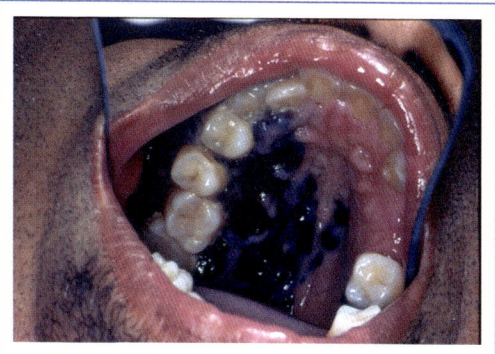

Figure 24.7   Malignant melanoma of the palate.
Courtesy: Haytham Al Bayaty.

- Treatment includes radical surgical resection.
- Radiation and chemotherapy are ineffective.
- Prognosis is poor; however, early detection improves the prognosis.

ADDISON'S DISEASE

Definition/Description

- Addison's disease is primary hypoadrenalism.
- This condition stimulates secretion of adrenocorticotropic hormone, which in turn induces melanocyte-stimulating hormone. The net result is the appearance of patchy pigmentation of the skin and oral mucosa.

Cause

- Hypoadrenalism may be due to the destruction of adrenal cortex by immune disorders, infection or malignancy.

Clinical Features

- In Addison's disease, brown patches on the gingival, buccal mucosa, tongue and palate are seen.
- Patients also have systemic findings such as abdominal pain, nausea, vomiting, weight loss and hypotension.

Diagnosis

- History, clinical findings and laboratory tests.

Management

- Oral pigmented patches do not require treatment.
- Systemic treatment for the disorder is necessary.

McCUNE-ALBRIGHT SYNDROME AND POLYOSTOTIC FIBROUS DYSPLASIA

Definition/Description

- McCune-Albright syndrome (MAS) is characterised by the clinical triad of fibrous dysplasia of bone, *cafe-au-lait* skin pigmentation and precocious puberty.
- Fibrous dysplasia of the polyostotic type involves multiple bones, including the jaws. Pigmentation of the oral tissues may also occur in this syndrome.
- Monostotic type of fibrous dysplasia, also known as 'Jaffe-Lichtenstein' syndrome, affects single bone.

Cause

- Both types are due to a defect in bone maturation during embryogenesis.
- Mutations in the regulatory GNAS-1 gene cause proliferation of the osteoprogenitor cells, resulting in the formation of fibrous matrix with woven bone.

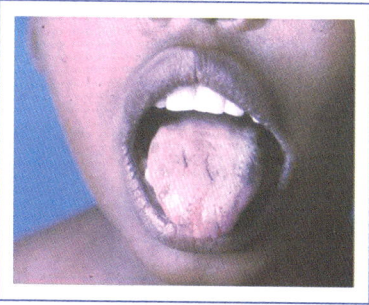

Figure 24.8 An African boy with fibrous dysplasia involving the facial skeleton. Note the brown patchy pigmentation of the tongue.
Courtesy: S. R. Prabhu.

Clinical Features

- In MAS, melanotic patches on the skin and oral mucosa (Figure 24.8) usually appear during early childhood.
- In both types, buccal, instead of lingual, expansion of the jaw bone is seen.

Diagnosis

- Radiographical appearance of the involved bones in both types show ground-glass appearance.
- Histopathological assessment is confirmatory for both types.

Management

- Recognition of MAS and prompt referral of the patient to an endocrinologist who is experienced in MAS management are essential.
- Bisphosphonates have beneficial effect for bony lesions.
- Fracture is the primary indication for surgical treatment of dysplastic lesions.

HAEMANGIOMA AND OTHER VASCULAR MALFORMATIONS

Definition/Description

- Haemangioma is a hamartomatous lesion. It is characterised by proliferation of endothelial cells.
- Vascular malformations are developmental malformations and do not show endothelial proliferation.
- Both haemangioma and vascular malformations occur in infancy. Haemangioma regresses as child grows, whereas vascular malformations persist throughout life.
- Tongue is the common site for both conditions. The lesion may be blue purple in colour and flat or slightly raised. Diascopy is positive in these patients.

VARIX AND THROMBUS

Definition/Description

- Varices are abnormally dilated veins, seen mostly in the elderly patients.
- Ventral surface of the tongue is the common site for varices. They appear as bluish-purple tortous elevations and blanch on pressure.
- Sometimes, a varix may contain a thrombus, in which case, it appears as a nodule and does not blanch on pressure. Such varices are common on the buccal mucosa and lips.

HAEMATOMA, PETECHIAE, ECCHYMOSIS AND PURPURA

Definition/Description

- Haematoma, petechiae, ecchymosis and purpura appear as flat or elevated coloured lesions. These are caused by extravasation of blood into the soft tissues. These lesions do not blanch on pressure. If the cause of these lesions is not associated with trauma, patient should be investigated for underlying blood disorders such as thrombocytopaenia or haemophilia.
- Colour of haematoma varies from red, purple, blue or bluish black, depending on the length of time the blood has been present in the soft tissue outside the blood vessels. Over a period of two weeks, colour returns to normal.

SUGGESTED READINGS

Wilson DF, Moore SR, Logan RM. Pigmented lesions. In: Prabhu SR, editor. *Textbook of Oral Medicine*. New Delhi, India: Oxford University Press; 2004. pp. 107–16.

Lamey P-J, Lewis MAO. Dermatoses and pigmentary disorders. In: Lamey P-J, Lewis MAO, editors. *A Clinical Guide to Oral Medicine*. London, U.K.: BDJ Books; 1999. pp. 57–62.

Cawson RA, Odell EW. Melanoma and other pigmented lesions. In: Cawson RA, Odell EW, editors. *Cawson's Essentials of Oral Pathology and Oral Medicine*. 8th ed. Edinburgh, Scotland: Churchill Livingstone; 2008. pp. 327–31.

Chapter 25

Mucosal warts and wart-like lesions

S. R. Prabhu

VERRUCA VULGARIS (ORAL WARTS)

Definition/Description

- Verruca vulgaris is a mucocutaneous warty lesion usually found on the lips, palate or attached gingiva.

Cause

- Human papillomaviruses (HPV) types 2, 4, 6 and 11 are the causative agents.

Clinical Features

- Skin lesions are common. In majority of cases, oral lesions are due to autoinoculation of the virus from the lesions on the fingers.
- Lesions of verruca vulgaris are nodular or cauliflower-like pedunculated white or pink lesions found on the lips, palate or the gingivae.
- In immunocompromised patients, multiple lesions may be found.

Diagnosis

- Clinical appearance of the lesions and microscopic findings.

Management

- Refer the patient to an oral surgeon.
- Surgical removal, cryosurgery and laser surgery are effective.

ORAL PAPILLOMA

Definition/Description

- Oral papilloma is a cauliflower-like, pedunculated or sessile, normal pink or whitish lesion that occurs on the oral mucosa.

Cause

- HPV types 6 and 11 are aetiologically associated with oral papillomas.

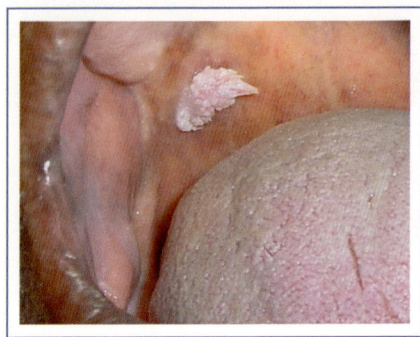

Figure 25.1   Oral papilloma at the junction of hard and soft palates. *Courtesy*: Haytham Al Bayaty.

Clinical Features

- Oral papilloma is a painless papillary lesion commonly located on the hard and soft palates (Figure 25.1) and uvula. Tongue and lips are involved less frequently.
- Papilloma is usually less than 1 cm in diameter and exhibits papillary projections, which are white or normal pink in colour.
- When traumatised, the lesion may bleed.
- Papilloma should be differentiated from other HPV-related lesions such as verruca vulgaris, condyloma accuminatum and focal epithelial hyperplasia.

Diagnosis

- Clinical examination and histological evaluation.

Management

- Refer the patient to an oral surgeon for surgical removal of the lesion.

CONDYLOMA ACUMINATUM

Definition/Description

- Condyloma accuminatum is a sexually transmitted disease caused by HPV.

Cause

- HPV types 6 and 11 transmitted to the oral cavity via orogenital contact.

Clinical Features

- Lesions of condyloma accuminatum are pink or white exophytic papillary growths located commonly on the lingual frenulum or soft palate. Other mucosal surfaces may also be involved.
- Usually, lesions are solitary and up to 3 cm in size.

Diagnosis

- History, clinical examination and histological evaluation.

Management

- Surgical removal or laser ablation.
- Topical podophyllin applications are useful.

FOCAL EPITHELIAL HYPERPLASIA

Definition/Description

- Focal epithelial hyperplasia is an HPV infection that involves oral mucosa. It is predominantly seen in children.

Cause

- HPV types 13 and 32.

Clinical Features

- Slightly raised multiple asymptomatic whitish-pink papules and plaques seen on the buccal and labial mucosae, predominantly in children.

Diagnosis

- Clinical appearance and asymptomatic nature of lesions in children.

Management

- No treatment is required. Lesions regress spontaneously.
- For aesthetic needs, surgical removal is recommended.

VERRUCOUS CARCINOMA

Definition/Description

- Verrucous carcinoma, also known as Ackerman's tumour, is a well-differentiated squamous cell carcinoma with a relatively better prognosis than squamous cell carcinoma.

Cause

- Although the cause is not clearly understood, tobacco habits (smoking and chewing) seem to be associated with verrucous carcinoma.
- HPV association has also been reported.

Clinical Features

- Verrucous carcinoma appears as a painless thick, white cauliflower-like lesion (Figure 25.2).
- Common intraoral sites of involvement include buccal mucosa, mandibular alveolar ridge, the gingivae and the tongue.
- Lip and floor of the mouth are also occasionally involved.
- Verrucous carcinoma generally does not metastasise to the regional lymph nodes.

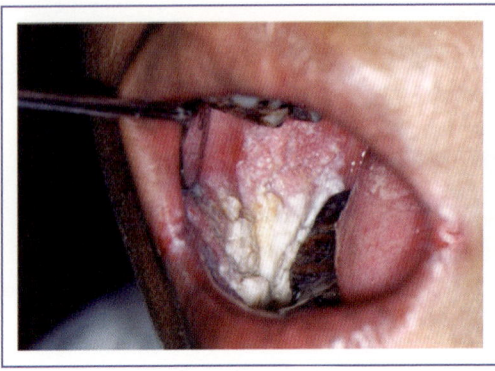

Figure 25.2 Verrucous carcinoma of the buccal mucosa.
Reproduced with permission from: Ramadas K, Lucas E, Thomas G, et al.
A Digital Manual for the Early Diagnosis of Oral Neoplasia. IARC, Lyon,
2008. Available from: http://screening.iarc.fr/atlasoral.php?lang=1

Diagnosis

• History, clinical and histological examination.

Management

• Surgery is the primary mode of treatment.

SUGGESTED READINGS

Laskaris G. Papillary lesions. In: Laskaris G, editor. *Pocket Atlas of Oral
    Diseases*. 2nd ed. Stuttgart, Germany: Georg Thieme Verlag; 2006.
    pp. 199–220.
Cawson RA, Odell EW. Common benign mucosal swellings. In: Cawson
    RA, Odell EW, editors. *Cawson's Essentials of Oral Pathology and Oral
    Medicine*. 8th ed. Edinburgh, Scotland: Churchill Livingstone; 2008.
    pp. 314–8.

Chapter 26

Oral malodour

N. Narayana

DEFINITION/DESCRIPTION

- Oral malodour or halitosis (sometimes referred to as bad breath) is a common symptom. It is a frequent or persistent unpleasant breath odour.
- Oral malodour is common on awakening in the morning (morning breath).

CAUSE

There are multiple causes of oral malodour. These include the following:

- Periodontal disease
- Smoking and ingested foods that have volatile component (e.g., garlic and onion)
- Alcohol
- Hydrogen-sulphide-producing bacteria resident in the tongue biofilm (e.g., *Veillonella, Actinomyces and Prevotella*)
- Poor oral hygiene
- Fermentation of food particles
- Poorly designed denture or bridge
- Dental plaque
- Tonsillitis
- Dental caries
- Mucosal ulcerative conditions
- Pericoronitis
- Blood clot in the tooth socket
- Dry mouth
- Sinus infection
- Nasal infections
- Oral cancer
- Starvation
- Systemic diseases such as diabetic acidosis, uraemia, hepatic disease, gastrointestinal disease and psychogenic factors.

CLINICAL FEATURES

- Majority of symptoms are behavioural issues:
  - Patients, usually adults, complain of unpleasant odour on the exhaled breath.

- Patients who do not have malodour may imagine it because of psychogenic reasons.
- Patients may cover the nose or face while talking.
- They may avoid or keep distance from other people.
- They may avoid social occasions.
- Usually, patients chew gum and use mints, mouthwashes or sprays to reduce malodour.
- Frequent tooth brushing is common among these individuals.
- They often clean their tongue vigorously.
- Those with systemic disorders may present signs and symptoms of the disease (e.g., diabetes, liver disease and kidney disease), causing oral malodour.

DIAGNOSIS

- By smelling exhaled air from the mouth (organoleptic method) and nose and comparing the two.
  - Oral malodour: Source is oral or pharyngeal.
  - Nasal malodour: Source is nasal passage or sinus.
  - Both oral and nasal malodour: Source is systemic.
- Use of Halimeter: Halimeter is an apparatus to measure volatile sulphur compounds (e.g., H_2S).
- Microbiological tests: BANA (benzoyl-arginine-naphthylamide) test or dark-field microscopy.

MANAGEMENT

- Treat any identifiable cause.
- Advise the patient to:
  - Avoid odiferous foods (e.g., onions and garlic).
  - Brush teeth after meals.
  - Keep good oral hygiene.
  - Rinse at least twice daily with chlorhexidine mouthwash.
  - Brush the tongue before going to bed.
  - Keep the mouth as moist as possible by using sugar-free chewing gum.
  - Use proprietary 'fresh-breath' preparations.
  - Leave dentures in hypochlorite or chlorhexidine solution outside the mouth at night.
- If intraoral causes are suspected, refer the patient to a dentist.
- If extraoral or systemic causes are suspected, refer the patient to a specialist.

SUGGESTED READINGS

Scully C, Felix DH. Oral medicine-update for the dental practitioner. Oral malodour. *Br Dent J*. 2005;199:498–500.

Oral and Dental Expert Group. Halitosis. *Therapeutic Guidelines: Oral and Dental*. Version 2. Melbourne, Australia: Therapeutic Guidelines Limited; 2012. pp. 97–100.

Chapter 27

Dry mouth and taste disorders

S. R. Prabhu and N. Narayana

DRY MOUTH (XEROSTOMIA)

Definition/Description

- Dry mouth (xerostomia) is the subjective sense of dryness of the mouth as a result of reduced salivary flow or alterations in the composition of saliva. This is a common salivary problem in the general population.

Cause

The causes of dry mouth include the following:

- Anxiety, drugs, dehydration, irradiation and salivary gland disease.
- Classes of drugs associated with dry mouth include cytotoxic drugs, anticholinergic drugs, psychoactive agents, sympathomimetic drugs and diuretics.
- Dehydration, as in diabetes mellitus, diabetes insipidus, chronic renal failure, hyperparathyroidism and starvation, may also cause dry mouth.
- Irradiation to the head and neck region causes salivary gland damage, which leads to hyposalivation, resulting in dry mouth.
- Salivary gland aplasia is a rare disorder. Mostly, salivary gland dysfunction is acquired. One of the important salivary gland diseases that causes dry mouth is Sjögren's syndrome (discussed below).

Clinical Features

- Patients may complain of the following:
  - Difficulty in swallowing, especially dry foods.
  - Difficulty in speaking.
  - Controlling dentures.
  - Unpleasant taste and oral malodour.
  - Dryness of the eyes, nasal and genital mucosae.
  - Lips adhere to one another.
  - Lipstick or food debris may be seen sticking to the teeth or soft tissues.
  - Saliva pooling in the floor of the mouth is absent.
  - Tongue is dry, lobulated and red, with partial depapillation.

♦ Increased susceptibility to oral candidiasis.
♦ Joint pains may point to Sjögren's syndrome.

Diagnosis

- History of dryness of mouth while resting, eating or swallowing.
- Enquiry should be made about the daily intake of fluids, snoring and mouth breathing.
- Medical and drug history.
- Sialometry: Allow the patient to sit quietly and dribble into a measuring container for more than 15 minutes. In normal individuals, saliva flow rate exceeds 1.5 mL/15 min (0.1 mL/min).
- Investigations may be required to confirm or exclude systemic disease.

Management

- Identify and eliminate the cause.
- Advise the patient to:
  ♦ Avoid agents that increase the dryness.
  ♦ Use frequent sips of water or ice chips.
  ♦ Use synthetic salivary substitutes.
  ♦ Use salivary stimulants such as chewing gum containing xylitol or sorbitol.
  ♦ Avoid cariogenic diet.
  ♦ Maintain high standards of oral hygiene and use topical fluoride agents.
- Prescribe sialogogues (pilocarpine) if hyposalivation leading to dry mouth is severe.
- Refer the patient to a specialist if systemic diseases are present.

DRY MOUTH IN SJÖGREN'S SYNDROME

Definition/Description

- Sjögren's syndrome is an autoimmune disorder that affects exocrine glands, including lacrimal and salivary glands, thus causing dry mouth and dry eyes.
- This syndrome is common in middle-aged or old women.

Cause

- An autoimmune disorder.
- Viral aetiology and genetic predisposition have also been implicated.

Clinical Features

- Two types of the disease are known: primary and secondary Sjögren's syndrome.
- Primary Sjögren's syndrome is characterised by dry mouth and dry eyes.
- Secondary Sjögren's syndrome is characterised by connective tissue disorder (rheumatoid arthritis) in addition to dry eyes and dry mouth.

- Dry eyes have the sensations of grittiness and itching.
- Inflammation of the conjunctiva and soft crusts at the angle of the eyes are seen.
- Lacrimal glands are swollen.
- Dry mouth.
- Tongue is dry, lobulated and red, with partial depapillation.
- Risk of dental caries is increased.
- Increased susceptibility to oral candidiasis.

Diagnosis

- History and clinical examination.
- For suspected Sjögren's syndrome, laboratory findings include the following:
    - ◆ Erythrocyte sedimentation rate.
    - ◆ Autoantibodies: antinuclear factor and rheumatoid factor.
    - ◆ Specific antinuclear antibodies: SS-A (Ro) and SS-B (La).
    - ◆ Sialometry.
    - ◆ Labial salivary gland biopsy.

Management

- Refer the patient to a specialist (rheumatologist).
- For oral complaints, refer the patient to a dentist.
- Management of dry mouth can be carried out by using salivary stimulants and salivary substitutes.

TASTE DISORDERS

Definition/Description

- Disorders of taste include unpleasant taste (cacogeusia), absence of taste (ageusia), diminished taste (hypogeusia), distorted taste (dysgeusia) and heightened taste (hypergeusia).

Cause

- Unpleasant taste is usually due to poor oral hygiene, oral and nasal infections, starvation, dry mouth and use of medications or certain foods.
- This is also associated with systemic disorders such as diabetes, depression, anxiety states, psychoses, mumps and gastrointestinal, respiratory, hepatic and renal diseases.
- Disorders that can result in taste dysfunction include lingual, facial or chorda tympani nerve damage, dry mouth, smoking, drugs, irradiation, psychotic disorders, ageing, nutritional disorders, brain tumours, head injuries, multiple sclerosis, Bell's palsy and loss of smell because of viral infection of the upper respiratory tract.

Clinical Features

- Alteration in taste can be in several forms: unpleasant taste, loss of taste, diminished taste, distorted taste or heightened taste.

- Those who have lost the sense of taste may also complain of loss of sense of smell.
- Those with other systemic diseases may also present signs and symptoms of the underlying disease.

Diagnosis

- History.
- The basic taste sensations are sweet, salty, sour and bitter. Taste may be tested by applying substances representing these four taste qualities in increasing concentrations on the tongue. The purpose is to detect the lowest concentration that can be recognised.
- Substances used are for the above diagnosis are as follows:
  - Glucose: 4%, 10% and 40%.
  - Sodium chloride: 2.5%, 7.5% and 15%.
  - Citric acid: 1%, 5% and 10%.
  - Quinine: 0.075% and 1%.
- The sensation of taste is observed 0.5 to 4 seconds after application of the various substances on the tongue. The test solution is applied alternatively to the left and right sides of the tongue with the help of a small piece of blotting paper. The lowest concentration that the patient recognises (threshold concentration) is recorded.

Management

- Identification and elimination of the cause.

METALLIC TASTE

Metallic taste is a common complaint. If it is the only complaint, the following possible causes need to be investigated.

1. Poor oral hygiene: Blood in the mouth in gingival inflammatory conditions causes metallic taste. Once the infection is eliminated, the taste improves.
2. Prescription drugs: These medicines include antibiotics such as tetracycline, allopurinol (used to treat gout), lithium (used to treat certain psychiatric conditions) and some cardiac medications. Antidepressants can also cause metallic taste because of their role in causing dry mouth.
3. Over-the-counter vitamins or medicines: Multivitamins with heavy metals (such as copper, zinc and chromium), cold remedies (such as zinc lozenges), prenatal vitamins and iron or calcium supplements can cause metallic taste.
4. Infections: Upper respiratory infections, cold and sinusitis change the sense of taste. Often, taste can be metallic.
5. Cancer treatment: Patients being treated for cancer with chemotherapy or radiation therapy may experience metallic taste.
6. Pregnancy: During the early stages of pregnancy, some women find that their sense of taste is metallic.
7. Dementia: People with dementia often have taste abnormalities.
8. Chemical exposures: Patients who are exposed to mercury or lead or who inhale high levels of these substances often complain of metallic taste.

SUGGESTED READINGS

Crispian S. *Oral and Maxillofacial Medicine: The Basis of Diagnosis and Treatment*. 2nd ed. Edinburgh, Scotland: Churchill Livingstone. pp. 79–85.

Prabhu SR. Clinical evaluation of taste sensation. In: Prabhu SR, editor. *Textbook of Oral Diagnosis*. New Delhi, India: Oxford University Press; 2007. pp. 68–9.

Viswanathan V, Nix P. Managing the patient presenting with xerostomia: a review. *Int J Clin Pract*. 2010;64:404–7.

Chapter 28

Oral mucosal burning and burning mouth syndrome

S. R. Prabhu and N. Narayana

ORAL MUCOSAL BURNING

Oral mucosal burning is a common symptom. Often, oral burning symptoms are associated with oral mucosal diseases such as lichen planus, candidiasis, geographic tongue, mucositis due to chemotherapy and radiation therapy for cancer, xerostomia and cranial nerve injury. Oral mucosal burning is also associated with menopause, diabetes, anxiety and the use of angiotensin-converting-enzyme inhibitors.

In this chapter, oral mucosal burning in the absence of any detectable abnormality is discussed. This clinical condition is called burning mouth syndrome (BMS).

BURNING MOUTH SYNDROME

Definition/Description

- Burning mouth syndrome is characterised by a burning sensation on the tongue or oral mucosa in the absence of detectable mucosal abnormality or any other organic disorder.

Cause

- Cause is not fully understood.
- Precipitating factors may include nutritional deficiencies (vitamins B_1, B_2 and B_6 and zinc deficiencies), hormonal changes associated with menopause, denture-related lesions, oral mucosal infections, xerostomia, hypersensitivity reactions, anxiety, medications and diabetes mellitus.

Clinical Features

- The patient experiences chronic pain in the form of burning sensation of moderate to severe intensity, which may vary throughout the course of the day.
- Onset of the burning sensation is spontaneous.

Three Types of Burning Mouth Sensation

- **Type 1:** Patient is free of pain on awakening but develops a burning sensation in the late morning, which gradually increases in severity and reaches peak intensity by evening.

- **Type 2:** Patient experiences continuous burning symptoms throughout the day.
- **Type 3:** Patient experiences intermittent burning symptoms, with pain-free intervals during the day.

Usually, pain involves the tip of the tongue and the anterior part of the dorsum of the tongue. Anterior hard palate and lower labial vestibule are other sites that may be involved. Dry mouth and taste disturbances are frequently associated.

Diagnosis

- History and clinical examination.
- Oral mucosa is clinically normal.
- Elimination of systemic disorder.
- Investigations for candidiasis and salivary gland dysfunction.
- Full blood count, iron studies, serum folate, vitamin B_{12} and fasting blood glucose.

Management

- Recognition of the condition is important.
- Symptomatic treatment includes topical diphenhydramine elixir, lidocaine hydrochloride jelly and viscous or low concentrations of capsaicin.
- If systemic cause is identified, refer the patient to a specialist.
- Tricyclic antidepressants have some beneficial effects.
- If burning persists after management of systemic or local oral conditions, diagnosis of BMS can be considered.

SUGGESTED READINGS

Grushka M, Epstein JB, Gorsky M. Burning mouth syndrome. *Am Fam Phys*. 2002;65:615–20.

Lamey PJ. Burning mouth syndrome. *Dermatol Clin*. 1996;14:339–54.

Narayana N. Burning mouth syndrome. In: Prabhu SR, editor. *Textbook of Oral Medicine*. New Delhi, India: Oxford University Press; 2004. pp. 60–2.

Chapter 29

Facial palsy and facial sensory loss

S. R. Prabhu

FACIAL PALSY

Definition/Description

- Facial palsy is also known as facial nerve palsy or facial paralysis.

Cause

- The most common cause of facial palsy is Bell's palsy. Bell's palsy may be due to unknown causes or associated with herpes simplex or herpes zoster infections.

Clinical Features

- Weakness or complete paralysis of all muscles of facial expression on one side of the face (Figure 29.1).
- Facial crease and nasolabial fold disappear.

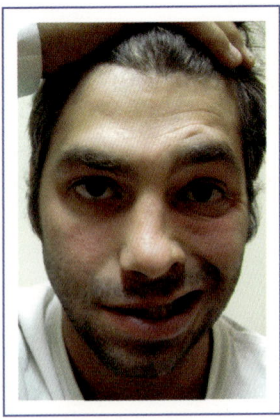

Figure 29.1   A person with Bell's palsy attempting to show his teeth and raise his eyebrow on his right side.

Reproduced with permission from: James Heilman. Available from: http://en.wikipedia.org/wiki/Bell%27s_palsy

- The forehead unfurrows.
- Corner of the mouth droops and eyelids do not close.
- Lower eyelid sags.
- The eye rolls upwards (Bell's phenomenon) on attempted closure.
- Tear production decreases, but tears tend to flow onto the cheek due to the loss of lid control.
- Food and saliva pool in the affected side of the mouth and may spill out from the corner.
- Facial sensation is preserved (however, some patient may complain of a feeling of numbness on the affected side).

Diagnosis

- History and neurological examination.
- Examination includes patients performing activities such as raising eyebrows, closing eyes and showing teeth.
- Magnetic resonance imaging studies are helpful in determining the possible association of neoplastic disease.

Management

- Most patients recover within a few weeks.
- For patients with severe symptoms, immediate treatment with corticosteroids is essential.
- Acyclovir is indicated.
- Eye care is necessary to avoid eye problems.
- In chronic cases, the use of Faradic stimulation may become necessary.
- For some patients, surgical intervention is necessary.

FACIAL SENSORY LOSS

Definition/Description

- Facial sensory loss refers to diminishing sensory response or complete loss of sensory response to stimuli.

Cause

- Trauma to the nerve from third molar surgery or trigeminal nerve injuries, pressure on the mental nerve from the denture, osteomyelitis or tumours, zygomatic or middle-third facial fractures, multiple sclerosis, brain tumours and psychogenic causes.

Clinical Features

- Diminished response or loss of response to pinprick of the facial skin.
- Corneal, facial or oral ulceration may occur due to loss of sensation.

Diagnosis

- History and clinical (neurological) examination.
- MRIs are useful in determining the association of neoplastic disease.

Management

• Elimination and treatment of the underlying causes.

SUGGESTED READINGS

Naidoo SK. VII nerve palsy: evaluation and management. *CME*. 2004;22:254–8. [Accessed 2015 Jul 15]. Available from: http://www.ajol.info/index.php/cme/article/ viewfile/43972/27489

Tiemstra JD, Khatkhate N. Bell's palsy: diagnosis and management. *Am Fam Physician*. 2007 Oct 1;76:997–1002.

Part IV

Topics of special relevance

Chapter 30

Oral and dental trauma

P. V. Abbott

TRAUMA TO THE MOUTH AND TEETH

Trauma to the mouth and teeth is a relatively common occurrence, and studies show that every second person will experience some form of dental trauma by the age of 14 years. Fortunately, the most common injuries are relatively minor (such as small fractures of tooth). Patients with minor injuries are not likely to seek urgent care from medical practitioners or hospitals; instead, they tend to wait until they see a dentist. However, there are many other injuries that are more severe, and in such cases, patients attend emergency services, seeking help.

Injuries to the mouth and teeth are usually a result of accidents; however, falls, fights and sport are also common causes. About one-third of oral trauma incidents occur during typical working hours of dentists, which implies that most injuries occur after-hours, when dentists may not be readily available. Hence, medical practitioners, especially those working in hospital or emergency services, are likely to regularly assess oral and dental injuries as a result of trauma and provide some initial management. The long-term prognosis of the damaged teeth is highly dependent on the emergency management and how quickly this management is provided.

Several classifications have been used in the dental literature to classify injuries to the mouth and teeth, but, for the sake of simplicity, they can be broadly categorised into the following four groups:

1. Soft tissue injuries
2. Fractures of the teeth
3. Displacement (luxation) of the teeth
4. Bone fractures

Each of these categories have subgroups, which have been outlined below, along with the typical presentation and first aid management that can be provided by medical practitioners. It is common for concurrent injuries to occur, that is, more than one injury occurring at the same time, and in particular, to the same tooth or to the adjacent tissues (Figure 30.1). Typical examples are a fracture of the tooth as well as displacement of the same tooth, or displacement of the tooth and laceration of the gum surrounding that tooth. When more than one type of injury occur, the more severe injury should take priority for first aid management.

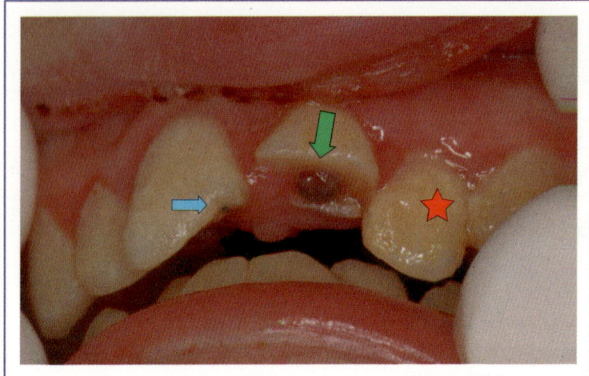

Figure 30.1 An example of concurrent injuries involving more than one injury to a tooth and injuries to several teeth at the same time. The maxillary right central incisor has a simple crown fracture (blue arrow), whereas the left central incisor has a complicated crown-root fracture, with exposure of the dental pulp (green arrow). The left lateral incisor (asterisk) has been laterally luxated, as the crown has been pushed towards the palate. *Courtesy*: Paul V. Abbott.

The following information and recommendations apply to the permanent dentition only and are not applicable to deciduous teeth (baby teeth) in young patients. The permanent teeth typically erupt in children from the age of about six years. The permanent teeth are larger and can be easily distinguished from the deciduous teeth by their size and the age of the patient. The child's parent(s) can usually advise whether the child has naturally lost the deciduous teeth and whether the injured teeth are the 'new teeth'.

Deciduous teeth with the injuries outlined below most likely require extraction. Attempts to reposition or replant deciduous teeth are likely to damage the underlying developing permanent tooth. Hence, it is advisable to not manipulate the deciduous teeth back to their original position.

If there is any doubt about whether the injured teeth are permanent or deciduous, then the best approach is to leave them 'as is' and refer the patient to a dentist for urgent evaluation and management.

SOFT TISSUE INJURIES

Soft tissue injuries usually occur in conjunction with other injuries to the teeth and mouth; however, at times, they may be the only injury. Three types of soft tissue injuries occur in the mouth. A brief description of all types and simple management methods that can be performed by a medical practitioner before the patient sees a dentist for further evaluation and dental management, are given below:

Laceration

- A tear or cut of the oral mucosa or lips: Usually, this is caused by a sharp object, but can also be caused by the teeth, especially if there are tooth fractures.
- If there are both a lacerated lip and a fractured tooth, then the fractured fragment may be embedded within the lip. Careful palpation and radiographic examination are required to assess this condition.

First Aid Management

- Administer local anaesthesia (e.g., lignocaine with 1:80,000 adrenaline).
- Clean the wound with gauze moistened with saline or chlorhexidine, and ensure that there are no tooth fragments or other foreign bodies in the wound.
- If any tooth fragments or foreign bodies are within the wound, then do not proceed with suturing; instead, refer the patient for urgent dental assessment and management.
- If no tooth fragments or foreign bodies are found in the wound, then suture the laceration with fine sutures (e.g., 4-0 silk suture).
- Instruct the patient to keep the area clean by using chlorhexidine mouthwash and/or gel.
- Advise the patient to see a dentist for further management. The wound should be checked by a dentist within 24 hours (assuming there are no other injuries that require more urgent dental assessment and management).

Subsequent Dental Management

- Sutures are typically removed five to seven days later.
- Chlorhexidine mouthwash or gel application is typically continued for up to 10 days. Healing is usually uneventful. However, occasionally, infections may occur and the tissue may have scarring.

Abrasion

- Scraping of the surface layer of the oral mucosa or lips, resulting in a 'raw' and bleeding surface.

First Aid Management

- Administer local anaesthesia (e.g., lignocaine with 1:80,000 adrenaline).
- Clean the wound with gauze moistened with saline or chlorhexidine. A brush may be needed to scrub the wound to remove foreign objects.
- Apply pressure to control haemorrhage.
- Instruct the patient to keep the area clean by using a chlorhexidine mouthwash and/or gel.
- Advise the patient to see a dentist for further management. The wound should be checked by a dentist within 24 hours (assuming there are no other injuries that require more urgent dental assessment and management).

Subsequent Dental Management

- Chlorhexidine mouthwash or gel application is typically continued for up to 10 days.
- Healing is usually uneventful; however, occasionally, infections may occur. Scarring is not common.

Contusion

- Bruising of the oral mucosa or lips.

First Aid Management

- There is no need for any invasive management of contusions.
- Ice packs can help to reduce discomfort and the duration of swelling.
- Instruct the patient to keep the area clean by using chlorhexidine mouthwash.
- Advise the patient to see a dentist for further management. The wound should be checked by a dentist within 24 hours (assuming there are no other injuries that require more urgent dental assessment and management).

Subsequent Dental Management

- Chlorhexidine mouthwash or gel application is typically continued for up to 10 days.
- Healing is usually uneventful. Infections and scarring are rare.

FRACTURES OF THE TEETH

Fractures of the teeth are the most common of the dental injuries. They may occur as a single injury or concurrently with other types of injuries (such as soft tissue injuries, displacement or luxation of the tooth and bone fractures). One or more teeth may be involved, depending on the cause and nature of the injury.

The maxillary anterior teeth are the most commonly injured teeth, with the two maxillary central incisors being injured far more often than the other anterior teeth.

The anterior teeth are usually damaged by 'direct trauma', which occurs when the teeth are hit by an object. Fractures of the posterior teeth are usually a result of 'indirect trauma', when the lower jaw is forced upwards and the mandibular teeth violently contact the maxillary teeth. This typically occurs when a force is applied to the lower border of the mandible (e.g., by a punch or a fall).

Fractures of the teeth are classified according to the extent of the fracture and the parts of the tooth involved. In particular, exposure of the dental pulp is important to note, as this creates a far more complex injury and needs comprehensive and urgent dental treatment.

The dental pulp is a soft tissue that exists inside the tooth. When the pulp is exposed, it appears as a pink or red tissue within the body of the tooth. It may bleed if probed or touched. The patient typically experiences pain because of the exposure. Patients complain of sensitivity (often severe) to temperature changes, such as cold air or drinks, and pain when the exposed pulp is touched.

Fractures of the tooth can generally be diagnosed by visual observation; however, if the fracture extends into the root or if it only involves the root, intraoral radiographs are required to diagnose the existence of the fracture and to determine its extent. Extraoral radiographs generally do not provide the details required to assess the fractures of the tooth.

The following are a simplified classification of the fractures of teeth and some simple management steps that can be performed by a medical practitioner before the patient sees a dentist for further evaluation and dental management. It should be noted that all fractures of teeth require comprehensive management by a dentist, which may involve intricate procedures (e.g., root canal treatment) and restoration of the teeth. Such treatment should not be unduly delayed.

Crown Fracture (With or Without Pulp Exposure)

- The crown of the tooth has a fracture (Figure 30.1).
- The fracture may involve only the enamel (outer layer) or the enamel and the dentine (inner layer).
- The dental pulp (soft tissue in the tooth, see above) may be exposed (Figure 30.1).

First Aid Management

- Crown fractures without pulp exposure are generally not urgent problems, because usually, the patient does not have pain. However, the patient should be advised to see a dentist as soon as possible for tooth restoration, as this would protect the underlying pulp and minimise the long-term consequences of the injury.
- Crown fractures with pulp exposure can be extremely painful for the patient; hence, such a patient should be referred immediately to a dentist for management.
- Little can be done to help a patient in this situation, unless some dental materials are available. In some cases, it might be possible to place a temporary filling material over the exposed pulp, but this is likely to exacerbate the pain. However, in most cases, it is not feasible to place the temporary filling material because the material is unlikely to stick to the tooth.

Subsequent Dental Management

- The fractured portion of the tooth requires restoration by a dentist. Various restorative techniques and materials may be used, depending on the location and extent of the fracture.
- When the pulp has been exposed, complex dental treatments, such as pulp capping, partial removal of the pulp and complete removal of the pulp with root canal treatment are required before tooth restoration.

Crown-Root Fracture (With or Without Pulp Exposure)

- The fracture involves the crown and the root of the tooth (Figure 30.1).

- The enamel, dentine and cementum (a layer covering the root) are all involved.
- The dental pulp may be exposed (Figure 30. 1).
- The tooth may appear to be loose or mobile — but only the fractured portion is loose in this situation.

First Aid Management

- Crown-root fractures are generally quite uncomfortable for the patient because the fractured portion of the tooth is held in position by the periodontal ligament; however, the fractured portion is loose and any movement of this fragment causes pain. Hence, urgent dental treatment is required.
- Crown-root fractures with pulp exposure can be extremely painful; hence, patients with such fractures should be referred immediately to a dentist for management.
- If a dentist is not readily available, the loose fragment can be temporarily stabilised by moulding a small piece of aluminium foil over the fractured tooth and several adjacent teeth (Figure 30.2). This temporary splint can be made by cutting a small piece of aluminium foil, folding it over several times to increase the thickness and rigidity and then moulding it over the teeth by using gentle digital pressure. This tends to discourage the patient from touching the loose fragment, which in turn reduces the pain.

Subsequent Dental Management

- The fractured portion of the tooth will require removal and restoration by a dentist. Various restorative techniques and materials may be used, depending on the location and extent of the fracture.
- When the pulp is exposed, root canal treatment is required before tooth restoration.

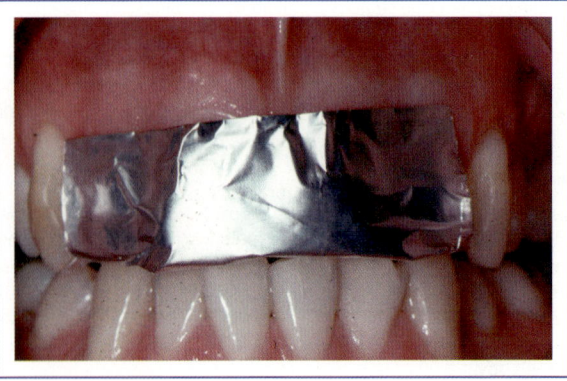

Figure 30.2 An example of a simple temporary splint using the aluminium foil that has been digitally adapted to cover the injured teeth.
Courtesy: Paul V. Abbott.

- Some teeth with crown-root fractures may require extraction, for example, when the fracture extends well into the root of the tooth.

Root Fracture

- The fracture is confined to the root.
- The cementum, dentine and pulp are all involved.
- The tooth may appear displaced from its normal position.

First Aid Management

- Root fractures are usually diagnosed radiographically. Therefore, these fractures may not be diagnosed by clinical examination unless the tooth appears to be displaced.
- If the tooth appears to be displaced, only the portion of the tooth coronal to the root fracture is actually displaced. In this case, the displaced fragment can be gently pushed back to its normal position. Then a piece of aluminium foil should be moulded over the tooth and several adjacent teeth to form a temporary splint (as explained in 'Crown-Root Fractures').
- Advise the patient to see a dentist as soon as possible for stabilisation and splinting of the fracture and further dental management.

Subsequent Dental Management

- Initially, the tooth will require stabilisation with a rigid splint to allow time for healing. Treatment is aimed at encouraging internal repair of the fracture, so that the dental pulp can produce dentine to hold the fragments together as long as the tooth is well-stabilised.
- Root fractures may heal in different ways and the response largely depends on the location of the fracture. Fractures located towards the apical end of the tooth root have the best prognosis, while those near the crown have the worst prognosis.
- Some teeth with root fractures may require root canal treatment, typically when the pulp does not survive and becomes infected.
- Some teeth with root fractures may require extraction; this depends on the location and extent of the fracture in the root.

DISPLACEMENT (LUXATION) OF THE TEETH

Teeth are attached to their bone sockets by the periodontal ligament. Hence, the tooth-bone interface is similar to other joints in the body. The periodontal ligament normally allows some tooth movement and provides a cushioning effect to help absorb the forces of biting and chewing.

When a tooth is subjected to trauma, the forces applied to the tooth may cause the periodontal ligament to be stretched or torn, resulting in loosening of the tooth (if stretched) or displacement (luxation) of the tooth from its normal position (if torn). Tooth displacement is similar to the dislocation injuries that occur in other joints of the body.

The nature of the injury depends on the direction and amount of force and also on the area of tooth where the force is applied. The force may cause a tooth to fracture, and it is common for the tooth to be both displaced and fractured. In such cases, the displacement injury should be the first priority for management, because it is important to return the tooth to its normal position in order to allow the blood supply to the dental pulp for recovery.

The general principles for managing displaced teeth are same as those for managing any other dislocated joint, that is, repositioning, stabilisation and rest. In addition, teeth may require specific dental treatment, depending on the overall situation and the particular injury. For example, some teeth may require root canal treatment to prevent a process known as external inflammatory root resorption, which can result in loss of the tooth if not treated appropriately, whereas other teeth may require restoration of a fracture. Hence, urgent referral to a dentist is essential for all displacement injuries.

Some medical practitioners advocate the application of various 'tissue glues' to temporarily stabilise displaced teeth after they have repositioned them. However, this is not recommended by dentists, because the adhesive material is difficult to remove (especially from loose teeth) and may interfere with the use of dental bonding materials that are used by dentists to splint these teeth. The need to clean the adhesive material from the teeth may exacerbate the already-traumatised periodontal ligament and thus delay or adversely affect the healing response.

Instead of using adhesive materials, a simple method to stabilise displaced teeth after repositioning is to use some aluminium foil moulded over the injured tooth and several adjacent teeth (Figure 30.2). This temporary splint can be made by cutting a small piece of aluminium foil, folding it over several times to increase the thickness and rigidity and then moulding it over the teeth by using gentle digital pressure. This will not hold the tooth in its exact original position but will discourage the patient from touching the tooth, which can result in further displacement. It should be considered only as a temporary measure, until a dentists stabilises the tooth with an appropriate splint.

In some situations, antibiotics should be prescribed, because antibiotics help to reduce the chances of inflammatory root resorption. Ideally, oral tetracycline (e.g., doxycycline) should be prescribed, because this drug has antibacterial and antiresorption effects.

If young age, an allergy or interaction with other drugs precludes the use of tetracycline, then oral penicillin can be used. However, not all injuries require antibiotics — only intrusion and avulsion injuries always require antibiotics. Medical practitioners can assist in these cases by early instigation of the antibiotic therapy (see below). Other luxation injuries may sometimes require antibiotics, but these injuries should be assessed by a dentist, who can then prescribe the necessary medicines.

The following are a simplified classification of displacement (luxation) injuries of teeth and some simple management that can be performed by a medical practitioner before the patient sees a dentist for further evaluation and dental management. As noted above, all patients with displacement injuries of the teeth require further and urgent comprehensive management by a dentist.

Concussion of a Tooth

- It is a mild injury to the periodontal ligament, where the tooth is tender to percussion or tapping.
- The tooth is not mobile and shows no other symptoms or signs.

First Aid Management

- No specific first aid management is required.
- Refer the patient to a dentist for further evaluation and management.
- Advise the patient to avoid biting with the tooth.
- Advise the patient to keep the tooth clean by using normal tooth brushing methods. A chlorhexidine mouthwash can also be recommended.

Subsequent Dental Management

- Healing after tooth concussion is usually uneventful and the tooth returns to normal function.
- Long-term monitoring is important to assess the pulp and the periodontal ligament.
- Some teeth may require root canal treatment in the future if the pulp does not survive and becomes infected.

Subluxation of a Tooth

- This is defined as loosening of the tooth, which shows abnormal mobility.
- The tooth is tender to percussion or tapping.
- Often, some bleeding is evident around the gingival margin (gum line).

First Aid Management

- No specific first aid management is required.
- Refer the patient to a dentist for further evaluation and management.
- Advise the patient to avoid biting with the tooth.
- Advise the patient to keep the tooth clean by using normal tooth brushing methods. A chlorhexidine mouthwash can also be recommended.

Subsequent Dental Management

- Healing after subluxation of a tooth is usually uneventful and the tooth returns to normal function.
- Long-term monitoring is important to assess the pulp and the periodontal ligament.
- Some teeth may require root canal treatment in the future if the pulp does not survive and becomes infected.

Extrusion of a Tooth

- In extrusion, the tooth becomes partially displaced out if its socket and appears to be longer than the adjacent teeth (Figure 30. 3).
- The patient is unable to bite their teeth together in the usual way because the extruded tooth is the first tooth to contact the opposing teeth on closure of the mouth.

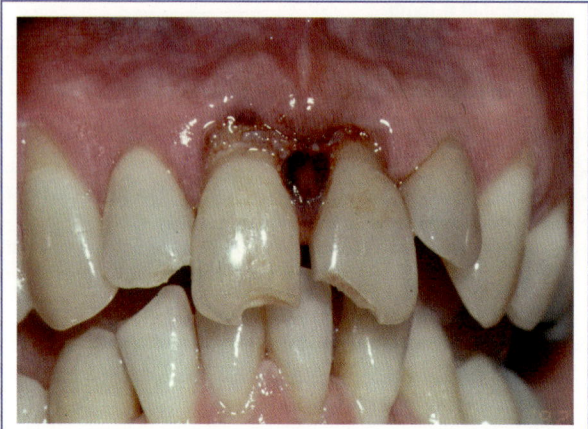

Figure 30.3 The two maxillary central incisors extruded from their normal position. Note the bleeding that has occurred around the gum line and between the teeth. Both of these teeth also have fractures of the crowns of the teeth (without pulp exposure).
Courtesy: Paul V. Abbott.

- The tooth is likely to be loose and there may be bleeding around the gingival margin (gum line).
- In some cases, lacerations of the gum or mucosa overlying the tooth may be seen.

First Aid Management

- Push the tooth back into its socket by applying gentle pressure in a vertical direction with the help of a finger. Local anaesthesia is not usually required for this procedure.
- Suture any lacerations associated with the tooth after administering local anaesthesia (see above); however, if there is no bleeding, lacerations may be left for the dentist to suture, once the teeth have been stabilised with a splint.
- Mould a piece of aluminium foil over the tooth and several adjacent teeth to form a temporary splint (see above).
- Refer the patient to a dentist for urgent and further evaluation and management.

Subsequent Dental Management

- Stabilisation with a splint is essential to allow the periodontal ligament and pulp to heal. A 'flexible' splint is usually used for 10 to 14 days to hold the tooth in position and to allow normal tooth movement during healing, as this encourages functional repair of the periodontal ligament and helps to avoid 'ankylosis' of the tooth. Ankylosis occurs if the ligament does not heal adequately.

- Long-term monitoring is important to assess the pulp and the periodontal ligament.
- Some teeth may require root canal treatment in the future if the pulp does not survive and becomes infected.

Lateral Luxation of a Tooth

- Displacement of a tooth in any direction other than axially is called lateral luxation. Typically, the crown of the tooth is displaced towards the palate (or into the mouth) and the root of the tooth is displaced labially (Figure 30.1). Occasionally, a tooth may be displaced in another direction.
- Lateral luxations always cause a fracture of the alveolar bone (Figure 30. 4).
- The patient is unable to bite teeth together in the usual way because the luxated tooth is the first tooth to contact the opposing teeth on closure of the mouth.

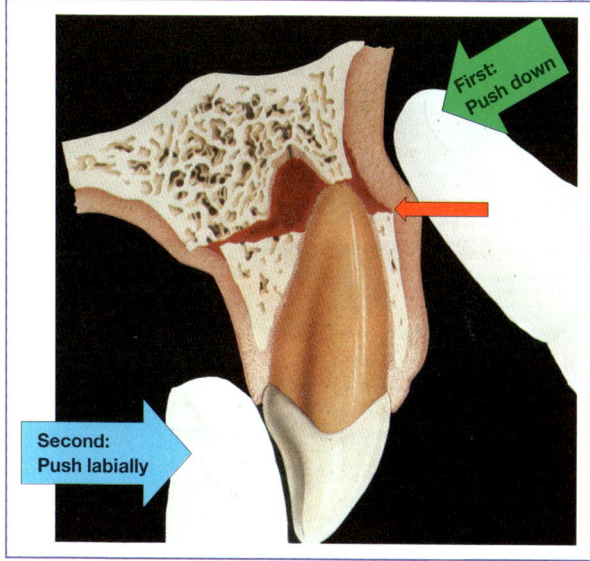

Figure 30.4 Diagrammatic representation of a laterally luxated tooth, viewed from the lateral side of the tooth. Note the typical bone fracture on the labial aspect of the alveolar socket wall (red arrow). The displaced tooth should be repositioned by first pushing downwards with a finger placed over the end of the tooth root (green arrow) and then by pushing labially with the thumb placed behind the crown of the tooth (blue arrow). The fractured bone will be repositioned along with the tooth, which will then require stabilisation with a splint.

Reproduced with permission from: Jens Andreasen. *Dental Trauma Guide*. 2007.

- The tooth is likely to be loose and there may be bleeding around the gingival margin (gum line).
- In some cases, lacerations of the gum or mucosa overlying the tooth may be seen.

First Aid Management

- The tooth needs to be repositioned back into its socket. However, care must be taken that the method used for repositioning does not cause any further damage the tooth root. The process of repositioning a tooth following typical lateral luxation (described above) is as follows:
  - Administer local anaesthesia (e.g., lignocaine with 1:80,000 adrenaline).
  - Place a thumb behind the crown of the tooth and a finger over the end of the tooth root (under the lip) (Figure 30.4).
  - Using the finger, apply a downwards pressure over the end of the tooth root, with the aim of pushing the tooth out of its socket (Figure 30.4). This is required to disengage the root tip from its displaced position over the fractured bone.
  - Then, use the thumb behind the crown to push the crown of the tooth towards the front of the mouth (Figure 30.4). It is common to feel the root tip 'click' back into place in its socket.
  - In summary, push the root downwards first and then push the crown labially.
- Suture any lacerations associated with the tooth; however, if there is no bleeding, lacerations may be left for the dentist to suture, once the teeth have been stabilised with a splint.
- Mould a piece of aluminium foil over the tooth and several adjacent teeth to form a temporary splint (see above) (Figure 30.2).
- Refer the patient to a dentist for urgent and further evaluation and management.

Subsequent Dental Management

- Stabilisation with a splint is essential to allow the periodontal ligament and pulp to heal. A 'rigid' splint is usually used for six weeks to hold the tooth and the associated fractured bone in position. If the tooth and bone are not adequately splinted, then fibrous healing is likely to occur and the tooth will remain mobile.
- Long-term monitoring is important to assess the pulp and the periodontal ligament.
- Many laterally luxated teeth require root canal treatment, because the pulp does not always survive and may become infected.
- Root canal treatment may also be required to prevent the development of inflammatory resorption of the tooth root. This resorption is a result of damage to the tooth root and infection of the root canal system.

Intrusion of a Tooth

- In intrusion, the tooth is pushed up into its socket, so it appears to be shorter than the adjacent teeth (Figure 30.5).

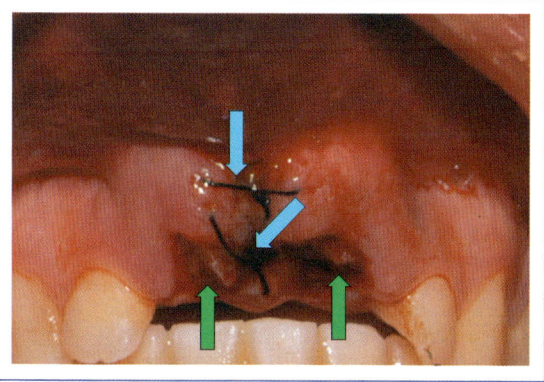

Figure 30.5 The two maxillary central incisors intruded into their sockets and the alveolar bone. The incisal edges of the teeth can be seen just inside the sockets (green arrows). Two sutures (blue arrows) have been placed to control bleeding before referral to a dentist for repositioning and splinting. *Courtesy*: Paul V. Abbott.

- The amount of intrusion varies. Some teeth may be intruded so far that they are barely visible in the mouth. Ideally, intraoral radiographs are required to assess these cases.
- Intrusion of a tooth causes crushing of the wall of the bone socket and usually causes a fracture of the alveolar bone.
- The region overlying the tooth root may appear swollen as a result of expansion of the socket, as the tooth is intruded.
- The tooth is likely to be loose, and there may be bleeding around the gingival margin (gum line).
- In some cases, lacerations of the gum or mucosa overlying the tooth may be seen.

First Aid Management

- Ideally, intruded teeth need to be repositioned to their normal place. However, repositioning is not urgent and the patient can wait for a dentist. It is not urgent because the intruded teeth do not interfere with biting. In addition, they can be difficult to grasp and manoeuvre and are not very stable once repositioned unless splinted by a dentist (i.e., temporary splinting with aluminium foil is not very effective in these cases). Hence, no specific first aid management is required.
- Suture any lacerations associated with the tooth after administering local anaesthesia (see above) (Figure 30.5). However, if there is no bleeding, lacerations may be left for the dentist to suture, once the teeth have been stabilised with a splint.
- Refer to a dentist for urgent and further evaluation and management.
- Antibiotics should be prescribed, as they help to reduce the chances of inflammatory root resorption. Ideally, oral tetracycline

(e.g., doxycycline) should be prescribed, because this drug has antibacterial and antiresorption effects. If young age, an allergy or interaction with other drugs precludes the use of tetracycline, then penicillin can be used.

Subsequent Dental Management

- Repositioning and stabilisation with a splint are essential to allow the periodontal ligament and dental pulp to heal. A 'rigid' splint is usually used for six weeks to hold the tooth and the associated fractured bone in position.
- Long-term monitoring is important to assess the periodontal ligament. Ankylosis of the tooth is a common sequelae of intrusion because of the damage that occurs to the root surface and to the periodontal ligament.
- Almost all intruded teeth require root canal treatment as the pulp does not survive and can become infected. Root canal treatment is also performed to prevent the development of inflammatory resorption of the tooth root. This resorption is a result of damage to the root and infection of the root canal system.

Avulsion of a Tooth

- In avulsion, the tooth is completely dislodged from its socket. It may still be in the mouth, but usually, it is knocked out of the mouth (Figure 30. 6).

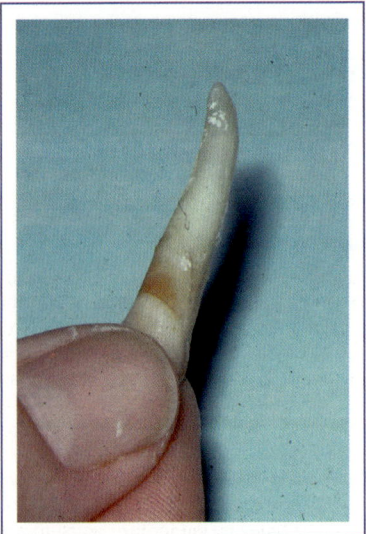

Figure 30.6 The correct way to handle an avulsed tooth, by holding only the crown of the tooth. Do not touch the root part of the tooth, if at all possible. *Courtesy*: Paul V. Abbott.

- The tooth socket will appear empty, and the patient, parent or companion may present with the tooth in hand or in a container. If the tooth is not produced, then visually examining the socket should be done to confirm that the tooth was knocked out and not intruded (see above).
- The tooth socket and the surrounding gum may bleed.
- In some cases, lacerations of the gum or mucosa overlying the socket may be seen.
- The patient will not have any pain but he or she may be quite distressed by the accident and the loss of the tooth.
- Time is extremely important when dealing with an avulsed tooth. The patient should be advised to see a dentist immediately for further treatment after the first aid management.
- Every minute counts in this situation, because the aim is to preserve the periodontal ligament, which attaches the tooth to the bone socket.
- The longer the tooth is out of its socket, the more the number of ligament cells that die. Therefore, the healing and long-term prognosis of the tooth are significantly affected by any delays.

First Aid Management

- Ideally, the tooth should be replanted into its socket as soon as possible to preserve the periodontal ligament that remains attached to the tooth root.
  - Local anaesthesia is not essential for replantation of the tooth but it helps in the overall management of the patient. It is required if any lacerations need suturing. Hence, it is usually advisable to administer local anaesthesia (e.g., lignocaine with 1:80,000 adrenaline).
  - Handle the tooth with care and avoid touching the root surface, that is, hold the tooth only by its crown portion (Figure 30.6). The crown is the whiter, shiny part, whereas the root is the yellow, longer, tapering part of the tooth.
  - Do not scrub or rub the tooth. Do not clean it with an antiseptic solution. If dirty, rinse the tooth gently only with saline. Do not use water.
  - If the tooth socket has a blood clot in it, then gently remove the clot with a pair of tweezers or gently irrigate it with saline by using a syringe, but take care not to touch the bony walls of the socket.
  - Gently seat the tooth into its socket, taking care not to scrape the root on the bony walls of the socket.
  - Suture any lacerations associated with the tooth; however, if there is no bleeding, lacerations may be left for the dentist to suture, once the teeth have been stabilised with a splint.
  - Mould a piece of aluminium foil over the tooth and several adjacent teeth to form a temporary splint (see above) (Figure 30. 2).
  - Refer to a dentist for immediate evaluation and further management.
  - Antibiotics should be prescribed, as they help to reduce the chances of inflammatory root resorption occurring. Ideally, oral tetracycline (e.g., doxycycline) should be prescribed, because

this drug has antibacterial and antiresorption effects. If young age, an allergy or interaction with other drugs precludes the use of tetracycline, then penicillin can be used.

- If it is not possible to replant the tooth or if you are unsure about the correct position, then it is important to store the tooth in a suitable medium that will help to keep the periodontal ligament cells alive until the tooth is replanted.
  - ◆ The best storage medium is tissue culture solution (balanced salt solutions), if available.
  - ◆ If tissue culture medium is unavailable, then the tooth can be stored in milk. Any milk solution is suitable, but do not use sour milk or yoghurt. The milk can be taken directly from the fridge.
  - ◆ Saline and saliva are the alternative suitable storage media, but they are not as effective as milk or tissue culture solutions.
  - ◆ Plastic wrap can also be used to keep the tooth moist if none of the above media is available. If you are using plastic wrap, ask the patient to spit into the plastic as their saliva will help keep the tooth moist.
  - ◆ Do not use water to store an avulsed tooth, because this will rapidly kill the periodontal ligament cells through lysis as a result of its incompatible osmolarity.
  - ◆ If you are using a storage medium, ensure that the tooth is fully submerged. Handle the container carefully so that the tooth root surface is not damaged during transport to a dentist.
  - ◆ Do not scrub or rub the tooth. Do not clean it with an antiseptic solution. If dirty, rinse the tooth gently only with saline. Do not use water.
  - ◆ Suture any lacerations associated with the tooth after administering local anaesthesia (see above); however, if there is no bleeding, lacerations may be left for the dentist to suture, once the tooth has been replanted and stabilised with a splint.
  - ◆ Refer the patient to a dentist for immediate evaluation and further management.
  - ◆ Antibiotics should be prescribed, as they help to reduce the chances of inflammatory root resorption. Ideally, oral tetracycline (e.g., doxycycline) should be prescribed, because this drug has antibacterial and antiresorption effects. If young age, an allergy or interaction with other drugs precludes the use of tetracycline, then penicillin can be used.

Subsequent Dental Management

- Stabilisation with a splint is essential to allow the periodontal ligament and pulp to heal. A 'flexible' splint is usually used for 10 to 14 days to hold the tooth in position and to allow normal tooth movement during healing, as this encourages functional repair of the periodontal ligament and avoids 'ankylosis' of the tooth. Ankylosis of the ligament does not heal adequately. However, if bone fractures are associated with avulsion, then a 'rigid' splint is required for six weeks.
- Long-term monitoring is important to assess the periodontal ligament. Ankylosis of the tooth is a common sequelae of avulsion

because of the damage that occurs to the root surface and to the periodontal ligament.

- Almost all avulsed teeth require root canal treatment as the pulp does not survive and can become infected. Root canal treatment is also performed to prevent the development of inflammatory resorption of the tooth root. This resorption is a result of damage to the root and infection of the root canal system.

BONE FRACTURES

Bone fractures can be simple fractures of the alveolar bone (i.e., the bone around the teeth) or may involve the maxilla or mandible. Bone fractures are often associated with displacement of teeth and/or tooth fractures. The fracture may also involve the tooth socket, which can lead to complications in the healing of the bone fracture, and the tooth itself.

The general principles for managing bone fractures of the jaw are the same as those for any other bone fracture, that is, repositioning, stabilisation and review. Fractures of the alveolar bone are usually stabilised by applying a splint to the teeth; hence, dental management is necessary. Fractures of the mandible and maxilla require much more comprehensive management, often including open reduction and the placement of plates and screws. Hence, these cases require referral to an oral and maxillofacial surgeon for management. The following are a simplified classification of bone fractures of the jaws and some simple management methods that can be performed by a medical practitioner before the patient sees a dentist or an oral and maxillofacial surgeon for further evaluation and dental management. All patients with bone fractures of the jaws require further and urgent comprehensive management by a dentist or an oral and maxillofacial surgeon.

Alveolar Bone Fractures

- Alveolar bone fractures may involve just one wall of the tooth socket or the entire alveolus.
- Fractures of the alveolar socket wall are typically associated with lateral luxation or intrusion injuries (see above for first aid management).
- Fractures of the entire alveolus show mobility of several teeth, which typically appear displaced (such as laterally luxated). However, it is the alveolus that has fractured, and so, several teeth move together as a 'block' when one tooth is tested for mobility.
- The patient is unable to bite teeth together in the usual way because the displaced teeth are the first teeth to contact the opposing teeth on closure of the mouth.
- Lacerations of the gum or mucosa overlying the displaced teeth are usually seen.

First Aid Management

- Ideally, the fractured bone segment needs to be repositioned.
- Administer local anaesthesia (e.g., lignocaine with 1:80,000 adrenaline).

- Repositioning the fractured segment can be achieved by grasping the teeth and moving the segment back into place. Often, a 'click' is felt as the teeth engage their sockets.
- Suture any lacerations; however, if there is no bleeding, lacerations may be left for the dentist to suture, once the bone and teeth have been stabilised with a splint.
- Mould a piece of aluminium foil over the loose teeth and several adjacent teeth to form a temporary splint (see above). This will have minimal effect but may help the patient avoid moving the fractured segment.
- Refer the patient to a dentist for urgent further evaluation and management.
- Advise the patient to avoid biting with the teeth.

Subsequent Dental Management

- Stabilisation with a splint is essential to allow the fractured bone to heal. A 'rigid' splint is usually used for six weeks to hold the fragments in position.
- Long-term monitoring is important to assess the teeth associated with the bone fracture, especially for the survival of the pulp and periodontal ligament.
- If the pulp does not survive, then root canal treatment may be required or some teeth may require extraction.
- If the periodontal ligament is significantly affected by the injury, then it may not heal and the tooth or teeth may require extraction.

Fractures of the Maxilla or Mandible

- Many different signs and symptoms may be present, depending on the position and extent of the fractures.
- The patient is not able to bite the teeth together in the usual way, especially with mandibular fractures, in which teeth on one side of the mouth may contact when biting but teeth on the other side have no contact.
- Submucosal haemorrhage is likely to occur in the mouth.
- Extraoral bruising is likely to occur.
- Palpation is likely to reveal a 'step defect' of the bone margin.
- The patient generally experiences considerable pain, especially on moving the jaws, biting, etc.
- Maxillary fractures may involve the mid-third of the face, the zygoma, the orbits, and/or other facial bones and structures.
- Some jaw fractures can be life-threatening, as the swelling and bleeding may compromise the airway.

First Aid Management

- Assess the patient for head injuries, loss of consciousness and airway patency. Stabilise the patient, as required.
- Pull the lower jaw forward to ensure that the airway is not compromised.
- A bandage may be applied under the jaw to keep it in a forward position and to support the fractured bone.
- Refer the patient to an oral and maxillofacial surgeon for urgent evaluation and management.
- Advise the patient to avoid biting.

Subsequent Dental Management

- Stabilisation with some form of splint or other rigid fixation (e.g., plates and screws) is essential to allow the fractured bones to heal. A 'rigid' splint is usually used for six weeks to hold the fragments in position. Plates are usually left *in situ* on a permanent basis, unless they cause subsequent problems (e.g., infection and pain).
- Long-term monitoring is important to assess the teeth associated with the bone fracture, especially for survival of the pulp and periodontal ligament.
- If the pulp does not survive, then root canal treatment may be required or some teeth may require extraction.
- If the periodontal ligament is significantly affected by the injury, then it may not heal and the tooth or teeth may require extraction.

MEDICATIONS

Analgesics or Nonsteroidal Anti-inflammatory Drugs

Patients may have some pain or discomfort immediately after trauma to the teeth, mouth and jaws. However, once the injuries have been appropriately managed (especially once they are fully stabilised with splints and sutures), there is little, if any, pain. Hence, pain management provided by medical practitioners after oral and dental trauma typically only needs to cover the period until the patient obtains comprehensive dental treatment. When considering medications, practitioners should consider whether the patient is likely to require general anaesthesia for the dental treatment. Typically, in adults, general anaesthesia is required only for fractures of the mandible and maxilla. Fractures of the alveolus, tooth displacements, tooth fractures and soft tissue injuries can usually be managed with local anaesthesia.

Following are the suggested medications for pain relief:

- ♦ Ibuprofen (orally): 400 mg 4 hourly, or
- ♦ Paracetamol (orally): 1000 mg 4 hourly

Antibiotics

As discussed above, antibiotics are not required for most injuries of the mouth and teeth. However, there are certain injuries (intrusions and avulsions of the permanent teeth; see above), for which antibiotics are recommended to reduce the possibility of inflammatory root resorption. Oral tetracycline is the first drug of choice (e.g., doxycycline). Alternatively, oral penicillin can be used in young patients or if tetracycline is contraindicated. Some other injuries may require antibiotics, but this should be decided by the dentist who manages the case.

Tetanus Toxoid Vaccine

The patient's tetanus status should be checked, especially for teeth that have been avulsed. If necessary, administer a booster vaccine.

SUGGESTED READINGS

Dental Trauma Guide [Internet]. San Diego, CA: International Association for Dental Traumatology; 2014 [updated 2014 Jul 2]. Available from: http:// www.dentaltraumaguide.org

Andreasen JO, Andreasen FM, Andersson L. *Textbook and Color Atlas of Traumatic Injuries to the Teeth*. 4th ed. Oxford, U.K.: Blackwell-Munksgaard; 2007.

Andreasen JO, Bakland LK, Flores MT, Andreasen FM, Andersson L. *Traumatic Dental Injuries: A Manual*. 3rd ed. Oxford, U.K.: Wiley-Blackwell; 2011.

Abbott PV. Dental first aid for the medical practitioner. *Mod Med Aust*. 1989;32:43–50.

Oral and Dental Expert Group. Management of dental problems for medical practitioners. *Therapeutic Guidelines: Oral and Dental*. Version 2. Melbourne, Australia: Therapeutic Guidelines Ltd; 2012.

Chapter 31

Oral mucosal infections

L. Samaranayake, H. M. H. N. Bandara
and S. R. Prabhu

BACTERIAL INFECTIONS OF THE ORAL MUCOSA

Necrotising Ulcerative Gingivitis

Definition/Description

- It is a rapidly progressive ulceration of the interdental papillae, caused predominantly by anaerobic gram-negative bacteria.

Cause

- Anaerobic bacteria: *Treponema vincentii, Fusobacterium fusiformis, Porphyromonas gingivalis, Leptotrichia buccalis* and *Prevotella intermedia.*
- Predisposing factors: Reduced general and local host resistance. Immunocompromised status, stress, heavy smoking and drinking and malnutrition.

Clinical Features

- Necrotic interdental papilla with crater-like ulcers (Figure 31.1 A).
- Gingival bleeding, pain and halitosis are common.
- In HIV/AIDS patients, necrotising ulcerative periodontitis (Figure 31.1 B) is often reported. In this condition, alveolar bone resorption, leading to tooth mobility, is present.

Diagnosis

- History and clinical examination.
- Identification of gram-negative organisms in smears.

Management

- Oral hygiene measures, oxygenating mouth rinses, antibiotics (e.g., penicillin and metronidazole) and symptomatic treatment for pain.
- Nutritional supplements are useful in building up host resistance.

Cervicofacial Actinomycosis

Definition/Description

- Actinomycosis is a chronic suppurative granulomatous infectious disease. Three clinical forms of the disease are cervicofacial (lumpy jaw), thoracic and abdominal actinomycosis.

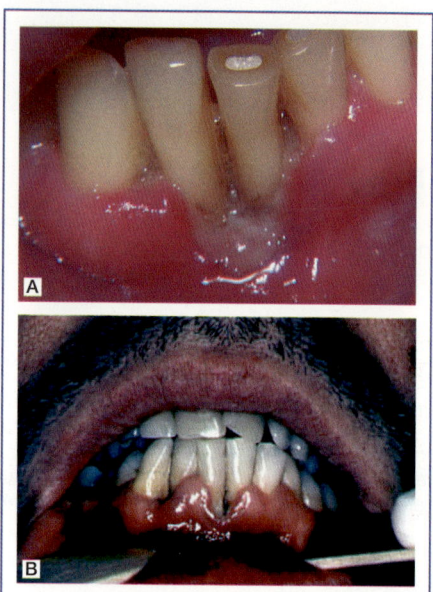

Figure 31.1 (A) Necrotising ulcerative gingivitis involving the lower anterior teeth. Crater-like ulcers of the interdental gingival papillae are characteristic. (B) Necrotising ulcerative periodontitis involving the periodontal tissues of the lower incisors.
Reproduced with permission from: (A) Dr. Steve Debbink, Dental Director, AIDS Resource Center of Wisconsin. Reproduced with permission from David Reznik. Available from: www.HIVdent.org (B) 1996–1997 John Valentine. Reproduced with permission from David Reznik. Available from: www.HIVdent.org

Cause

- Actinomycosis is caused by the bacteria called *Actinomyces*. These are commensal organisms present in the oral cavity and less commonly in the gastrointestinal tract.
- Pathogenic species of *Actinomyces* involved in human infection include *A. israelii, A. naeslundii, A. viscosus* and *A. odontolyticus*. *Actinomyces* are gram-positive, anaerobic or microaerophilic filamentous branched bacteria. Infection may result from oral trauma, dental surgery or dental caries.

Clinical Features

- Cervicofacial actinomycosis is the most common type of infection, comprising 50% to 70% of the reported cases.

- Initially, infection is characterised by chronic soft tissue swelling in the jaw, frequently at the border of the mandible. Pain is not a prominent feature. This is followed by the discharge of pus containing granules with sulphur-like appearance (called sulphur granules) from the sinus tracts. Cervical lymphadenopathy is not common.

Diagnosis

- History of oral trauma or dental manipulation.
- Clinical examination of the swelling, sinuses, and pus discharge (sulphur granules).
- Imaging studies (X-rays, computed tomographic scan and magnetic resonance imaging) are helpful but offer only nonspecific information.
- Fine-needle aspiration and culture studies of the discharge.

Management

- Intravenous administration of antibiotics and surgical exploration are recommended.
- Penicillin is the drug of choice. Tetracycline and erythromycin are employed for the patients allergic to penicillin.

Gangrenous Stomatitis (Noma or Cancrum Oris)

Definition/Description

- It is a progressive and mutilating disease of the orofacial structures. It occurs in young children in certain parts of Africa and Asia.

Cause

- Microbes: *Fusobacterium nucleatum* (an anaerobic fusiform bacteria), *Treponema vincentii* and *Bacteroides asaccharolyticus* (previously *B. melaninogenicus*).
- Predisposing factors: Malnutrition, stress and exanthematous disease.

Clinical Features

- Usually, it begins as necrotising ulcerative gingivitis and spreads rapidly to the adjacent soft tissues.
- Sore mouth, profuse salivation and intense halitosis.
- Disease enters advanced stage in just two to three days.
- Extraoral skin shows blue-black discolouration, followed by a gangrenous phase, which is characterised by the appearance of slough and a perforating wound, resulting in the exposure of the teeth and bone (Figure 31.2).

Diagnosis

- Clinical findings are indicative of the disease.

Management

- In acute stages of the disease, hospitalization, administration of intravenous fluids and the use of antibiotics such as penicillin or sulphonamides are indicated.

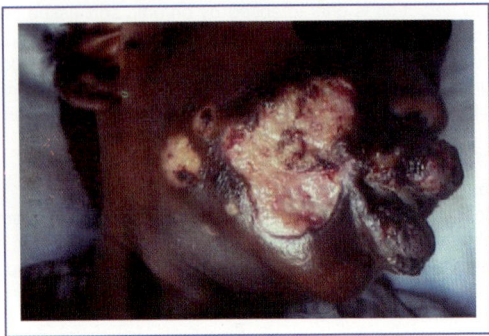

Figure 31.2 Gangrenous stomatitis (noma) in an African child. Infection usually starts as necrotising ulcerative gingivitis and spreads rapidly to the associated orofacial structures.
Courtesy: Lakshman Samaranayake.

- Local care of the wound and feeding are essential.
- Reconstructive surgery is recommended for healed cases.

Tuberculosis

Definition/Description

- It is a chronic granulomatous infection caused by *Mycobacterium tuberculosis*.
- Primary oral tuberculosis is rare in immunocompetent individuals.

Cause

- Acid-fast bacillus *M. tuberculosis*.
- Predisposing factors: Poor socioeconomic and hygienic conditions, nutritional deficiencies and immunosuppression.

Clinical Features

- Pulmonary tuberculosis is the commonest form of the disease.
- Tuberculosis ulcers of the oral tissues solely due to primary infection are rare.
- Occasionally, secondary tuberculosis ulcers of the oral mucosa occur in untreated pulmonary tuberculosis.
- Lateral borders and dorsum of the tongue (Figure 31.3) are the common sites for oral tuberculosis ulcers.
- Oral tuberculosis ulcers are irregular in shape and typically show undermined margins and mucous-like material in the base of the ulcer. Often, these ulcers are clinically mistaken for carcinoma.
- Systemic features include weight loss, night sweats, fever and cough and haemoptysis.

Diagnosis

- History, clinical examination, X-ray of the chest and sputum cultures of acid-fast bacilli.

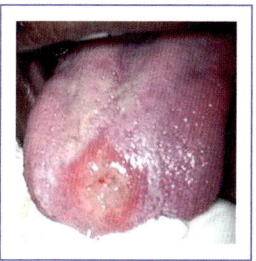

Figure 31.3 Tuberculous ulcer of the dorsum of the tongue.
Reproduced with permission from: Ajay GN, Laxmikanth C, Prashanth SK. Tuberculous ulcer of tongue with oral complications of oral antituberculosis therapy. *Indian J Dent Res*. 2006;17:87–90.

- Diagnosis of oral tuberculosis ulcer can be confirmed by staining the biopsy samples for the presence of acid-fast mycobacterium by using Ziehl-Neelsen stain.

Management

- Remission of oral tuberculosis ulcers occurs with systemic antituberculosis treatment.

Leprosy (Hansen's Disease)

Definition/Description

- It is a contagious and mutilating dermatological disease caused by *M. leprae*. Two major clinical types of leprosy exist: tuberculoid and lepromatous leprosy.

Cause

- *M. leprae* is the causative organism.

Clinical Features

- Symptoms and signs of leprosy are usually confined to the skin and cutaneous nerves.
- In tuberculoid leprosy, hyperaesthesia or paraesthesia of the areas supplied by the trigeminal nerve can occur. The facial skin may also present hypopigmented and anaesthetic patches.
- Lepromatous leprosy is characterised by the destruction of the nasomaxillary complex, resulting in saddle nose, atrophy of the anterior nasal spine and premaxillary bone recession (Figure 31.4).
- Skin lesions on the face may present erythematous and anaesthetic patches.

Diagnosis

- History, clinical examination and lepromin skin test for microbiological identification of *M. leprae*.

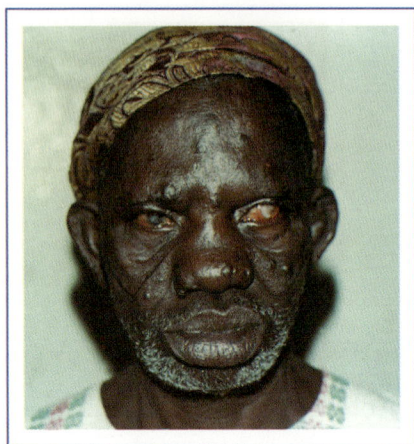

Figure 31.4 A patient with lepromatous leprosy. Note the saddle nose and associated general facial disfigurement and blindness. Oral mucosal involvement of the infection is rare.
Courtesy: Lakshman Samaranayake.

Management

- Multidrug therapy with dapsone, rifampicin and clofazimine is recommended to control the spread of leprosy.
- The damage already caused by the disease cannot be reversed.

Syphilis

Definition/Description

- Syphilis is a spirocheatal disease. Two forms of the disease exist: acquired and congenital syphilis.
- Acquired syphilis is a sexually transmitted disease, whereas congenital syphilis is transmitted from the infected mother to the child *in utero*.
- Acquired syphilis exhibits three stages: primary, secondary and tertiary. In all three stages of the disease, oral lesions may be seen in different clinical forms.

Cause

- Spirochaete: *Treponema pallidum*.

Clinical Features

Primary syphilis

- In primary syphilis, an ulcerative lesion called chancre occurs at the site of entry of the spirochaete.
- The upper lip in men and the lower lip in women are the common sites of chancre. Rarely, tongue, tonsils and pharynx can also be involved.

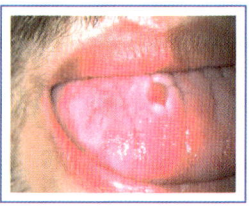

Figure 31.5 Primary syphilis: Chancre of the tongue in an individual who has had unprotected orogenital contact with his partner. Clinical suspicion of syphilis was confirmed by serology.

Reproduced with permission from: Ramoni S, Cusisni M, Gaiaini F, Crosti C. Syphilitic chancres of the mouth: three cases. *Acta Derm Venereol*. 2009;89:648–9. doi:10.2340/00015555-0709.

- Chancre occurs between 10 days and 90 days after the exposure. It is a solitary painless ulcer that exhibits rolled or raised borders and punched-out appearance (Figure 31.5). Chancre is often mistaken for carcinoma.
- Cervical lymph node enlargement with rubbery consistency is common in the early stages of oral infection.
- Chancre usually heals without treatment in about four to five weeks of its appearance.
- Chancre is an infective lesion.

Secondary syphilis

- In secondary syphilis, mucocutaneous patches occur.
- Oral involvement is due to haematogenous spread of spirochaetes and oral lesions appear as maculopapular mucosal patches.
- Oral lesions are flat and linear. Usually, they are covered by a grey membrane. Often, these coalesce and form serpiginous lesions called 'snail-track' ulcers (Figure 31.6).

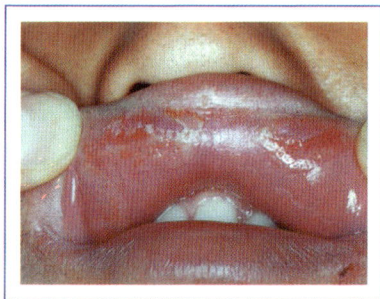

Figure 31.6 Mucous patches (on the patient's right) and a snail-track ulcer (left) of the labial mucosa in a patient with secondary syphilis.
Courtesy: Lakshman Samaranayake.

- Ulcerative lesions heal spontaneously within two to six weeks.
- At the time of presentation, patients present copper-coloured coin-like skin rashes, fever and generalised lymphadenopathy.
- Serology is positive in this stage.
- Mucous patches are infective lesions.

Tertiary syphilis

- Approximately, untreated secondary syphilis may progress into tertiary syphilis in one-third of the patients.
- In this stage of the disease, oral gummatous ulceration occurs, resulting in perforation of the tissue. This is usually seen on the hard palate.
- Unlike the ulcers of the primary and secondary syphilis, spiro-chaetes are not found in the gummata. In rare instances, syphilitic glossitis, leading to syphilitic leukoplakia, may be seen in tertiary syphilis. Syphilitic leukoplakia is considered to be a potentially malignant lesion.

Congenital syphilis

- Congenital syphilis is a severe, disabling, and often life-threatening infection seen in infants.
- A pregnant mother with untreated syphilis can transmit the disease through the placenta to the unborn infant.
- Nearly 50% of infected infants die, but in those who survive, congenital syphilis typically manifests after two years of birth. These children present with gummatous ulcers, involving the nose, septum and hard palate.
- Other orofacial and dental and features include centrally notched, widely spaced maxillary central incisors and poorly developed multiple rounded rudimentary cusps in molars (mulberry molars). Ocular lesions leading to interstitial keratitis, deafness and frontal bossing are also consistent features of congenital syphilis.

Diagnosis

- Diagnosis of acquired syphilis
    - A detailed history of the sexual and social lifestyle of the individual.
    - The presence of *T. pallidum* in smears taken from chancre and ulcers can be detected by dark-ground illumination method. However, current opinion is that this test should be avoided because of the risk of nosocomial transmission and the possible confusion with other treponemes of the normal oral flora.
    - For oral mucous patches of secondary syphilis and gummata of the tertiary syphilis, microscopical examination of the biopsy samples yields useful information.
- Tests used to confirm syphilis include Venereal Disease Research Laboratory test (VDRL test), rapid plasma reagin test, enzyme immunoassay, the *T. pallidum* particle agglutination assay (TPPA test) and the microhaemagglutination assay for *T. pallidum* antibodies (MHA-TP assay).

- Diagnosis of congenital syphilis
  - History of the mother regarding possible infection with syphilis during pregnancy, clinical examination of the child, including dental examination, eye examination and cerebrospinal fluid examination for detection of *T. pallidum*, and serological tests for syphilis.

Management

- Oral lesions of the primary and secondary stages of syphilis respond to the systemic antibiotic treatment. Antibiotics are also effective in treating congenital syphilis.
- Gummata are irreversible and require surgical correction.

Gonorrhoea

Definition/Description

- Gonorrhoea is a sexually transmitted disease caused by *Neisseria gonorrhoeae*. Occasionally, oral and pharyngeal lesions of gonorrhoea are reported.

Cause

- The causative organism is *N. gonorrhoeae*, a gram-negative bacterium.
- Oral involvement of the disease can occur due to orogenital contact with an infected person. Incubation period is 2 to 10 days.

Clinical Features

- Gonorrhoea is characterised by urethritis, painful urination (dysuria) and genital mucopurulent discharge.
- Gonococcal stomatitis and pharyngitis may occur with erythematous and oedematous lesions on the pharynx and uvula.
- In some cases, ulcerative lesions on the tongue may also occur.
- Occasionally, temporomandibular joint involvement is reported in patients with gonococcal arthritis.

Diagnosis

- History, clinical examination, and Gram stain and culture of the genital discharge or blood.

Management

- Antibiotics: Ampicillin, erythromycin and ciprofloxacin.

Scarlet Fever

Definition/Description

- Scarlet fever is a streptococcal infection. It involves the throat, tonsils and skin.

Cause

- Bacterium: *Streptococcus pyogenes*.

Clinical Features

- Fever of sudden onset, sore throat, headache, cervical lymph-adenopathy, vomiting, erythematous skin rash on the limbs and tonsillar exudates.
- Altered taste sensation and presence of furred or red tongue (strawberry tongue) are the oral features seen in patients with scarlet fever.

Diagnosis

- History and clinical examination.
- Throat swab for microbial identification and culture.
- Serology for antistreptolysin O titre.

Management

- Antibiotics, antipyretics and bed rest.

VIRAL INFECTIONS OF THE ORAL MUCOSA

Primary Herpetic Gingivostomatitis

Definition/Description

- It is a relatively common infection of the gingival tissues and oral mucosa caused predominantly by herpes simplex virus (HSV) type 1.

Cause

- In up to 90% of cases, HSV type 1 is involved, whereas in less than 10% of cases, HSV type 2 is aetiologically involved.
- Transmission of the infection is by contact with mucosal lesions or infected saliva.
- Incubation period is about five days.

Clinical Features

- Children are commonly affected.
- Multiple vesicles occur on the gingival and other mucosal surfaces, which rupture, leaving shallow painful ulcers with erythematous haloes and greyish-yellow bases (Figure 31.7).
- Gingivae are swollen and oedematous.
- Systemic symptoms such as fever, malaise and anorexia may be present.
- Cervical lymph nodes are enlarged.

Diagnosis

- History and clinical findings.
- Antibody titre estimation during the active phase and convalescent period (three to four weeks after the infection) is helpful. Antibody titre is high during the convalescent period, indicating recent infection.

Management

- No treatment is necessary because the infection is self-limiting.

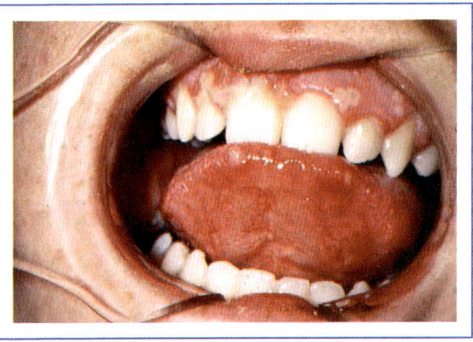

Figure 31.7   Primary herpetic gingivostomatitis in a child. Note vesiculoulcerative lesions on the gingivae and the tip of the tongue.
Courtesy: D. F. Wilson.

- Symptomatic treatment may be required in some patients.
- For immunocompromised patients, it is advisable to treat the patient with oral and topical antiviral agent (e.g., acyclovir).

Secondary (Recurrent) Herpetic Infection (Herpes Labialis)

Definition/Description

- Secondary herpetic infection commonly affects lips. The condition is called herpes labialis (commonly known as 'cold sore').
- Infection is usually recurrent.
- Vesicular lesions are located on the lip, at the mucocutaneous junction of the mouth.

Cause

- Herpes labialis is caused by the reactivation of HSV (type 1 in most cases), which remains dormant in the sensory ganglia of the trigeminal nerve after the primary infection.
- Predisposing factors for the reactivation of the dormant virus includes sunlight or cold, psychological stress, menstruation, trauma, common cold and immune suppression.

Clinical Features

- Recurrent herpetic infection has a prodromal phase. During this period, itching and tingling sensation occur a day before the appearance of multiple vesicles on the lip and sometimes also on the side of the nose (Figure 31.8).
- Vesicles rupture, become encrusted and heal without scarring.
- Intraoral involvement of recurrent herpetic infection is rare in immunocompetent individuals.

Diagnosis

- History and clinical examination.

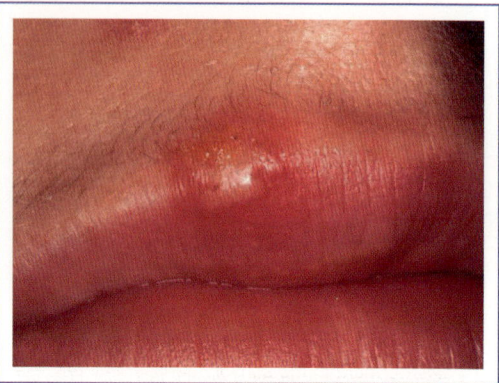

Figure 31.8 Clinical presentation of herpes labialis on the mucocutaneous junction of the upper lip.
Courtesy: Lakshman Samaranayake.

Management

- Application of 5% acyclovir cream during the prodromal phase is effective in lessening the clinical course of the infection.
- The virus is present in the vesicles and saliva. Gloves must be worn during the examination in order to avoid herpetic whitlow on the fingers.

Chickenpox

Definition/Description

- Chickenpox is a common childhood viral infection of the skin and mucous membranes.

Cause

- Varicella-zoster virus (VZV) (also known as human herpes virus type 3).

Clinical Features

- Symptoms include fever, malaise and skin rash, and vesicles on the trunk and face.
- Painful oral vesicles and ulcers may occur in these patients.
- Intraoral lesions are commonly seen on the palate, pillars of the fauces and uvula.

Diagnosis

- History and clinical features.
- Confirmatory laboratory tests include electron microscopical identification of the virus from vesicular fluid. (This is not done routinely.)
- Serology for specific IgM antibodies in acute and convalescent periods.

Management

- This is a self-limiting infection. Symptomatic treatment may be necessary.
- Vaccine to prevent chickenpox is available.

Shingles (Herpes Zoster)

Definition/Description

- Shingles is a mucocutaneous infection caused by the reactivation of VZV in adults.

Cause

- Reactivation of the VZV in those who have had chickenpox in childhood causes shingles.
- VZV remains dormant in the sensory ganglia until reactivated. In the trigeminal region, the ophthalmic division is most frequently affected. Second and third divisions of the trigeminal nerve may also be involved, giving rise to painful vesicular lesions in the maxillary and mandibular regions, respectively.

Clinical Features

- During the prodromal phase, the pain in the region is deep-seated and unilateral, often mimicking the pain of dental origin.
- This is followed by vesicles seen unilaterally along the distribution of the branches of the trigeminal nerve.
- Shallow ulcers result due to the rupture of vesicles.
- On the skin, these vesicles rupture and form crusts.
- If the maxillary division is involved, ulcerations are located on the hard and soft palates. If the mandibular division is involved, the skin of the lower part of the face shows vesicles and ulceration (Figure 31.9).

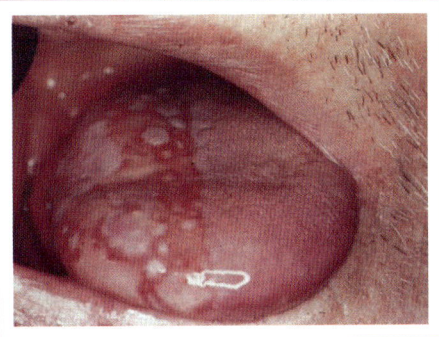

Figure 31.9 Herpes zoster infection of the tongue. Note the sharp midline demarcation of the lesion (due to the reactivation of the virus travelling via the lingual branch of the trigeminal nerve).
Courtesy: Lakshman Samaranayake.

- Corneal ulceration results from the ophthalmic nerve involvement.
- Systemic symptoms may include fever and malaise.
- Shingles is a very painful condition. Its complication may cause postherpetic neuralgia.
- Ramsay Hunt syndrome is a complication of shingles. It may occur in some individuals and is characterised by the appearance of vesicles on the uvula, palate, anterior tongue and auricle. This may be accompanied by transient facial palsy.

Diagnosis

- History and clinical features.
- Laboratory investigations, such as cytological or serological examinations.

Management

- Uncomplicated cases do not need any specific treatment. Symptomatic treatment of pain is required.
- Antiviral medications such as acyclovir, famciclovir and valacyclovir are effective in improving the symptoms if instituted within the first three days of the appearance of eruptions.
- In postherpetic neuralgia, antidepressant such as amitriptyline is effective.

Hand, Foot and Mouth Disease

Definition/Description

- Hand, foot and mouth disease occurs in children, particularly in the areas where the infection is epidemic.

Cause

- Causative virus is a member of the Coxsackie virus group.

Clinical Features

- Small blisters appear on the dorsal and lateral aspects of the fingers and toes and rashes appear on the hands and feet. Oral ulcers develop on the tongue and buccal mucosa.
- Systemic symptoms are generally mild.

Diagnosis

- History and clinical features.

Management

- It is a self-limiting condition. Symptomatic treatment may be necessary.

Herpangina

Definition/Description

- Herpangina is a viral infection of the oropharynx.

Cause

- It is caused by Coxsackie virus.

Clinical Features

- Systemic features include sore throat, fever, malaise and lymphadenopathy.
- Oral involvement includes blisters, erosions and round ulcers, mainly on the soft palate.

Diagnosis

- History of illness and clinical appearance of lesions confined to soft palate and pharynx provide useful diagnostic clues.

Management

- Treatment is largely symptomatic.

Infectious Mononucleosis

Definition/Description

- Infectious mononucleosis is a viral disease that is predominantly seen in young adolescents. It is also known as glandular fever or kissing disease.

Cause

- It is caused by Epstein-Barr virus. The infection is usually transmitted through close contact with the infected person or contaminated objects.

Clinical Features

- Infection is characterised by fever, sore throat, malaise and cervical lymphadenopathy.
- Hepatosplenomegaly, anaemia and meningitis may occur in rare cases.
- Oral manifestation of the disease includes blood blisters on the palate.

Diagnosis

- History and clinical findings.
- White blood cell count shows leukocytosis.
- Identification of heterophile antibody that can agglutinate sheep red blood cells (Paul-Bunnell test) and Epstein-Barr virus antibody titres (IgM and IgG) are confirmatory.

Management

- Disease is self-limiting.
- Alcohol consumption should be avoided until the patient recovers fully.
- Symptomatic treatment of fever and rest are adequate.

Cytomegalovirus Infections

Definition/Description

- Cytomegalovirus (CMV) infections mainly involve salivary glands. Oral involvement is uncommon.

- In immunocompromised patients and those receiving immunosuppressive medications, oral ulcers due to CMV infection are often noted.

Cause

- Causative agent is CMV.

Clinical Features

- Usually, a single ulcer is present. Tongue and buccal mucosa are the preferred sites. Ulcers mimic major aphthae.

Diagnosis

- History, clinical examination, viral culture and serology.

Management

- Systemic antiviral treatment is effective in reducing the symptoms.

FUNGAL INFECTIONS OF THE ORAL MUCOSA

Pseudomembranous Candidiasis (Thrush)

Definition/Description

- Pseudomembranous candidiasis is an acute candidal infection that results in superficial pseudomembranous white lesions of the oral mucosa. This condition is also known as thrush.

Cause

- Important pathogenic candidal species include *Candida albicans*, *C. tropicalis*, *C. glabrata*, *C. parapsilosis*, *C. guilliermondii*, *C. krusei*, *C. dubliniensis* and *C. stellatoidea*.
- Oral pseudomembranous candidiasis is caused mainly by *C. albicans*.
- Predisposing factors that render the host to candidal infection include infancy or old age, pregnancy, prolonged use of wide-spectrum antibiotics, corticosteroids, cytotoxic drugs and immunosuppressive agents, radiation, poorly maintained dentures, self-administered intravenous recreational drugs, primary and acquired immunodeficiency states (HIV/AIDS), acute and chronic leukaemia, lymphoma, diabetes, hypothyroidism, Addison's disease and iron deficiency.

Clinical Features

- Oral pseudomembranous candidiasis typically shows white curd-like mucosal plaques (Figure 31.10), which can be easily rubbed off with gauze, which leaves a raw erythematous and bleeding base.
- Some patients may complain of bad taste and mucosal burning sensation.

Diagnosis

- Clinical findings are suggestive of candidal infection.

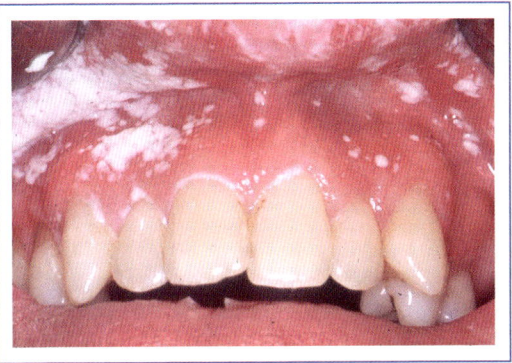

Figure 31.10   Pseudomembranous candidiasis (thrush) in an HIV-infected young adult. Note the fungal invasion of gingival crevice.
Courtesy: Lakshman Samaranayake.

- Microscopical identification of large number of organisms in smears.
- Culture studies or serology.

Management

- Antifungal treatment with topical application of nystatin or amphotericin B.
- Identification and elimination of predisposing factors.
- Systemic antifungal treatment may be required for candidiasis of the gastrointestinal tract and other mucosal sites.

Erythematous (Atrophic) Candidiasis

Definition/Description

- It is a *Candida*-associated infection of the oral mucosa, resulting in a red lesion on the dorsum of the tongue or hard palate.

Cause

- Erythematous candidiasis is a consequence of the long-term use of topical or systemic antibiotics or corticosteroids.
- In elderly full-denture wearers, erythematous candidiasis is a common feature.

Clinical Features

- Lesion on the tongue is an asymptomatic depapillated centrally located erythematous patch on the dorsum of the tongue (Figure 31.11 A).
- Similar patch can also occur in the centre of the palate, particularly in HIV-positive patients (Figure 31.11 B).
- In denture wearers with *Candida*-associated stomatitis, angular cheilitis is also common.

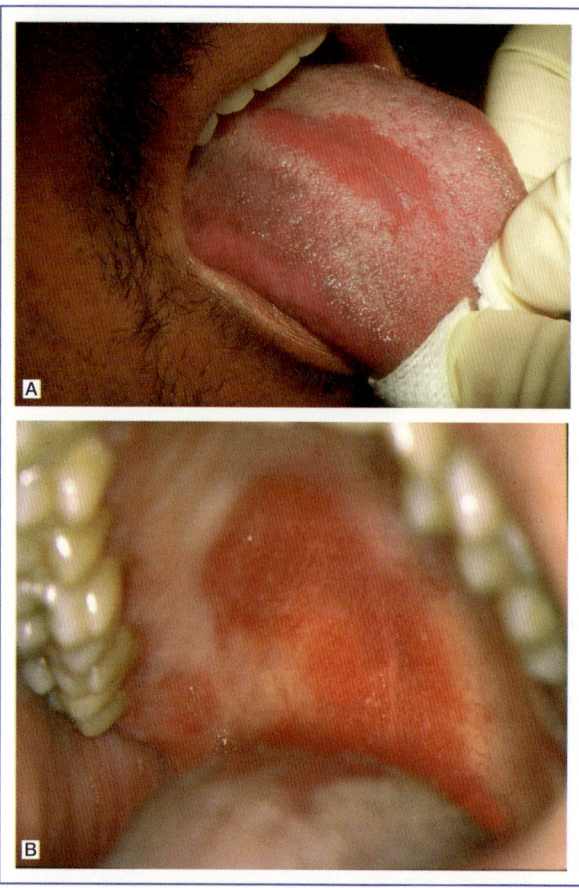

Figure 31.11 (A) Erythematous candidiasis of the dorsum of the tongue in an HIV-infected individual. (B) Erythematous candidiasis of the dorsum of the tongue and the palate in an HIV-Infected individual.
Reproduced with permission from: (A) David Reznik. Available from: www.HIVdent.org (B) Lakshman Samaranayake.

Diagnosis

• History, clinical examination and microscopical identification of the *Candida* from smears obtained from the erythematous lesions. Often, candidal presence in these lesions can be very scanty.

Management

• Topical antifungal agents such as nystatin and amphotericin B are effective. Fluconazole is recommended for HIV/AIDS patients.

- Identification and management of the underlying disease or contributing factor should be carried out for successful antifungal treatment.

Hyperplastic Candidiasis (Candidal Leukoplakia)

Definition/Description

- Hyperplastic candidiasis refers to a predominantly fixed white lesion of the oral mucosa, associated with *Candida*.
- This lesion, also known as candidal leukoplakia, is considered as a potentially malignant disorder because of the risk it carries for malignant transformation.

Cause

- *C. albicans* is associated with this lesion. Majority of patients include habitual tobacco users in the form of smoking or chewing.

Clinical Features

- Lesions of hyperplastic candidiasis present as raised white lesions usually fixed to the underlying mucosa. These lesions cannot be rubbed off.
- Sometimes, these are small, palpable and translucent whitish areas. Larger lesions are dense and opaque plaques (Figure 31.12) and are rough in surface texture.
- Cheek mucosa posterior to the labial commissures are the preferred sites.
- Approximately 9% to 40% of these lesions have been reported to transform into oral squamous cell carcinomas, if not treated early.

Diagnosis

- Diagnostic steps include a detailed history, clinical examination and microscopical evaluation of the samples obtained from the lesional biopsy.

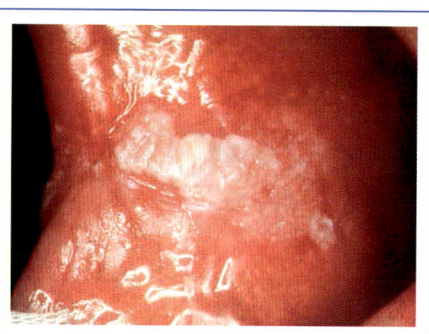

Figure 31.12   Classic appearance of chronic hyperplastic candidiasis of the labial commissures of the mouth.
Courtesy: Lakshman Samaranayake.

Management

- Topical antifungal treatment with nystatin or amphotericin B is effective in some patients.
- Systemic use of fluconazole is recommended for patients with chronic infections and for those who do not respond to nystatin and amphotericin B applications.
- Smaller lesions may be surgically removed.
- Patients with recalcitrant hyperplastic lesions should be kept under regular surveillance if they are resistant to therapy.

Candida-Associated Denture Stomatitis (Denture Sore Mouth)

Definition/Description

- *Candida*-associated denture stomatitis is a chronic candidal infection of the mucosa in denture wearers.

Cause

- Chronic infection with *Candida* in denture wearers.
- Contributing factors include poor denture hygiene, ill-fitting dentures, xerostomia and systemic factors such as diabetes, Sjögren's syndrome and iron-deficiency anaemia.

Clinical Features

- The condition is asymptomatic in some denture wearers, but complaints of occasional soreness of the denture-bearing mucosal surface are common.
- Three clinical forms of lesions may be seen, mainly on the hard palate. The denture-bearing mucosa may show erythema and oedema (Figure 31.13 A), diffuse and confluent erythema and oedema, or papillary hyperplasia and inflammation of the palatal mucosa (Figure 31.13 B).
- Mucosa in contact with the lower denture is not involved in this process.

Diagnosis

- A detailed history and clinical examination of the mucosal lesions.
- Examination of the denture is also necessary because a poorly maintained denture can harbour yeasts and bacteria in the plaque biofilms on the fitting surface of dentures.

Management

- Patient should be advised to maintain denture hygiene.
- Dentures should not be worn by patients at night (bedtime).
- Dentures should be soaked in sodium hypochlorite or chlorhexidine solution to eliminate candidal hyphae.
- If dentures are ill-fitting, a review of denture fitness to relieve trauma is required.
- Patient should be advised to have a low-carbohydrate diet.
- Medication includes systemic antifungal treatment for a week with nystatin or amphotericin B, and myconazole topical applications on the fitting surface of the denture.

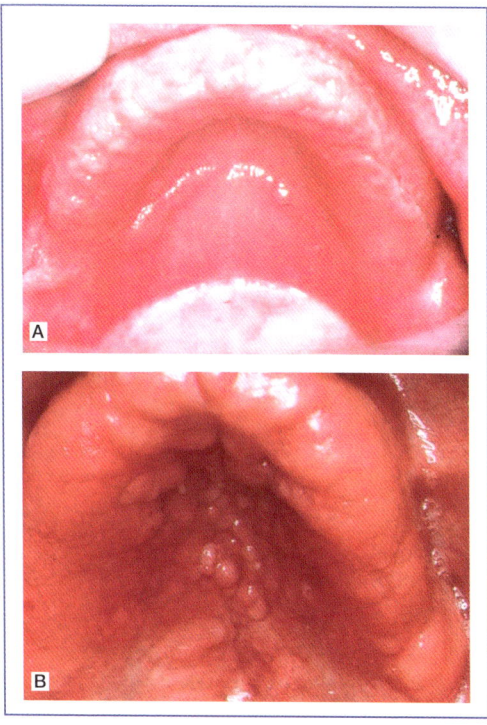

Figure 31.13 (A) *Candida*-associated denture stomatitis showing the erythematous and oedematous denture-bearing (palatal) mucosa. (B) *Candida*-associated denture stomatitis showing palatal papillary hyperplasia.
Courtesy: Lakshman Samaranayake.

Median Rhomboid Glossitis (Glossal Central Papillary Atrophy)

Definition/Description

- Median rhomboid glossitis refers to an area of papillary atrophy that is rhomboid in shape and located centrally on the dorsum of the tongue anterior to the circumvallate papillae.

Cause

- Candidal infection is the major cause.
- Smoking, prolonged use of corticosteroid inhalers and remnants of tuberculum impar may also be associated with this condition.

Clinical Features

- Central papillary atrophy on the dorsum of the tongue is asymptomatic in majority of cases.

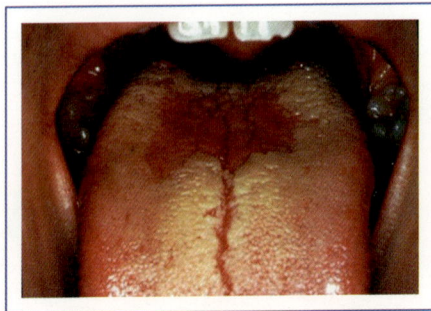

Figure 31.14 Median rhomboid glossitis. The classic rhomboid erythematous lesion located anterior to the circumvallate papillae.
Courtesy: Lakshman Samaranayake.

- The lesion shows atrophy of lingual filiform papillae and is located centrally and anterior to the circumvallate papillae (Figure 31.14).
- Lesion is smooth, raised or lobulated. Occasionally, patients may complain of mild burning sensation and bad taste.
- Patients often have cancer phobia.

Diagnosis

- History and clinical examination.
- Smear obtained and stained with specific stains may show candidal hyphae.

Management

- No specific treatment is necessary, unless the lesion is strongly positive for *Candida*.
- Maintenance of oral hygiene is necessary.
- If patient is cancer-phobic, reassurance is required.

Angular Stomatitis (Angular Cheilitis or Perleche)

Definition/Description

- Angular cheilitis refers to sore, red and fissured angles of the mouth, which may be associated with candidal infection, particularly in full-denture wearers.

Cause

- *C. albicans* infection in full-denture wearers.
- Occasionally, mixed infection with *Staphylococcus aureus* may be present.
- Reduced vertical dimension of the mouth may be a contributing factor.

Clinical Features

- In majority of cases, patient is a full-denture wearer with poor denture hygiene.

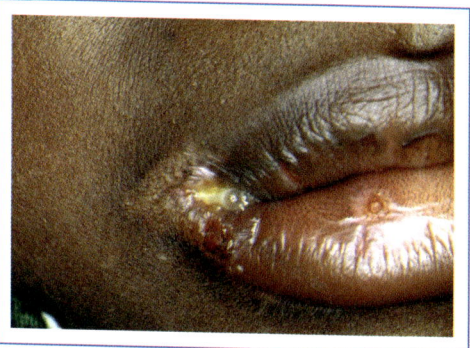

Figure 31.15   Angular stomatitis.
Courtesy: Lakshman Samaranayake.

- Bilaterally, at the angle of the mouth, red, fissured lesions occur. These are painful and may bleed on opening the mouth widely (Figure 31.15).
- Often, saliva drools through these cracks onto the skin.
- Patient may show signs of iron deficiency or pernicious anaemia.

Diagnosis

- History and clinical examination of the mouth and dentures.
- Smear stained with fungal stains shows fungal involvement. Bacteria such as *S. aureus* may also be detected, particularly when yellow crusting at the angles of the mouth is visible.
- It is advisable to check for anaemia and any other underlying contributing disorder.

Management

- Topical antifungal therapy with nystatin or amphotericin B, attention to denture hygiene and vertical dimension and investigation and treatment of other underlying contributing factors (e.g., anaemia).
- If staphylococcal infection is also present, an antibacterial preparation, such as fusidic acid and neomycin, is required. Chlorhexidine mouthwash is recommended.

Linear Gingival Erythema

Definition/Description

- Linear gingival erythema refers to a localised or generalised erythematous band of approximately 2 mm width, which extends along the gingival margins in immunocompromised individuals.

Cause

- Lesion is associated with mixed candidal and bacterial infection in patients with immune deficiency (e.g., in HIV/AIDS patients).

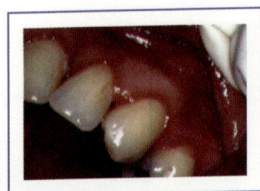

Figure 31.16 Linear gingival erythema. Note the linear red band surrounding the gingival margins.
Reproduced with permission from: David Reznik. Available from: www. HIVdent.org

Clinical Features

- The condition shows the presence of asymptomatic, linear red bands of approximately 2 mm width around the marginal gingiva. These bands may be localised, involving gingival margins of one or two teeth, or generalised (Figure 31.16).
- Erythematous bands are not induced by dental plaque and generally do not respond to the removal of debris or dental plaque.

Diagnosis

- History and clinical examination.
- Patient's immune status should be checked.

Management

- Antifungal treatment and attention to the underlying disorder.

Aspergillosis

Definition/Description

- Aspergillosis is an infection caused by the species of the genus *Aspergillus*.

Cause

- Pathogenic species such as *A. fumigatus*, *A. niger* and *A. flavus*.

Clinical Features

- The respiratory tract, external auditory canal, nasopharynx, cornea, gastrointestinal tract and, occasionally, skin may be the primary sites of infection.
- Oral infection is generally seen in the disseminated form of the disease.
- Paranasal sinuses are frequently involved in aspergillosis. Those with impaired immune responses are prone to develop aspergillosis.
- Though rare, oral involvement of the soft palate can occur as an ulcerative lesion surrounded by a ring of blackened necrotic tissue.

Diagnosis

- Identification of the organisms and culture studies are the confirmatory tests.
- Specimens are obtained from sputum and biopsy material.

Management

- Amphotericin B is the treatment of choice.
- Intravenous antifungal treatment and surgical debridement of the lesions may be necessary in those with immunocompromised status.

Histoplasmosis

Definition/Description

- Histoplasmosis is a fungal disease caused by *Histoplasma capsulatum* and *H. duboisii*.

Cause

- *H. capsulatum*, a dimorphous fungus.

Clinical Features

- Disease presents in three forms: acute primary histoplasmosis, progressive disseminated histoplasmosis and chronic cavitary histoplasmosis.
- In progressive disseminated form of the disease, oral manifestations are common.
- Lesions may be papular, ulcerative, nodular or verrucous in appearance. Any mucosal area may be involved. Lesions may extend onto the pharynx. Sore throat is a common complaint.

Diagnosis

- Identification of the fungus from the infected material and culture studies.

Management

- Systemic amphotericin B and supportive treatment.

SUGGESTED READINGS

Darwazeh AMG. Common infections of the oral mucosa. In: Prabhu SR, editor. *Textbook of Oral Medicine*. New Delhi, India: Oxford University Press; 2004. pp. 142–55.

Samaranayake L. *Essential Microbiology for Dentistry*. 4th ed. London, U.K.: Churchill Livingstone; 2012. pp. 307–24.

Samaranayake L, Parathitiyawa N. Infections of the oral mucosa. In: Warnakulasuriya S, Tilakaratne WM, editors. *Oral Medicine and Pathology: A Guide to Diagnosis and Management*. New Delhi, India: Jaypee Brothers Medical Publishers; 2014. pp. 361–82.

Cawson RA, Odell EW. Diseases of the oral mucosa: introduction and mucosal infections. *Cawson's Essentials of Oral Pathology and Oral Medicine*. 8th ed. London, U.K.: Churchill Livingstone; 2013. pp. 206–17.

Chapter 32

Cysts, tumours and tumour-like growths of the jaws

S. R. Prabhu and D. F. Wilson

CYSTS OF THE JAW BONES

Radicular and Residual Cysts

Definition/Description

- A radicular (periapical) cyst is an inflammatory cyst associated with the apex of the root of a nonvital tooth.
- A residual cyst, on the other hand, is usually a radicular cyst of the jaw that persists after the tooth is extracted, leaving the cyst behind. Hypothetically, residual cysts can also originate from inflammatory reactivation of the embryonic epithelial cell in the area of the healing tooth socket after tooth extraction.
- Radicular cysts are the most common cysts of the jaw bones.
- Residual cysts are more common among older people.

Cause

- Both types of cysts have an inflammatory cause.

Clinical Features

- A radicular cyst is usually asymptomatic and may cause a slowly progressive swelling of the jaw in the affected region.
- The tooth involved is nonvital, but multirooted teeth may show vitality if the radicular cyst involves only one root of the tooth.
- Radiographically, a radicular cyst is located at the apex of the tooth (Figure 32.1 A). A residual cyst occurs at the site of a previously extracted tooth (Figure 32.1 B).
- The lesions are radiolucent and unilocular and tend to have sharply defined borders.

Diagnosis

- History, clinical examination and radiographical and microscopic findings.

Management

- Refer the patient to a dentist for appropriate treatment.
- Radicular cyst: Surgical removal or endodontic treatment of the affected tooth. If the tooth is not restorable, then it should be extracted.
- Residual cysts: Surgical removal or radiographical monitoring.

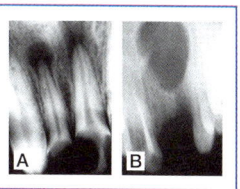

Figure 32.1 Radiographs of (A) radicular (periapical) cyst and (B) residual cyst. Reproduced with permission from: Charles Dunlap. Available from: https://dentistry.umkc.edu/Practicing_Communities/asset/Jcysts.pdf

Dentigerous and Eruption Cysts

Definition/Description

- Dentigerous cyst refers to a developmental odontogenic cyst that is attached to the neck of the unerupted tooth and encompasses the tooth crown.
- An eruption cyst is a developmental soft tissue cyst of dental origin that forms over an erupting tooth. This is mostly seen in children in relation to the erupting permanent teeth. The majority of eruption cysts are simply dentigerous cysts that have come to assume an extraosseous position.

Cause

- Dentigerous cyst is a result of cystic change in the embryonic enamel organ epithelium after enamel formation is complete.
- Causes of eruption cyst may include trauma, infection or lack of space for eruption of the tooth.

Clinical Features

- Dentigerous cysts are slow growing but can grow to a large size within the jaw. Over a period of time, the cyst may cause swelling of the jaw bone.
- The tooth with which the cyst is involved is within the jaw bone; hence, there will be clinical evidence of a missing tooth in the dental arch.
- Initially, dentigerous cysts are asymptomatic.
- If infected, the cyst can cause painful and tender swelling.
- Radiographically, a dentigerous cyst is a unilocular radiolucency that contains the crown of an unerupted or impacted tooth (Figure 32.2).
- The most commonly involved tooth is the mandibular third molar.
- An eruption cyst clinically appears as a circumscribed, fluctuant, often translucent swelling of the alveolar ridge over the site of an erupting tooth.
- Because of the haemorrhage (due to trauma), an eruption cyst may appear as a purple-coloured, dome-shaped lesion (Figure 32.3).

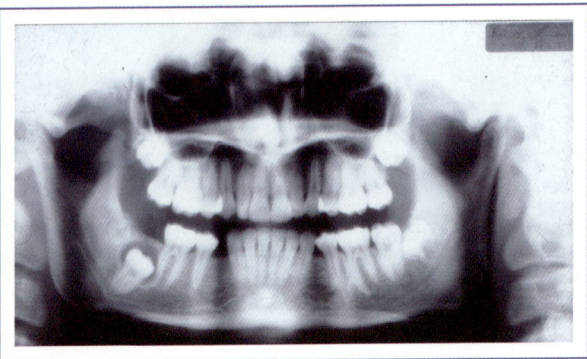

Figure 32.2 Radiographs of dentigerous cyst. Note a well-defined radio-lucency around the neck of an unerupted second right mandibular molar. *Courtesy*: David Wilson.

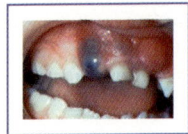

Figure 32.3 Eruption cyst. Purple colour is due to the haemorrhage derived from repeated trauma from mastication.
Reproduced with permission from: Charles Dunlap. Available from: https://dentistry.umkc.edu/Practicing_Communities/asset/Jcysts.pdf

Diagnosis

- History regarding noneruption of the tooth, clinical examination and radiographical findings.
- The clinical and radiographical findings of dentigerous cyst can be similar to those of ameloblastoma and odontogenic keratocysts, particularly if the lesion occurs in association with an unerupted mandibular third molar. Histological evaluation of all dentigerous cysts is recommended to confirm the diagnosis and to rule out the possibility of keratocyst or ameloblastoma.
- Eruption cysts are diagnosed on history and clinical grounds.

Management

- Refer the patient to an oral surgeon.
- Surgical removal of the dentigerous cyst with or without the tooth involved.
- The majority of eruption cysts disappear on their own. They do not require any treatment. If they bleed or are infected, surgical treatment to expose the tooth and drain the contents is required.

Odontogenic Keratocyst

Definition/Description

- Odontogenic keratocyst (OKC) is a benign, aggressive, odonto-genic developmental cystic lesion, usually seen in the second and third decades. It is also referred to as odontogenic keratocystic tumour.

Cause

- OKC is caused by a developmental cystic lesion. OKC is often described as a benign neoplasm because of its ability to exhibit relatively aggressive intraosseous growth.

Clinical Features

- OKC has a predilection for the posterior part of the mandible, including the ramus, but can occur anywhere in the jaws.
- Initially, the lesion is asymptomatic. Over time, the tumour can grow larger, causing swelling of the jaw.
- Radiographically, keratocysts can present as unilocular or multi-locular radiolucent lesions of variable sizes. Cortical expansion is seen in larger lesions. Some lesions may be associated with an unerupted tooth (Figure 32.4).

Diagnosis

- History, clinical examination and radiographical and microscopical evaluations.

Management

- Refer the patient to an oral maxillofacial surgeon.
- Surgery is recommended. However, the rate of recurrence of this tumour is high.

Multiple Keratocysts (Basal Cell Naevus Syndrome)

- This is a rare condition that is characterised by multiple keratocysts (Figure 32.5 A), multiple basal cell naevi (Figure 32.5 B), bifid ribs and intracranial calcifications. It occurs early in life.

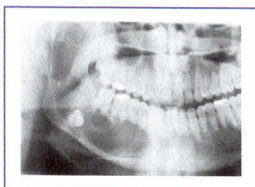

Figure 32.4 Odontogenic keratocyst. Radiographical differential diag-nosis includes dentigerous cyst and ameloblastoma.
Reproduced with permission from: Charles Dunlap. Available from: https://dentistry.umkc.edu/Practicing_Communities/asset/Jcysts.pdf

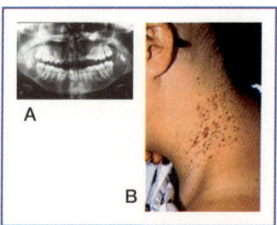

Figure 32.5 Basal cell naevus syndrome: (A) Radiograph shows multiple cysts and (B) clinically, basal cell naevi are seen on the neck.
Reproduced with permission from: Charles Dunlap. Available from: https://dentistry.umkc.edu/Practicing_Communities/asset/Jcysts.pdf

- Naevoid basal cell carcinomas of the skin are common in patients with this syndrome.

JAW TUMOURS

Ameloblastoma

Definition/Description

- A benign locally aggressive tumour of the odontogenic origin, usually seen in adults.

Cause

- Residual embryonic odontogenic epithelium in the jaws undergoes benign neoplastic or hamartomatous change.

Clinical Features

- Peak clinical incidence is in the third to fifth decades.
- It is a slow-growing and locally aggressive benign tumour.
- The mandibular molar region is a common site of occurrence, but these lesions can arise anywhere in the jaws. An unerupted third molar may be associated with the tumour.
- Expansion of the jaw may be seen in longstanding or more aggressive cases.
- Large lesions may present cortical perforation.
- Significant swelling of the affected jaw and face may be observed in advanced cases (Figure 32.6).
- Radiographical features: Unilocular or multilocular radiolucent appearances (Figure 32.7). The lesion may be associated with an unerupted impacted tooth.
- Displacement and/or root resorption of adjacent teeth is common.

Diagnosis

- History, clinical examination, radiography and histopathological evaluation.

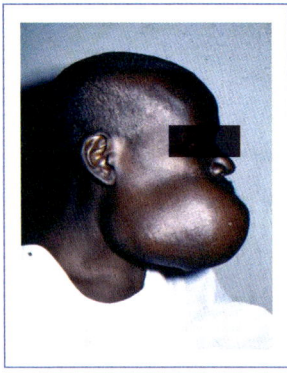

Figure 32.6 Ameloblastoma of the mandible.
Courtesy: S. R. Prabhu.

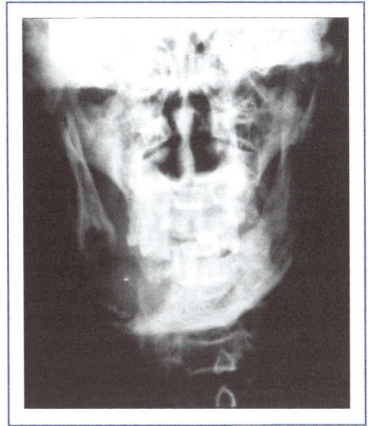

Figure 32.7 Right mandibular multilocular radiolucency in a patient with ameloblastoma.
Courtesy: S. R. Prabhu.

Management

- Surgical removal of the tumour is recommended.
- Refer the patient to an oral and maxillofacial surgeon.

Ameloblastic Fibroma

Definition/Description

- A benign odontogenic tumour of the jaw bones with a predilection for young individuals in their first or second decades.
- The lesion is generally regarded as a hamartoma.

Cause

- Proliferation of residual embryonic odontogenic epithelium and mesenchyme.

Clinical Features

- Slow-growing, painless tumour, with a site predilection for the posterior region of the mandible.
- Radiographical features include unilocular or mutilocular radiolucency associated with an unerupted tooth.

Diagnosis

- History, clinical examination, radiographical features and microscopical evaluation.

Management

- Surgery is recommended.
- Refer the patient to an oral and maxillofacial surgeon.

Odontomes (Odontomas)

Definition/Description

- Odontomes, also referred to as odontomas, are hamartomatous lesions of the jaw bones, which are composed of enamel, dentine, cementum and pulp. There are two basic types: complex odontome and compound odontome. It is common for a lesion to present radiographical and histological features of both forms.

Cause

- Odontomes are hamartomatous lesions derived from mixed (epithelial and mesenchymal) odontogenic tissues.

Clinical Features

- Odontome is usually seen in young adults.
- Asymptomatic lesions are discovered incidentally on radiographs.
- Large lesions cause jaw expansion and swelling.
- Radiographically, odontomes are seen predominantly as localised radiopaque lesions.
- Complex odontomes are more common in the mandibular molar region, whereas compound odontomes are usually located in the anterior maxillary region.
- Complex odontome is a mixture of dental tissues, with no anatomical resemblance to the teeth (Figure 32.8).
- Compound odontomes contain several small tooth-like structures (Figure 32.9 A and B).

Diagnosis

- History, clinical examination, radiographical features and microscopical evaluation.

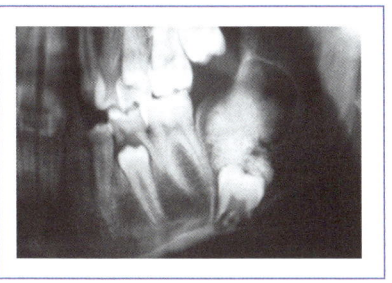

Figure 32.8 Radiograph of a complex odontome in the mandible. Reproduced with permission from: Ramadas K, Lucas E, Thomas G, et al. *A Digital Manual for the Early Diagnosis of Oral Neoplasia*. IARC, Lyon, 2008. Available from: http://screening.iarc.fr/atlasoral.php?lang=1

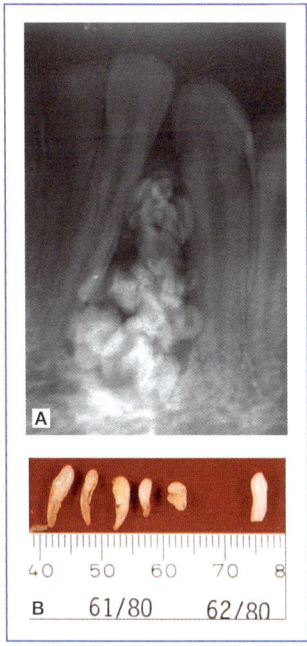

Figure 32.9 (A) Radiograph of the compound odontome with multiple teeth-like structures (denticles). (B) Surgically removed teeth from a compound odontome.
Reproduced with permission from: (A) Charles Dunlap. Available from: https://dentistry.umkc.edu/Practicing_Communities/asset/OdontTumors.pdf (B) D. F. Wilson.

Management

- Surgical removal is recommended.
- Refer the patient to an oral and maxillofacial surgeon.

Cementoblastoma (Cementoma)

Definition/Description

- Cementoblastoma, also known as cementoma, is an odonto-genic tumour of cementum. It occurs after the completion of root formation.

Cause

- Developmental tumour arising from cementoblasts.

Clinical Features

- Tumour occurs on and around the root of the mandibular poste-rior teeth. Radiographically, it appears as a round radiopaque mass attached to the end of the root. This is a slow-growing lesion.

Diagnosis

- History, clinical examination and radiographical and microscopical evaluations.

Management

- Surgical removal is recommended.
- Refer the patient to an oral and maxillofacial surgeon.

Osteoma

Definition/Description

Osteoma is a benign tumour of mature, compact or cancellous bone.

Cause

- Cause is not known.
- Traumatic, embryological and infective causes have been implicated.

Clinical Features

- Slow-growing, painless and usually a solitary lesion.
- Skull bones and facial bones, including maxilla and mandible, are occasionally involved; the maxillary sinus is the preferred site.
- Endosteal osteoma may occasionally present symptoms.
- Radiographically, osteoma appears as a well-circumscribed scle-rotic mass.
- In Gardner syndrome, osteomas are multiple (Gardner syndrome is characterised by intestinal polyposis, multiple osteomas and fibromas, epidermal cysts and impacted permanent and supernu-merary teeth).

Diagnosis

- Radiographical and histological evaluations of the lesion.

Management

- Local excision is recommended.
- Refer the patient to an oral and maxillofacial surgeon.

Osteosarcoma

Definition/Description

- Osteosarcoma is a malignant neoplasm that commonly originates from the medullary portion and occasionally from the outer surface of the bone.

Cause

- Genetic alterations resulting in overexpression of oncogenes and inactivation of tumour suppression genes.
- It can occur in previously irradiated bone, Paget's disease of bone, fibrous dysplasia and giant cell tumours of bone.

Clinical Features

- 5% to 7% of all osteosarcomas occur in the maxillofacial skeleton.
- Osteosarcoma occurs in patients in their third or fourth decade of life.
- Mandible is the preferred site.
- Slight male predilection.
- Swelling and pain are consistent features. Depending on the location of the lesion, patients may experience other symptoms such as paraesthesia, loosening of teeth, nasal obstruction and epistaxis.
- Radiograph shows a mixture of radiolucency and radiopacity. Extracortical bone produces a typical 'sunburst' appearance.
- Root resorption is common.

Diagnosis

- History, clinical examination and radiographical and histological evaluations.

Management

- Surgery and surgery with chemotherapy are preferred over the use of radiotherapy. Recurrence and metastasis are common.
- Patient needs to be referred to an oncologist. Treatment requires a multidisciplinary approach.

Burkitt's Lymphoma

Definition/Description

- Burkitt's lymphoma is a B-cell malignant neoplasm that occurs in children in an endemic form in the sub-Sahara region and in a sporadic form outside of Africa.

Cause

- 95% of the endemic form of Burkitt's lymphoma in Africa is associated with Epstein-Barr virus, whereas the sporadic Burkitt's lymphoma has only 15% association with Epstein-Barr virus.
- The third type of Burkitt's lymphoma occurs in patients with immunodeficiency, which is also associated with Epstein-Barr virus.

Clinical Features

- Children between the ages of three and eight years are commonly affected in the endemic form, whereas older children (between the ages of 10 and 12 years) are commonly affected in the sporadic form.
- Jaw lesions are common; maxilla is the preferred site in the endemic form, whereas ileocecal region of the bowel is affected commonly in the sporadic form.
- Jaw lesions show extensive osteolytic changes. The earliest sign is loosening of the teeth. Teeth float in the tumour mass.
- Expansion of the jaw and protrusion of the tumour mass into the mouth are rapid. Bilateral Burkitt's lymphoma (i.e., involvement of all four quadrants of the jaws by the tumour) may occur.
- Early radiographical signs show a loss of lamina dura and enlargement of the crypts of developing teeth in children. Focal areas of radiolucency and the displacement of teeth are also common findings on the extraoral radiographical views.

Diagnosis

- History, clinical examination and radiographical and histological evaluations.

Management

- The disease is fatal if not treated within first six months of diagnosis. Intensive chemotherapy yields good results.
- Refer the patient to an oncologist or maxillofacial surgeon.

Multiple Myeloma

Definition/Description

- Multiple myeloma is a malignant neoplastic proliferation of plasma cells with bone marrow involvement.

Cause

- Monoclonal malignant proliferation of plasma cells.

Clinical Features

- Vertebrae, ribs, skull, pelvis, scapula and clavicle are the skeletal sites that are involved.
- Mandible and maxilla are occasionally involved.
- Male predilection exists.
- Affected individuals are usually older than 40 years.
- Bone pain, pathological fractures, anaemia, hypercalcaemia and renal failure are common.
- Radiological appearance includes multiple well-defined, punched-out radiolucencies of the bone (evident on skull views but usually not evident on bone scan).

Diagnosis

- History, clinical examination, radiological examination and histological examinations.

Management

- Chemotherapy and supportive therapy are useful modalities of treatment. Bisphosphonates also have beneficial effects.
- Refer the patient to an oncologist.

TUMOUR-LIKE LESIONS OF THE JAWS

Fibrous Dysplasia

Definition/Description

- Fibrous dysplasia (FD) is characterised by localised replacement of normal bone by fibrous connective tissue that contains abnormal bone.

Cause

- The cause is unknown.

Clinical Features

- FD is a localised abnormality that can involve one (monostotic) or multiple (polyostotic) bones.
- Monostotic FD frequently affects the maxilla-facial skeleton.
- Initial development of FD causes facial swelling and asymmetry.
- Diagnosis is often done in infancy and childhood.
- Slow-growing lesion, which may become arrested, coinciding with the onset of puberty, is indicative.
- FD may show slight female preponderance.
- Maxilla-to-mandible ratio of FD is 2:1, with site predilection for the posterior part of the jaw.
- FD is usually asymptomatic, but pain may be a presenting symptom.
- In polyostotic FD, in addition to the bone involvement, *café au lait* pigmentation of the skin may also be present. This condition is called McCune-Albright syndrome. Patients with this condition may also present other symptoms of multiple endocrinopathies (such as precocious puberty, pituitary adenoma and hyperthyroidism).
- Occasionally, headaches, loss of vision, proptosis, diplopia, loss of hearing, anosmia, nasal obstruction, epistaxis and sinusitis-like symptoms may be present due to the encroachment by the lesion of anatomic spaces or foramina.

Radiographical Features

- Panoramic, reverse Towne, posterior-anterior and lateral skull views are adequate to identify FD lesions in the mandible. For maxillary lesions, computed tomography is useful.
- Radiographical features are variable: The most common feature is the 'ground glass' appearance of the lesion. The lesion lacks a sharply demarcated border and blends into the surrounding normal bone.

Diagnosis

- History, clinical examination and radiographical and histopathological features of the lesion are important.

- Histologically, the marrow is replaced by cellular fibrous tissue and the bone trabeculae are small and irregular in shape.

Management

- Refer the patient to an oral and maxillofacial surgeon. Surgery is the only mode of treatment. Cosmetic reduction of the lesion in the jaws is adequate in most cases.
- Radiation therapy is contraindicated, since there are cases that have developed postradiation osteosarcomas.

Cherubism

Definition/Description

- It is a hereditary condition characterised by painless, bilateral, symmetrical expansion of the jaws.

Cause

- An autosomally dominant hereditable condition.

Clinical Features

- Predominantly seen in males.
- Children aged two to five years are affected.
- Lesions may be confined to both mandible and maxilla.
- There is a site predilection for mandibular angle, ascending ramus and maxillary tuberosity. In maxillary involvement, the eyes are displaced upwards, revealing scleral show.
- Radiographically, the involved bone shows multilocular radiolucency.
- Primary teeth may be loose and permanent teeth are displaced.

Diagnosis

- History, clinical examination and radiological and histological evaluations.

Management

- Surgical curettage is the treatment of choice.
- Refer the patient to an oral and maxillofacial surgeon.

Ossifying Fibroma or Cementifying Fibroma

Definition/Description

- Ossifying fibroma (cementifying fibroma) is a slow-growing, benign neoplasm of the jaw bones, occurring most often in the mandible. It is composed of bone and/or cementum that develop within fibrous connective tissue.

Cause

- Cause of ossifying fibroma or cementifying fibroma is unknown, but developmental and traumatic causes have been suggested.

Clinical Features

- Ossifying fibroma is a slow-growing, painless benign neoplasm.
- Common in the third or fourth decade of life.
- Female predilection has been reported (male:female, 1:5).
- Mandible is the preferred site.
- Involvement of the molar-premolar area is common.

Radiographical Features

- Initially, it presents as a well-demarcated radiolucent lesion.
- At later stages, it has mixed radiolucent and radiopaque appearance.
- Displacement of the mandibular canal may occur in long-standing lesions.

Diagnosis

- History, clinical examination and radiographical and histological evaluations are useful.

Management

- Surgical removal of the tumour is the treatment of choice.
- Refer the patient to an oral and maxillofacial surgeon.
- Ossifying fibroma shows a tendency to recur.
- Radiotherapy is contraindicated because of the possibility of malignant transformation of the lesion.

Brown Tumour of Hyperparathyroidism

Definition/Description

- Excess parathyroid hormone in hyperparathyroidism can stimulate osteoclast-mediated bone resorption, which may produce a focal bone lesion called brown tumour of hyperparathyroidism.

Cause

- Primary and secondary hyperparathyroidism.

Clinical Features

- Jaw lesions of brown tumour are common.
- Well-defined unilocular or multilocular radiolucent lesions are seen.
- Mandible is commonly involved.
- Female predilection has been reported.
- Pain may be a feature.
- Radiographically, well-defined radiolucency is seen.
- Patient presents symptoms associated with hypercalcaemia, and laboratory findings suggest impaired renal function.

Diagnosis

- History, clinical examination and radiographical features.
- Laboratory tests are recommended for hyperparathyroidism.

Management

- If hyperparathyroidism is confirmed, the condition must be treated.
- The jaw lesions resolve without any further treatment.

SUGGESTED READINGS

Dunlap C. *Abnormalities of Teeth*. Kansas, MO: UMKC School of Dentistry; 2004. Available from: http://dentistry.umkc.edu/Practicing_Communities/asset/AbnormalitiesofTeeth.pdf

Dunlap C. *Odontogenic Tumors: The Short Version*. Kansas, MO: UMKC School of Dentistry; 2001. Available from: http://dentistry.umkc.edu/Practicing_Communities/asset/OdontTumors.pdf

Dunlap C. *Cysts of the Jaws*. Kansas, MO: UMKC School of Dentistry; 2000. Available from: http://dentistry.umkc.edu/Practicing_Communities/asset/Jcysts.pdf

Cawson RA, Odell EW. Cysts of the jaw bones. *Cawson's Essentials of Oral Pathology and Oral Medicine*. 8th ed. Edinburgh, Scotland: Churchill Livingstone; 2008. pp. 115–32.

Cawson RA, Odell EW. Odontogenic tumours and tumour-like lesions of the jaws. *Cawson's Essentials of Oral Pathology and Oral Medicine*. 8th ed. Edinburgh, Scotland: Churchill Livingstone; 2008. pp. 136–54.

Chapter 33

Oral manifestations of systemic diseases

S. R. Prabhu

ORAL MANIFESTATIONS OF GASTROINTESTINAL DISEASES

Gastroesophageal Reflux Disease

- Regurgitation of acidic gastric content can reduce the pH in the oral cavity to less than 5.5. This acidic environment begins to dissolve the enamel surface.
- The palatal aspects of the maxillary anterior teeth and premolars are commonly affected. Erosive lesions on the tooth surface appear smooth, shiny and yellow. Erosive lesions are sensitive to cold.
- Xerostomia, burning mouth syndrome and halitosis are common in gastroesophageal reflux disease.
- Dental erosion can be managed by appropriate restorative treatment by dentists.
- Patient referral to a dentist is recommended.

Bulimia Nervosa and Anorexia

- Bulimia nervosa is characterised by recurrent binge-eating episodes. The bulimic individual (usually a female) consumes abnormally large amounts of food in a relatively short period of time, followed by purging. The vomit is acidic, which causes damage to the teeth. Dental and oral aspects in bulimia nervosa include the following:
  - ◆ Dental erosion and xerostomia, which are common, increase the rate of dental caries.
  - ◆ Parotid enlargement is often reported.
  - ◆ Dental erosion requires dental restorative treatment. With normalisation of nutritional status, xerostomia and parotid gland enlargement disappear.
- Refer the patient to a dentist for dental treatment.

Crohn's Disease

- Oral manifestations in Crohn's disease include diffuse labial, gingival or mucosal swelling, cobblestoning of the buccal mucosa and gingivae, aphthous ulcers, mucosal tags, angular cheilitis and oral granulomas.
- Oral lesions usually resolve with systemic treatment of the underlying disease.

- Intralesional injections of corticosteroids (triamcinolone acetonide) may be necessary for labial swellings.
- Patient referral to a dentist is recommended.

Ulcerative Colitis

- Oral manifestations in ulcerative colitis can occur during the periods of exacerbation of the disease. These include aphthous ulceration or superficial haemorrhagic ulcers, angular stomatitis and pyostomatitis vegetans.
- Oral lesions usually respond to systemic treatment of ulcerative colitis.
- Local or systemic corticosteroids or dapsone yield good results.
- In some cases, treatment of ulcerative colitis may cause oral side-effects, such as xerostomia.

Coeliac Disease

- Oral manifestations in coeliac disease include glossitis, angular cheilitis, bleeding tendencies, oral mucosal ulcers, dental enamel hypoplasia, delayed eruption and oral mucosal signs of anaemia.
- Oral manifestations respond to the treatment of the underlying disorder. For successful management of the disease, gluten should be avoided in food.

Irritable Bowel Syndrome

- Psychogenic oral symptoms such as facial pain and temporomandibular disorder symptoms may be present in patients with irritable bowel syndrome.
- Oral manifestations may respond to the treatment of the underlying condition, but the response is variable.

Alcoholic Liver Disease

- Oral manifestations in alcoholic liver disease include jaundice of the oral mucosa, advanced periodontal disease, parotid enlargement, sweet and musty oral malodour and bleeding tendencies.
- For the management of oral symptoms and signs, referral of the patient to a dentist is recommended.
- Patient must be advised to stop alcohol consumption.

Liver Cirrhosis

- Oral manifestations of liver cirrhosis include jaundice of the oral mucosa (soft palate and sublingual region), bleeding tendencies and poor oral hygiene.
- Patient referral to a dentist for oral complaints is recommended.

ORAL MANIFESTATION OF CARDIOVASCULAR DISEASES

Angina Pectoris and Myocardial Infarction

- During the attack of angina or myocardial infarction, the patient may complain of acute pain in the jaw.
- Jaw pain may resolve as soon as the chest pain is brought under control.

Congenital Heart Disease

- Oral manifestations of congenital heart disease may include delayed tooth eruption, frequent positional anomalies of teeth and hypoplastic enamel. Mucosa may show pallor.
- In these patients, a high risk for dental caries exists and an increase in the occurrence of periodontal disease is common.
- For the management of oral conditions, patient referral to a dentist is recommended.

Rheumatic Fever or Infective Endocarditis

- Many clinicians believe that patients with rheumatic fever may have an increased risk of developing infective endocarditis after invasive dental treatment. They recommend that these patients should be given antibiotic prophylaxis before invasive dental procedures such as tooth extraction, implant placement, subgingival probing and scaling, endodontic treatment, placement of matrix and orthodontic bands, and intraligamentary local anaesthetic injections.
- Recommended prophylaxis includes 2 g of oral amoxicillin one hour before the procedure and, for penicillin-sensitive patients, 1.5 g of erythromycin one hour before the procedure, followed by 0.5 g six hours later.
- In some countries (e.g., the U.K.), prophylactic treatment is not recommended before dental invasive treatment.

Hypertension

- There are no specific oral manifestations of hypertension.
- The practitioner should be aware of the oral side-effects of anti-hypertensive drugs. These include xerostomia, gingival hyperplasia (with nifedipine), salivary gland swelling (with clonidine) and increased postoperative bleeding (with aspirin).
- Calcium channel blockers can cause mucosal lichenoid reactions and gingival swellings.

ORAL MANIFESTATIONS OF RESPIRATORY DISEASES

Chronic Obstructive Pulmonary Disease

- There are no significant oral manifestations of chronic obstructive pulmonary disease.
- Blue bloaters may show signs of cyanosis of the lips or intraoral mucosal structures.

Lung Abscess and Bronchiectasis

- Periodontal disease and halitosis are common in these diseases.

Pulmonary Tuberculosis

- Primary tuberculosis of the oral soft tissues is extremely rare; however, secondary involvement of the oral tissues can occur.
- Lesions of the secondary infection may include painless tuberculous ulcers on the dorsum or lateral borders of the tongue.
- The edges of tuberculous ulcers are undermined.

- Cervical lymphadenopathy is present.
- Tuberculous ulcers are chronic ulcers.
- Ulcers disappear once the systemic infection is treated with antituberculosis medication.

Cystic Fibrosis

- In cystic fibrosis, disorders of the salivary glands can give rise to xerostomia.
- Gingivitis and swelling of the lips are reported in these patients.
- Altered amounts of calcium and phosphates are present in saliva. This may promote higher calculus formation and enamel defects.

ORAL MANIFESTATIONS OF CHRONIC KIDNEY FAILURE AND NEPHROTIC SYNDROME

- In chronic renal failure and nephrotic syndrome, patients may present any of the following oral symptoms and signs:
    - ♦ Mucosal pallor due to anaemia.
    - ♦ Orange colouration of the mucosa due to deposition of carotene-like pigments.
    - ♦ Xerostomia with or without candidiasis.
    - ♦ Metallic taste.
    - ♦ Ammonia-like salivary odour.
    - ♦ Uraemic stomatitis, and in severe cases, burning sensation and ulceration.
    - ♦ Petechiae and gingival bleeding.
    - ♦ Necrotising ulcerative gingivitis.
    - ♦ Radiological findings include a 'ground glass' appearance of the alveolar bone.

ORAL MANIFESTATIONS OF ENDOCRINE AND METABOLIC DISEASES

Hyperthyroidism

- In hyperthyroidism, there is an increased risk for periodontal disease and premature eruption of teeth.

Hypothyroidism

- Untreated neonatal (congenital) hypothyroidism may result in an altered development of the jaws, malocclusion, delayed tooth eruption and a protruding tongue (cretinism).
- In older children and adults, hypothyroidism may result in macroglossia, glossitis, salivary gland swelling and an increased risk of dental caries and periodontal disease.
- In rare instances, oral lichen planus may be seen in hypothyroid patients.
- Adults with hypothyroidism may show delayed tooth eruption, an enlarged tongue, periodontal disease, alteration in taste sensation and delayed wound healing.

Hypopituitarism

- Delayed eruption of teeth is a feature of hypopituitarism.

Hyperpituitarism (Acromegaly)

- Mandibular prognathism, malocclusion, diastema, enlarged tongue and ankylosis of roots are common in acromegaly.

Diabetes Insipidus

- In patients with diabetes insipidus, osseous infiltrates are often found on the skull and jaws. These infiltrates can be identified on conventional dental radiographs.
- Loose teeth are often reported in diabetes insipidus. These may be due to Langerhans cell histiocytosis of the gingival tissues.
- Due to excessive thirst, children with diabetes insipidus drink large amounts of water (fluoridated at optimal level), which can result in dental fluorosis.

Diabetes Mellitus

- People with poorly controlled diabetes have an increased risk of periodontal disease and impaired salivary gland function.
- Diabetic patients may present with candidiasis, taste dysfunction, salivary dysfunction, burning mouth syndrome and generalised atrophy of the tongue.
- Delayed wound healing is a major consequence of diabetes mellitus.

Addison's Disease (Adrenal Insufficiency)

- Pigmentation of the oral mucosa is a feature of Addison's disease.
- Pigmentation can appear on any intraoral site, but in a majority of patients, the dorsum of the tongue and buccal mucosa are involved.
- Pigmented lesions are brown, diffuse and patchy in distribution.

Cushing Syndrome (Adrenocortical Excess)

- A Cushingoid person presents with a moon face and frontal balding.

Hypocalcaemia

- Chvostek's sign is a facial manifestation of severe hypocalcaemia (tetany). Chvostek's sign is characterised by involuntary twitching of the facial muscles, which are elicited by a light tapping of the facial nerve just anterior to the external auditory meatus.
- Tetany is characterised by paraesthesia of the lips, tongue, fingers and feet, carpopedal spasm, generalised muscle aching and spasms of the facial musculature.

Hypercalcaemia

- Jaw bone demineralisation, loss of lamina dura and osteitis fibrosa cystica (von Recklinghausen's disease of bone) may be seen in patients with hypercalcaemia.

ORAL MANIFESTATIONS OF THE NERVOUS SYSTEM

Stroke

- Oral and facial manifestations of stroke include slurred speech, difficulty in swallowing, unilateral paralysis of the oral and facial musculature, deviation of the tongue and loss of sensory stimuli of the oral tissues. These symptoms may occur after an episode of stroke.

Epilepsy

- Facial twitching is a feature of petit mal seizures. Patients taking phenytoin may present with hyperplasia of the maxillary and mandibular anterior gingival tissues.
- Oral soft tissue injuries (e.g., ulcers of the tongue) due to trauma received during seizures may be detected.

Parkinson's Disease

- Other than excessive salivation, there are no specific oral manifestations of Parkinson's disease.

Multiple Sclerosis

- Patients with multiple sclerosis (MS) may experience facial pain, and the disorder can trigger trigeminal neuralgia or facial palsy.
- Patients may complain of facial anaesthesia or numbness of the lower lip.
- Xerostomia and associated oral findings are common.

Myasthenia Gravis

- Oral manifestations of myasthenia gravis include facial weakness, sensation of stiffness of the mouth, inability to whistle, myasthenic snarl, chewing difficulty, regurgitation of fluids through the nose and choking.
- Patients of myasthenia gravis also experience inability to keep the head in balance.

ORAL MANIFESTATIONS OF HAEMATOLOGICAL DISEASES

Anaemia

- In all forms of anaemia, the oral mucosa is pale.
- Atrophic glossitis is a feature of **megaloblastic anaemia**. The dorsum of the tongue is smooth, bald and red. There may be accompanying erythematous candidiasis.
- In **iron-deficiency anaemia**, the dorsum of the tongue appears bald and red. Patients often complain of a burning sensation.
- In **Plummer-Vinson syndrome**, oral ulcerations, erythroplakic patches or squamous cell carcinomas may occur. Pharyngeal involvement is also common in these patients.
- Patients with **haemolytic anaemia** may show mucosal pallor and jaundice due to haemolysis. Dental radiographs may show increased radiolucency with lamellar striations due to hyperplasia of the bone marrow.
- In **sickle-cell anaemia**, an increased widening, a decreased number of trabeculations and signs of osteoporosis of the jaw bones may be evident on radiographs. In these patients, trabeculae between the teeth appear horizontal, giving a 'step ladder' appearance, and lamina dura may be more distinct and dense. Delayed

eruption of teeth and dental hypoplasia may be seen in patients with sickle-cell anaemia.
- Bimaxillary protrusion and alveolar enlargement, giving rise to chipmunk facies, is a feature of **thalassaemia major**. Vaso-occlusive events may precipitate ischaemic necrosis in the bone.

Thrombocytopaenia

- In thrombocytopaenia, oral mucous membranes may show purpuric spots. Often, these are accompanied by purpuric spots on the skin.
- Spontaneous gingival bleeding is also a feature of a severe form of thrombocytopaenia.

Haemophilia

- Spontaneous bleeding from oral soft tissues may occur in the severe form of the disorder.
- Excessive bleeding from trauma or surgery, including tooth extraction, is common in these patients.

Leukaemia

- Patients with acute or chronic leukaemia may reveal ulceration of the mucosa, gingival enlargement (due to leukaemic infiltrate), petechiae and ecchymosis of the mucous membrane.
- Gingival enlargement is common in myelogenous leukaemia.
- Lymhadenopathy is common in all forms of leukaemia.
- Acute oral infections are common. These infections must be promptly treated and their recurrence must be prevented.

Multiple Myeloma

- Oral manifestations of multiple myeloma include enlargement of the tongue due to amyloid deposition.
- Oral symptoms may include paraesthesia and pain of the jaw bones.
- Radiographs of the jaw bones or the skull show characteristic single or multiple 'punched out' radiolucencies.

Non-Hodgkin's Lymphoma

- Oral manifestations of non-Hodgkin's lymphoma include Waldeyer's tonsillar ring, oropharynx and soft palate.
- Salivary glands may also be involved.
- Involvement of the gingiva, palate, alveolar ridge, buccal sulcus and floor of the mouth has also been reported.
- Petechiae, fungal infections, viral infections, mucosal ulcers and oral paraesthesia are common.

ORAL MANIFESTATIONS OF IMMUNE SYSTEM DISORDERS

Allergic Mucositis

- Allergic contact dermatitis involving mucosa can be termed allergic (contact) mucositis.

- Allergic mucositis can manifest as lichenoid patches of the mucosa or as swelling of the tongue or lips because of inflammatory oedema.
- Allergies to lipstick, toothpaste, food items, spices and chewing gums containing artificial cinnamon have been reported to cause allergic contact mucositis.

Angioedema

- Angioedema (formerly known as angioneurotic oedema) is characterised by rapid swelling of the dermis, subcutaneous tissue, mucosa and submucosal tissues.
- Clinical features of allergic angioedema include acute and pronounced labial and periorbital swelling.
- Swelling can also extend to the tongue, pharynx and neck, causing respiratory obstruction.

Sjögren's Syndrome

- Oral manifestations of Sjögren's syndrome include disturbances in taste sensation, a fissured tongue, candidal infections and extensive dental decay due to xerostomia.
- A risk of development of lymphoma of the parotid glands exists at a later stage of the primary disease.

Temporal Arteritis

- The features of temporal arteritis include scalp tenderness, headaches, pulseless temporal arteries, ulcers on the scalp, thickened and tender temporal arteries and visual disturbances, including blindness in the advanced cases.

Wegener's Granulomatosis

- Nasal and oral manifestations include bloody nasal discharge, a depressed nasal bridge, ulcers on the palate and pharynx (painless or painful), strawberry gingivitis, underlying bone destruction accompanied by loosening of the teeth and nonspecific ulcerations throughout oral mucosa.

Behcet's Disease

- Aphthous-like oral ulcers may occur in Behcet's disease.

Human Immunodeficiency Virus Infection or Acquired Immune Deficiency Syndrome

- Specific conditions in the mouth caused by human immunodeficiency virus (HIV) infection have not been reported.
  - Conditions seen in HIV-infected patients occur due to immunocompromised status.
  - Oral conditions include the following:
    - Candidiasis
    - Herpes simplex virus infections
    - Ulcerative gingivitis or ulcerative periodontitis
    - Linear gingival erythema

- Hairy leukoplakia
- Kaposi's sarcoma
- Hodgkin's and non-Hodgkin's lymphoma
- Cytomegalovirus infections
- Human papillomavirus infections
- Aphthous-like ulcerations
- Salivary gland swelling

Detailed description of the above-listed conditions can be found in Chapter 37 (Oral lesions in HIV infection).

SUGGESTED READINGS

Chi AC, Neville BW, Krayer JW, Gonsalves WC. Oral manifestations of systemic disease. *Am Fam Physician*. 2010;82:1381–8. [accessed: 2015 Aug]. Available from: http://www.aafp.org/afp/2010/1201/p1381.html

Casiglia JM. Oral manifestations of systemic diseases. Medscape [Internet]. Atlanta (GA): WebMD LLC; 2013. [accessed: 2015 Aug]. Available from: http://emedicine.medscape.com/article/1081029-overview

Sroussi H, Prabhu A, Epstein J. Which antibiotic prophylaxis guidelines for infective endocarditis Should Canadian dentists follow? *J Can Dent Assoc*. 2007;73:401–5.

Chapter 34

Drug-induced oral adverse reactions, including medication-related osteonecrosis of the jaw

S. R. Prabhu

DRUGS ASSOCIATED WITH XEROSTOMIA

- Class of drugs that can induce xerostomia include antihistamines, antidepressants, antipsychotics, antihypertensive agents, anticholinergics and decongestants.
- Xerostomia is common in the elderly patients taking multiple medications.

DRUGS ASSOCIATED WITH NONSPECIFIC ULCERATIONS AND MUCOSITIS

- Medications that can cause nonspecific ulcerations and mucositis include methotrexate, 5-fluorouracil, melphalan, doxorubicin, barbiturates, dapsone, sulphonamides, tetracyclines, indomethacin, salicylates, naproxen, methyldopa, penicillamine, phenylbutazone, propranolol, thiazides, tolbutamide, alendronate, captopril and phenytoin.
- By direct contact with the mucosa, aspirin and hydrogen peroxide can cause nonspecific ulcerations.

DRUGS ASSOCIATED WITH MUCOSAL SWELLINGS

- Medications that can induce mucosal swellings include penicillins and penicillin derivatives, cephalosporins, barbiturates, aspirin, sulpha drugs and angiotensin-converting-enzyme inhibitors.
- Drugs can induce hypersensitivity reactions or disorders mediated by immunoglobulin E and mast cells, which can range from focal swellings to full-blown anaphylaxis.

DRUGS ASSOCIATED WITH VESICULOBULLOUS LESIONS

- Medications that can cause vesiculobullous oral lesions can be classified under different clinical categories as shown below:
    - Pemphigus-like lesions: Medications associated with such lesions include ampicillin, captopril, cephalexin, ethambutol, heroin, ibuprofen, penicillamine, phenobarbital, practolol, propranolol and rifampin.

- ◆ Pemphigoid-like lesions: Class of drugs associated with these lesions include antirheumatics, cardiovascular medications, antibiotics and sulphonamides.
- ◆ Erythema multiforme-like lesions: Class of drugs associated with these lesions include antibiotics, barbiturates, protease inhibitors and nonsteroidal anti-inflammatory drugs (NSAIDs).

DRUGS ASSOCIATED WITH LICHEN PLANUS-LIKE (LICHENOID) REACTIONS

- Class of medications that can cause lichenoid (lichen planus-like) reactions include antibiotics, anticonvulsants, antidiabetics, antifungals, antihistamines, antihypertensives, antimalarials, antiretrovirals, calcium-channel blockers, chemotherapeutics, immunomodulators, NSAIDs, psychiatric drugs, barbiturates and protease inhibitors.

DRUGS ASSOCIATED WITH LUPUS ERYTHEMATOSUS-LIKE ORAL LESIONS

- Medications that can cause lupus erythematosus-like oral lesions include carbamazepine, chlorpromazine, griseofulvin, hydantoins, hydralazine, isoniazid, lithium, methyldopa, penicillamine, primidone, quinidine, reserpine, streptomycin, thiouracils and trimethadione.

DRUGS ASSOCIATED WITH MUCOSAL PIGMENTATIONS

- Drugs that can cause mucosal pigmentation include amiodarone, antimalarials, busulfan, clofazimine, cyclophosphamide, oestrogen, imatinib, ketoconazole, minocycline, chlorpromazine and zidovudine.

DRUGS ASSOCIATED WITH GINGIVAL ENLARGEMENT

- Drugs that can cause gingival enlargement include calcium-channel blockers, cyclosporine, phenytoin and sodium valproate.

DRUGS ASSOCIATED WITH ALTERATIONS IN TASTE

- Taste changes are common, especially among the elderly patients who take multiple medications. Some drugs can alter the food taste, causing a metallic, salty or bitter taste in the mouth.
- Drugs causing taste disturbances include angiotensin-converting-enzyme inhibitors, aspirin, diclofenac, diltiazem, metronidazole and sulphonamides.

MEDICATION-RELATED OSTEONECROSIS OF THE JAW

Definition/Description

- Medication-related osteonecrosis of the jaw (MRONJ) is said to be present in patients with the following conditions[1]:
  - ◆ Current or previous treatment with antiresorptive or antiangiogenic agents.
  - ◆ Exposed bone or bone that can be probed through an intraoral or an extraoral fistula(e) in the maxillofacial region and has persisted for more than eight weeks.

♦ No history of radiation therapy for the jaws or obvious metastatic disease of the jaws.

Cause

- Antiresorptive medications:
  - ♦ Bisphosphonates (BPs): Intravenous BPs given once in a year are used to manage cancer-related conditions, skeletal-related events associated with bone metastasis of solid tumours (lung, breast and prostate malignancies) and lytic malignant lesions, such as multiple myeloma.
  - ♦ Oral BPs are used for osteoporosis and osteopaenia, Paget's disease of bone and osteogenesis imperfecta.
  - ♦ Evidence suggests that the use of oral BPs for a minimum of three years is required for the development of osteonecrosis of the jaw.
  - ♦ RANK Ligand inhibitor (denosumab): It is an antiresorptive medication that inhibits osteoclast function and associated bone resorption. It is effective in reducing skeletal-related events related to metastatic bone disease of solid tumours.
  - ♦ Antiangiogenic medications: These medications (e.g., zoledronic acid) inhibit angiogenesis and cause avascular necrosis.

MRONJ occurs exclusively in the jaw bones. Factors implicated in the pathogenesis of MRONJ include the following:

- Altered bone remodelling or oversuppression of bone resorption
- Suppression of innate or acquired immunity
- Vitamin D deficiency
- Soft tissue BP toxicity
- Inflammation or infection

Oral Health-Associated Risk Factors

- Dentoalveolar surgery is the major risk factor for MRONJ.
- Trauma during intubation, fractures, dentures, pre-existing dental inflammatory disease and mandibular tori disease.

Clinical Features

- Areas of exposed and necrotic jaw bone may remain asymptomatic for months.
- Lesions may become symptomatic when surrounding soft tissues are inflamed.
- Pain and swelling are experienced in the affected area; these symptoms are more frequently in the mandible than in the maxilla (2:1 ratio).
- Secondary infection with or without pus may be present. Chronic maxillary sinusitis may be the presenting symptom when the maxilla is involved.
- Numbness or heavy sensation may be reported in the affected area.

- An irregular mucosal ulceration with exposed bone in the jaw, persisting for longer than eight weeks, is typical clinical finding.
- Exposed bone is yellow-white in colour, with smooth or ragged borders (Figure 34.1), sometimes with associated extraoral or intraoral sinus tracts.
- Halitosis is seen in patients with MRONJ.
- Radiographical findings in advanced cases show poorly defined areas of moth-eaten radiolucencies in the affected jaw. Computed tomography and magnetic resonance imaging are also useful imaging studies.

Diagnosis

- The patient's history and clinical examination are recommended for diagnosis.
- Diagnostic criteria include the following:
  - Patient presents an area of exposed bone in the jaw, persisting for more than eight weeks.
  - Patient must present no history of radiation therapy for the head and neck region.
  - Patient must be receiving or must have taken BP medication.
  - Some investigators recommend measuring the levels of serum C-terminal collagen peptides (biomarkers of bone turnover) to stratify patients' risk of bisphosphonate-associated osteonecrosis of the jaw (BONJ) before dental surgery. Values less than 100 pg/mL are considered high risk. Too much variability is a problem associated with this method of investigation.
- Differential diagnosis include the following:
  - Alveolar osteitis
  - Sinusitis

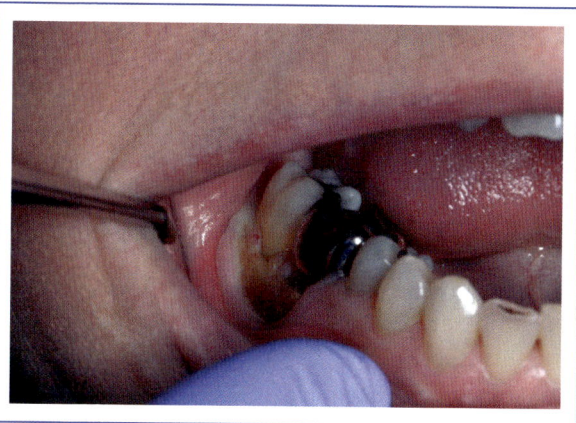

Figure 34.1 Bisphosphonate-associated osteonecrosis of the lower jaw in a patient who has received intravenous bisphosphonate.
Courtesy: Nagamani Narayana.

- Gingivitis or periodontitis
- Chronic sclerosing osteomyelitis
- Osteoradionecrosis, if patient taking antiresorptive or antiangiogenic medication has also undergone radiation therapy for head and neck cancer.

Management

- Use of antimicrobial mouth rinses, topical antifungals and systemic antibiotics are necessary to prevent infection.
- Discontiuing bisphosphonates and avoidance of surgical procedures in the mouth are recommended.
- Referral of the patient to an maxillofacial surgeon for surgical debridement and resection of the necrotic bone is recommended.

RECOMMENDATIONS FOR MEDICAL AND DENTAL PRACTITIONERS

Recommendations for medical practitioners and dental practitioners are as follows[2]:

Before Bisphosphonate Prescription

- The medical practitioner should discuss with the patient the following:
  - Benefits of BP (or use of other antiresorptive or antiangiogenic agents) treatment.
  - Risk of adverse events, including osteonecrosis of the jaw.
  - Risk and/or benefit of other treatment options.
  - Option of dental treatment, if in doubt.
- The dental practitioner should make the patient dentally fit, so that the patient has a low chance of future extractions.

Patients on Bisphosphonates

- The medical practitioner should take the following steps:
  - If the medical practitioner is suspicious of osteonecrosis of the jaw in the patient, then he or she should refer the patient to an appropriate dental specialist for further investigation.
- The dental practitioner should take the following steps:
  - Be aware of the dosage of antiresorptive or antiangiogenic medication and other risk factors.
  - Avoid extractions or other jaw bone surgery.
  - If surgery is unavoidable, then obtain informed consent from the patient.
  - Perform extractions with minimal trauma and suture the socket.
- In patients with established MRONJ, systemic antibiotics for three weeks or more and antimicrobial mouth rinses may be necessary. This approach reduces the infection and pain. Surgical debridement of the necrotic bone assists in the healing process.
- Hyperbaric oxygen therapy is also beneficial.
- For patients taking oral antiresorptive medication (in particular, BPs) for three years or more, some clinicians recommend a drug holiday of at least three months before dentoalveolar surgery and throughout the healing period.

REFERENCES

1. American Association of Oral and Maxillofacial Surgeons. Medication-related osteonecrosis of the jaw: update. Rosemont, IL: AAOMS; 2014. Available from: http://aaoms.org/docs/position_paper/mronj_position_paper.pdf
2. Sambrook P, Oliver I, Goss A. Bisphosphonates and osteonecrosis of the jaw. *Aust Fam Physician*. 2006;35:801–3.

SUGGESTED READINGS

Pejcic A. Drug-induced oral reactions. In: Virdi MS, editor. *Emerging Trends in Oral Health Sciences and Dentistry*. Rijeka, Croatia: InTech; 2015. doi: 10.5772/59261.

Berenson JR, Stopek AT. Medication related osteonecrosis of the jaw in patients with cancer [Internet]. [Place unknown]: UpToDate, Inc; 2015 [updated 2015 Aug 18]. Available from: http://www.uptodate.com/contents/medication-related-osteonecrosis

Chapter 35

Oral health in pregnancy

S. C. Yeoh

PREGNANCY AND ORAL HEALTH

- Maternal periodontal disease has been associated with preterm birth as well as infant low birth weight.[1] In addition, high carriage of cariogenic bacteria in mothers can increase the risk of dental caries in the child.[2] All pregnant women should be educated on these risks and encouraged to seek professional dental advice. Maintenance of good oral hygiene is paramount.
- Several oral soft tissue lesions are associated with pregnancy, including gingivitis and 'pregnancy tumours'.
- Pregnant women can safely undergo routine dental treatment, including intraoral radiography, periodontal treatments, restorations and extractions. However, these are often deferred until the second trimester.

COMMON ORAL PROBLEMS IN PREGNANCY

Tooth Erosion

Pregnant women are often at risk of tooth erosion, particularly if they experience morning sickness with vomiting and/or acid reflux.[3] Enamel erosion can lead to tooth sensitivity and wear.

Patients should be encouraged to reduce the risk of tooth erosion by adopting the following practices:

- Appropriate use of antiemetic medication and antacids to reduce the frequency of exposure of the teeth to gastric acid.
- Use a sodium bicarbonate mouth rinse immediately after vomiting (one teaspoon of sodium bicarbonate in a cup of water).[4]
- Chew sugar-free gum to stimulate saliva flow to help neutralise and wash away acid.
- Avoid brushing the teeth immediately after vomiting, as this may increase the risk of tooth erosion.
- Supplementing routine oral hygiene regime with a fluoride mouth rinse and products such as GC Tooth Mousse™ may protect eroded or sensitive teeth.[5]

Dental Caries

- Pregnant women are at a higher risk of developing dental caries than the general population. This may be due to increased intraoral

acidity, sugary dietary cravings and nausea or vomiting, making oral hygiene practices difficult.[6]
- If left untreated, dental caries can lead to serious consequences, including development of abscesses and facial cellulitis.

Studies have shown that mothers who have a high level of caries also increase the risk of development of dental caries in their children.[2]

Patients should be encouraged to continue with good oral hygiene practices throughout pregnancy. Patients should adopt the following practices:

- Brush the teeth twice a day with fluoride-containing toothpaste.
- Floss twice a day.
- Limit consumption of a high-sugar diet.
- Go for a regular dental check-up.

Gingivitis

- Gingivitis is the inflammation of the gums. It is commonly seen in pregnant women because of fluctuations in pregnancy hormones, in combination with a decreased immune response and alterations in the oral flora.
- Gingivitis affects up to 75% of pregnant women.[3] Studies have shown that approximately 50% of women with gingivitis experience a significant exacerbation during pregnancy.[6]
- Vigorous oral hygiene practices reduce the severity of gingivitis. Patients should be encouraged to seek professional dental care.

Periodontitis

- Periodontal disease, more specifically, periodontitis has been linked to poor pregnancy outcomes. Periodontitis is a destructive infection that affects the gingival tissues, thus leading to underlying bone destruction and loosening of teeth.
- Bacteria infiltrate the periodontium-producing toxins, which stimulate a chronic inflammatory response.[7] Recurrent bacteraemia may trigger the release of inflammatory cytokines [interleukins and prostaglandins (PGs)], which may affect pregnancy.[8]
- Elevated levels of these inflammatory markers have been detected in the amniotic fluid of women with periodontitis and who give preterm birth compared with healthy controls.[9]
- Oral bacteria have been detected in the amniotic fluid and placenta of women with preterm labour and periodontitis.[10] It has been postulated that the inflammatory cytokines released may initiate labour. In addition, the release of PGE_2 is thought to restrict placental blood flow, resulting in intrauterine growth restriction and low birth weight.[11]

The American Academy of Periodontology recommends that all women who are pregnant or are planning to become pregnant should undergo a periodontal examination and any necessary treatment.[12]

Signs of gingivitis and periodontitis include the following:

- Bleeding gums, especially when brushing teeth
- Swelling and redness of the gingival tissues
- Halitosis
- Mobile teeth

Mobile Teeth

- Even in the absence of periodontal disease, teeth have been noted to become slightly mobile during pregnancy. This is thought to be the effect of an increased level of pregnancy hormones, which affect the periodontium.[13] This type of tooth mobility is temporary and generally resolves once the baby is delivered.
- In cases where tooth mobility is related to periodontitis, patients should be referred to a dentist for further management.

Pregnancy Oral Tumour

- Pregnancy oral tumour or pyogenic granuloma is a vascular oral soft tissue lesion that occurs in approximately 5% of pregnancies. It is thought to develop because of an increased level of progesterone, in combination with local factors such as bacteria and inflammatory stimulants.
- Clinically, these lesions generally appear on the gingival tissues; however, they may affect any part of the oral mucosa. Typically, the lesions are exophytic and erythematous and bleed readily. Clinically, these lesions mimic pyogenic granulomas (Figure 35.1). They most commonly form during the first trimester, enlarge quickly and often regress after the baby is born.

Management often entails monitoring during pregnancy and excision if the lesion becomes symptomatic or does not regress after delivery. These lesions commonly recur if they are removed during pregnancy.[14]

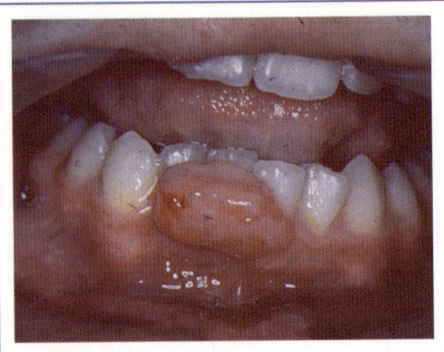

Figure 35.1 Pregnancy tumour.
Courtesy: David Wilson.

DENTAL CARE DURING PREGNANCY

Screening and Prevention

- All pregnant women should be encouraged to upkeep good oral hygiene habits, including tooth brushing and flossing twice a day.
- Patients should be advised to avoid or limit the amount of sugar consumption and follow the given general dietary advice.
- Preventive dental cleaning and six-monthly checkups during pregnancy are not only safe but also recommended.
- Agents such as topical chlorhexidine [The US Food and Drug Administration (FDA) category B] are safe to use during pregnancy and breastfeeding. Studies have shown that use of these agents can lower the maternal oral bacterial load and reduce the transmission of cariogenic bacteria to infants.[15]

Radiographs

- Routine radiographs usually taken during annual examinations can usually be postponed until after the birth.
- Dental radiographs may be taken during pregnancy, if required, for acute diagnostic purposes. When possible, radiography should be delayed until after the first trimester.
- The American College of Radiology has stated that 'no single diagnostic X-ray has a radiation dose significant enough to cause adverse effects in a developing embryo or foetus'. In addition, the reported teratogenic risk of radiation exposure from oral films is 1000 times less than the natural risk of spontaneous abortion or malformation.[16]
- Additionally, patients can be reassured that the use of modern digital intraoral radiographs will also limit the risk of radiation exposure to the unborn baby.

Routine Dental Treatment

- Pregnant patients should be encouraged to continue with their routine dental care regimes, including dental appointments.
- Urgent dental treatment should be performed at any stage of pregnancy. Routine dental work should be ideally performed during the second trimester of pregnancy.
- Women in the third trimester may be at a risk of vena caval compression if laid supine in the dental chair.
- Brief appointments, frequent repositioning and use of a pillow to prop the patient, thus avoiding the supine position, may be helpful in making the process more comfortable.

Medications for Dental Procedures

- Lignocaine (FDA category B) combined with epinephrine (FDA category C) is the most common local anaesthetic used for dental treatment. This is considered safe to use during pregnancy when dosed appropriately.
- Sedatives such as benzodiazepines should be avoided. The use of nitrous oxide during pregnancy remains controversial.

Management of Acute Dental Conditions

- If antibiotics are indicated, penicillin, amoxicillin, cephalexin and clindamycin (all FDA category B) are considered safe to use during pregnancy.

Severe dental infections can lead to facial cellulitis, which requires hospitalisation for intravenous antibiotics. Analgesics such as paracetamol (FDA category A) can be used safely at all stages of pregnancy.

Suggestions for Addressing Dental Work Needs

- The Australian Dental Association recommends that pregnant women should eat a balanced diet, brush their teeth thoroughly with a fluoride toothpaste twice a day and floss daily.
- Women should undergo preventive examination and cleaning during pregnancy.
- They should defer any elective dental work until the second trimester or until after the delivery, if possible.
- While in the dental chair, patients should be encouraged to maintain healthy circulation by keeping their legs uncrossed.
- Patients should be advised to bring a pillow to their appointment to help keep themselves comfortable in the dental chair.

REFERENCES

1. Clothier B, Stringer M, Jeffcoat MK. Periodontal disease and pregnancy outcomes: exposure, risk and intervention. *Best Pract Res Clin Obstet Gynaecol*. 2007;21:451–66.
2. Berkowitz RJ. Acquisition and transmission of mutans streptococci. *J Calif Dent Assoc*. 2003;31:135–8.
3. American Dental Association Council on Access, Prevention and Interprofessional Relations. *Women's Oral Health Issues*. Chicago, IL: American Dental Association; 2006 [assessed 2015 Jan 01]. Available from: http://www.ada.org/sections/professionalResources/pdfs/healthcare_womens.pdf
4. Kumar J, Samelson R, editors. *Oral Health Care During Pregnancy and Early Childhood: Practice Guidelines*. New York, NY: New York State Department of Health; 2006 [cited 2015 Jan 01]. Available from: http://www.health.state.ny.us/publications/0824.pdf
5. Lewis CW, Milgrom P. Fluoride [published correction appears in Pediatr Rev, 2003;24(12):429]. *Pediatr Rev*. 2003;24:327–36.
6. Hey-Hadavi JH. Women's oral health issues: sex differences and clinical implications. *Women Health Prim Care*. 2002;5:189–99.
7. American Academy of Periodontology. *Periodontal (Gum) Diseases*. Chicago, IL: American Academy of Periodontology. [assessed 2015 Jan 10]. Available from: http://www.healthymouthshealthylives.org/en/about-the-partnership/partner-profile-page/American%20Academy%20of%20Periodontology/2012
8. Boggess KA, Edelstein BL. Oral health in women during preconception and pregnancy: implications for birth outcomes and infant oral health. *Matern Child Health J*. 2006;10(5 suppl):S169–74.
9. Dörtbudak O, Eberhardt R, Ulm M, Persson GR. Periodontitis, a marker of risk in pregnancy for preterm birth. *J Clin Periodontol*. 2005;32:45–52.

10. Goepfert AR, Jeffcoat MK, Andrews WW, et al. Periodontal disease and upper genital tract inflammation in early spontaneous preterm birth. *Obstet Gynecol*. 2004;104:777–83.

11. Offenbacher S, Lieff S, Boggess KA, et al. Maternal periodontitis and prematurity. Part I: obstetric outcome of prematurity and growth restriction. *Ann Periodontol*. 2001;6:164–74.

12. Task Force on Periodontal Treatment of Pregnant Women, American Academy of Periodontology. American Academy of Periodontology statement regarding periodontal management of the pregnant patient. *J Periodontol*. 2004;75:495.

13. Scheutz F, Baelum V, Matee MI, Mwangosi I. Motherhood and dental disease. *Community Dent Health*. 2002;19:67–72.

14. Sills ES, Zegarelli DJ, Hoschander MM, Strider WE. Clinical diagnosis and management of hormonally responsive oral pregnancy tumour (pyogenic granuloma). *J Reprod Med*. 1996;41:467–70.

15. Silk H, Douglass A, Douglass J, Silk L. Oral health during pregnancy. *Am Fam Physician.* 2008;77:1139–44.

16. Livingston HM, Dellinger TM, Holder R. Considerations in the management of the pregnant patient. *Spec Care Dentist*. 1998;18:183–8.

Chapter 36

Dental sleep medicine: Sleep bruxism and oral appliance therapy for snoring and obstructive sleep apnoea

R. Balasubramaniam

SLEEP BRUXISM

Definition/Description

- Bruxism is defined as repetitive activity of the jaw muscles and is characterised by clenching or grinding of the teeth and/or bracing or thrusting of the mandible.
- Bruxism during sleep is known as sleep bruxism (SB).
- SB has no gender difference. It typically peaks during childhood and decreases with age.
- SB affects 8% of the adult population.

Risk Factors

- Risk factors for SB include cigarette smoking; consumption of caffeine, alcohol and recreational drugs such as ecstasy, cocaine and amphetamines; medications such as selective serotonin reuptake inhibitors and haloperidol; and sleep-disordered breathing, including snoring and obstructive sleep apnoea (OSA).
- SB increases the risk for tooth wear and fracture, muscle fatigue and pain, headache and temporomandibular disorders.
- Orofacial pain is reported in 66% to 84% of patients with SB.

Clinical Features

- Tooth-grinding noise, reported by bed partner
- Tooth wear
- Masticatory muscle pain, especially in the morning
- Masseter muscle hypertrophy
- Morning headache

Pathophysiology

- SB events commonly occur in the second and third sleep stage transitions from nonrapid eye movement to rapid eye movement sleep cycles.

- The prevailing hypothesis is that rhythmic masticatory muscle activity is associated with autonomic sympathetic cardiac activity and sleep arousals.
- In a subgroup of SB patients, life stressors may result in jaw motor activity.
- Genetics appears to play a role in SB, whereby a 4.25 times increased risk of SB has been seen to be associated with single nucleotide polymorphism of the C-allele carrier of the serotonin 2A receptor.
- Occlusal disharmony (so-called bad bite) does not cause and is no longer considered to be directly associated with SB.
- SB may have a protective role, whereby it is thought to occur to overcome upper airway obstruction.

Diagnosis

Clinical Assessment

- Clinical diagnosis of SB is based on the observation of signs and symptoms such as abnormal tooth wear, hypertrophy of masseter muscles, fatigue, discomfort or pain of jaw muscles. Reporting of observed SB events by a parent or bed partner is helpful. Nevertheless, tooth wear is not considered a distinctive sign of SB.

Ambulatory Monitoring

- Ambulatory monitors can detect the electromyogram events associated with SB; however, without audio-video recording, these devices cannot exclude orofacial movements unrelated to SB, such grimacing and swallowing.
- Ambulatory monitoring does not have the validity for the diagnosis of SB.

Sleep Laboratory Recording

- The gold standard for SB diagnosis is a full-night polysomnography with audio-video recording, which enables the monitoring of electro-encephalographical, electrocardiographical, electromyographical and respiratory signals during sleep.
- The use of polysomnography is not necessary for routine clinical care of SB.

Management

Treatment strategies for SB may be divided into the following:
- Behavioural therapies
    - There is moderate evidence for the effectiveness of biofeedback and cognitive behavioural therapy for SB.
- Occlusal therapies
    - Occlusal appliances are useful for decreasing SB for approximately 2 weeks; however, they may protect teeth from attrition caused by SB in the long term.
    - Mandibular advancement appliances may decrease SB by up to 70% in the short term. No long-term data on safety or efficacy are available.
- Pharmacological therapies

♦ Clonazepam, clonidine, gabapentin and botulinum toxin injections into the masticatory muscles may decrease SB in the short term.

ORAL APPLIANCE THERAPY FOR SNORING AND OBSTRUCTIVE SLEEP APNOEA

Definition/Description

- Obstructive sleep apnoea (OSA) is characterised by snoring and collapse of the pharyngeal airway during sleep, resulting in partial reduction (hypopnoea) or complete cessation (apnoea) of the airflow despite breathing effort.
- Thirty percent of adults suffer from chronic snoring, and 9% men and 5% women suffer from OSA. Patients with OSA typically report snoring, gasping and snorting, excessive sleepiness, fatigue, tiredness and morning headache.
- OSA has been linked to systemic hypertension, myocardial infarction, stroke, congestive heart failure, atrial fibrillation, carotid artery atherosclerosis, diabetes, excessive daytime sleepiness, impaired quality of life and increased mortality.
- Continuous positive airway pressure (CPAP) is a highly effective treatment modality and is considered the gold standard; however, its long-term compliance is poor. Other treatments include weight loss, postural modification, upper airway surgery and orthognathic surgery.

Guidelines for Oral Appliance Therapy

- Oral appliances are not as effective as CPAP.
- Oral appliances may be used to treat mild to moderate OSA patients who prefer oral appliance over CPAP and those who do not respond to CPAP, who are not appropriate candidates for CPAP or who fail treatment attempts with CPAP or treatment with behavioural measures, such as weight loss or change of sleep position.

Mechanism of Action of Oral Appliances

- There are two types of oral appliances: (1) mandibular advancement devices (MADs) and (2) tongue-retaining devices.
- MADs advance and retain the mandible in a forward position, preventing the tongue and soft palate from collapsing against the posterior pharyngeal wall (Figure 36.1). This enlarges the velopharyngeal airway and, to a lesser extent, the oropharyngeal and hypopharyngeal airways.
- Tongue-retaining devices are less commonly used. They protrude and hold the tongue forward via a suction mechanism. They are an alternative treatment, typically used in edentulous patients.

Candidates for Treatment

Patients require healthy teeth and periodontal tissues to retain a MAD. Similarly, screening for underlying temporomandibular disorders is necessary to avoid exacerbation of this condition as a consequence of mandibular advancement.

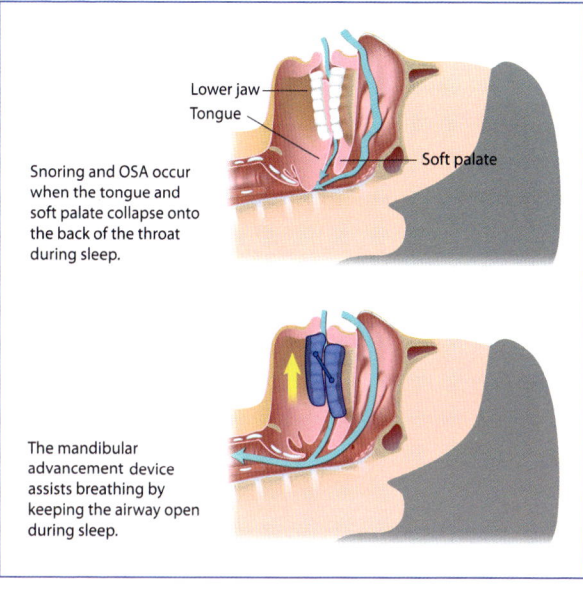

Lower jaw

Tongue

Soft palate

Snoring and OSA occur when the tongue and soft palate collapse onto the back of the throat during sleep.

The mandibular advancement device assists breathing by keeping the airway open during sleep.

Figure 36.1   Mandibular advancement devices advance and retain the mandible in a forward position, preventing the tongue and soft palate from collapsing against the posterior pharyngeal wall and hence improving the patency of the upper airway.

Reproduced with permission from: Alila Medical Media.

- Patient-specific factors that improve success include the following:
  - ◆ Younger patients
  - ◆ Smaller neck circumferences
  - ◆ Women
  - ◆ Lower-body mass index
  - ◆ Supine-dependent OSA patients

Efficacy of Mandibular Advancement Devices

- MADs are considered an effective treatment option for snoring and mild to moderate OSA when measured by the apnoea-hypopnoea index. They are less effective for the treatment of severe OSA (Table 36.1).
- When compared with CPAP, MADs are less effective when measured by apnoea-hypopnoea index. However, most patients prefer MADs over CPAP, because MADs are easy to use and more comfortable (Table 36.2).
- MADs improve sleepiness, daytime tiredness and lethargy.
- MADs have a favourable effect on systolic, diastolic and arterial blood pressure.

Table 36.1 Randomised, crossover, placebo-controlled studies on mandibular advancement devices for obstructive sleep apnoea*#

Reference	N	AHI_{base}	AHI_{appl}	Success rate %	Response rate %	Comments
Metha et al, 2001	24	30	14	38	25	For AHI = 5
				54	17	For AHI = 10
Gotsopoulos et al, 2002	73	27	12	36	37	For AHI = 5
Johnston et al, 2002	20	38	23	30	10	For both AHI = 5 and 10
Barnes et al, 2004	80	21	14	–	–	Tablet placebo; CPAP arm
Naismith et al, 2005	73	24	12	36	–	For AHI = 5
				55	–	For AHI = 10
Vanderveken et al, 2008	35	14	6	49	11	For AHI = 5 Thermoplastic
Deane et al, 2009	27	27	12	27	41	For AHI = 5 TRD

*AHI_{base} = Apnoea-hypopnoea index before treatment; AHI_{appl} = Apnoea-hypopnoea index after treatment; CPAP = Continuous positive airway pressure; N = Number of subjects; TRD = Tongue-retaining devices.
#Success rate is the reduction of AHI_{base} to a value less than that defined for obstructive sleep apnoea and response rate is the reduction of AHI_{base} by greater than 50% than that defined for obstructive sleep apnoea

Adapted from Hoffstein V. Review of oral appliances for treatment of sleep-disordered breathing. *Sleep Breath*. 2007;11:1–22.

Table 36.2 Randomised, crossover studies of mandibular advancement devices compared with continuous positive airway pressure for obstructive sleep apnoea*

Reference	N	AHI_{base}	AHI_{appl}	AHI_{CPAP}	Comments
Ferguson et al, 2006	19	20	10	4	68% satisfied with MAD
Clark et al, 1996	21	34	20	11	MAD preferred
Ferguson et al, 1997	20	25	14	4	65% preferred MAD
Randerath et al, 2002	20	18	14	4	MAD easier to use
Engleman et al, 2002	48	31	15	8	Neither treatment preferred
Tan et al, 2002	24	22	8	3	MAD preferred
Barnes et al, 2004	80	21	14	5	CPAP more difficult use; however, more effective

*AHI_{base} = Apnoea-hypopnoea index before treatment; AHI_{appl} = Apnoea-hypopnoea index after treatment with oral appliance; AHI_{CPAP} = After treatment with continuous positive airway pressure; CPAP = Continuous positive airway pressure; N = Number of subjects; MAD = Mandibular advancement devices

Adapted from Hoffstein V. Review of oral appliances for treatment of sleep-disordered breathing. *Sleep Breath.* 2007;11:1–22.

- There is some emerging evidence that MADs are equally effective as CPAP in decreasing cardiovascular mortality among patients with severe OSA.
- MADs are superior to CPAP with regards to improvement of general health outcomes.

Side-effects of Mandibular Advancement Devices

- Most of the side-effects of MAD use are minor and transient. These include excessive salivation, dry mouth, teeth discomfort, gingiva irritation, masticatory muscle tenderness and temporomandibular joint discomfort.
- More severe and persistent side-effects include temporomandibular joint arthralgia, masticatory myofascial pain and occlusal changes.

SUGGESTED READINGS

Anandam A, Patil M, Akinnusi M, Jaoude P, El-Solh AA. Cardiovascular mortality in obstructive sleep apnoea treated with continuous positive airway pressure or oral appliance: an observational study. *Respirology*. 2013;18:1184–90.

Balasubramaniam R, Klasser G, Cistulli P, Lavigne G. The link between sleep bruxism, sleep disordered breathing and temporomandibular disorders: an evidence-based review. *J Dent Sleep Med*. 2014;1:27–37.

Balasubramaniam R, Klasser GD. Sleep Bruxism: what orthodontists need to know. In: Kandasamy S, Greene CS, Rinchuse DJ, Stockstill JW, editors. *TMD and Orthodontics: Essential Information for the Clinician*. 1st ed. Switzerland: Springer International Publishing; 2015.

Kryger MH, Roth T, Dement WC. *Principles and Practice of Sleep Medicine*. 5th ed. Philadelphia, PA: Saunders/Elsevier; 2011.

Kushida CA, Morgenthaler TI, Littner MR, et al. Practice parameters for the treatment of snoring and obstructive sleep apnea with oral appliances: an update for 2005. *Sleep*. 2006;29:240–3.

Lobbezoo F, Ahlberg J, Glaros AG, et al. Bruxism defined and graded: an international consensus. *J Oral Rehab*. 2013;40:2–4.

Ngiam J, Balasubramaniam R, Darendeliler MA, Cheng AT, Waters K, Sullivan CE. Clinical guidelines for oral appliance therapy in the treatment of snoring and obstructive sleep apnoea. *Aust Dent J*. 2013;58:408–19.

Chapter 37

Oral lesions in HIV infection

J. Hill and S. R. Prabhu

FUNGAL INFECTIONS

Candidiasis

Candidiasis, also known as candidosis, is a common opportunistic fungal infection caused by an overgrowth of the *Candida* species already present in the mouth. There are three frequently encountered forms of the disease: pseudomembranous candidiasis (thrush), erythematous candidiasis (atrophic candidiasis) and angular cheilitis.

Pseudomembranous Candidiasis (Thrush)

- Pseudomembranous candidiasis or thrush is most commonly caused by *C. albicans* and is characterised by the presence of creamy-white curd-like plaques on the buccal mucosa, tongue and other intraoral mucosal surfaces (Figure 37.1 A and B).
- Lesions are easily rubbed off with gauze, leaving a red or bleeding surface.

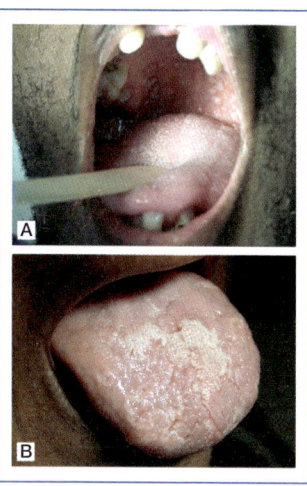

Figure 37.1 (A and B) Oral pseudomembranous candidiasis. *Courtesy*: Jeffrey Hill.

Diagnosis is based on the medical history and clinical appearance of the lesions. Useful tests include potassium hydroxide preparation and fungal culture.

Management of pseudomembranous candidiasis includes topical application of antifungal agents. These include nystatin oral gel eight hourly for 10 to 14 days. In severe cases, systemic use of nystatin 400,000 to 600,000 units Q6h for two weeks is effective. Patients should be instructed to hold the medicine in the mouth for several minutes before swallowing. Other systemic agents in use are fluconazole, itraconazole and amphotericin B.

Erythematous Candidiasis (Atrophic Candidiasis)

- Erythematous candidiasis is most commonly caused by *C. albicans*. It presents as a red, flat lesion on the dorsal surface of the tongue (Figure 37.2) and/or the hard palate, or on the edentulous ridge beneath removable dental appliances.
- Oral burning with salty or spicy food or acidic beverages is one of the common complaints among these patients.

Diagnosis is based on the medical history and clinical appearance of the lesion. Estimation of virological status and identification of *C. albicans* in a potassium hydroxide preparation are useful.

Management of erythematous candidiasis includes the use of antifungal agents, as listed for pseudomembranous candidiasis above.

Angular Cheilitis

- Angular cheilitis refers to the inflammation of one or both angles of the mouth.

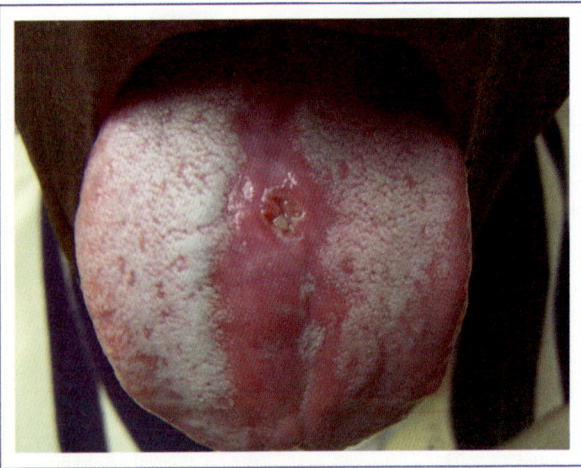

Figure 37.2 Erythematous candidiasis of the tongue with ulceration.
Courtesy: Jeffrey Hill.

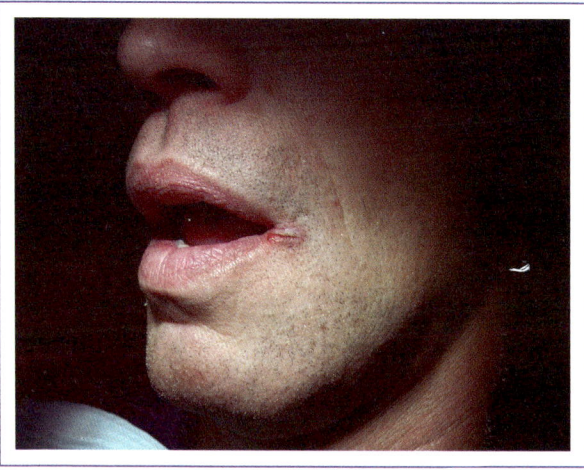

Figure 37.3   Angular cheilitis. Note the fissuring of the angle of the mouth. *Courtesy*: Jeffrey Hill.

- Angular cheilitis is caused by *C. albicans* and is characterised by erythema and/or fissuring of the corners of the mouth (Figure 37.3).
- Nutritional deficiencies (e.g., vitamin B complex and iron) and loss of proper dentition may be the contributing factors.
- Patients complain of restricted opening of the mouth, with pain and bleeding on mouth opening.
- If left untreated, angular cheilitis can remain for a long period of time.

   Diagnosis is based on the medical history and clinical presentation. Cytology and studies of fungal culture are useful.
   Management includes the use of topical application of nystatin-triamcinolone ointment on the affected areas after meals and at bedtime or application of miconazole 2% cream Q12h on the affected area for two weeks.

Linear Gingival Erythema

- Linear gingival erythema (LGE), also known as 'red-band gingivitis', is seen as a 2- to 3-mm-wide red band along the gingival margin (Figure 37.4).
- Gingival bleeding is a common feature. Although exact aetiology is not known, often candidal association has been reported with LGE.

   Diagnosis is based on the medical history and clinical appearance.
   Management of LGE includes debridement by dental professional, rinses with a 0.12% chlorhexidine gluconate suspension twice a day for two weeks and improved at-home oral hygiene.

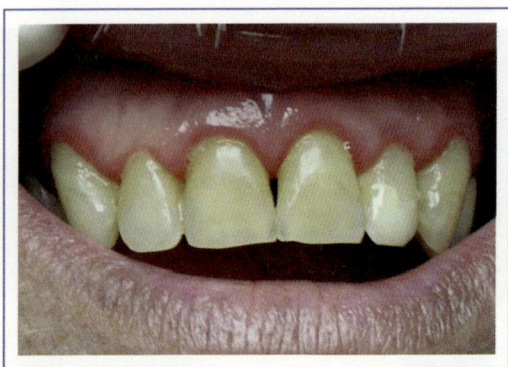

Figure 37.4 Linear gingival erythema presenting as red band along gingival margins.
Courtesy: Jeffrey Hill.

BACTERIAL INFECTIONS

Gingival and Periodontal Diseases

Bacterial gingival and periodontal diseases associated with HIV infection include necrotising ulcerative gingivitis (NUG) and necrotising ulcerative periodontitis (NUP).

Necrotising Ulcerative Gingivitis and Necrotising Ulcerative Periodontitis

- NUG and NUP reflect the same process of disease. In the former, gingival tissue destruction is present, whereas in the latter, periodontal ligament and alveolar bone destruction are defining features.
- NUG and NUP are caused by a mixed bacterial flora. Other associated factors include malnutrition, smoking, stress, trauma and preexisting gingivitis.
- NUP is a marker of severe immune suppression. Systemic findings such as fever, malaise and lymphadenopathy may be present.

Clinical features of NUG include necrotic ulcerations of the interdental areas (Figure 37.5 A), gingival bleeding, pain and foul breath. NUP is commonly a progression of NUG and is further characterised by alveolar bone destruction, resulting in loose teeth (Figure 37.5 B).

Diagnosis is based on the medical history and clinical grounds.

Management of NUG and NUP includes mechanical debridement (scaling and root planing) by the dentist and use of antibiotics (metronidazole and amoxicillin and clavulanate). Pain management is important. Oxidising mouthwash such as 3% hydrogen peroxide is effective against anaerobic microorganisms. Chlorhexidine (0.12%) mouth rinses and nutritional supplements are recommended.

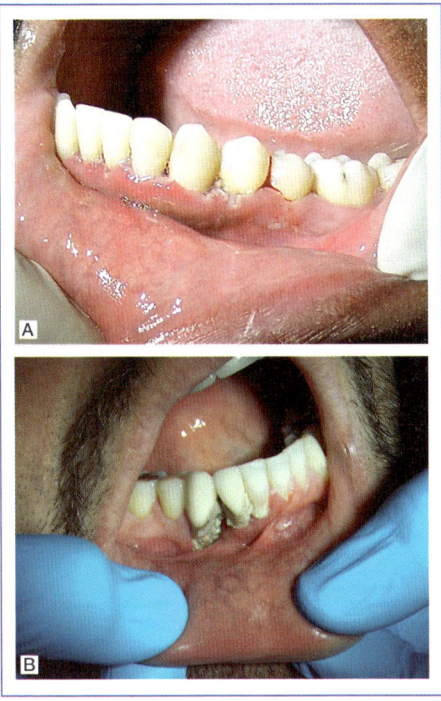

Figure 37.5   (A) Necrotising ulcerative gingivitis showing characteristic ulcers of the interdental papillae and (B) necrotising ulcerative periodontitis showing destruction of periodontal tissues.
Courtesy: Jeffrey Hill.

VIRAL INFECTIONS

Oral Hairy Leukoplakia

- Oral hairy leukoplakia (OHL) is caused by Epstein-Barr virus (EBV) and is characterised by white, corrugated lesions on the lateral surface of the tongue (Figure 37.6).
- OHL is asymptomatic and may be unilateral or bilateral.
- OHL lesions cannot be rubbed off.
- Presence of OHL is an indication of immunodeficiency.
- OHL has prognostic value in predicting the future development of AIDS in HIV-infected people.

Diagnosis is based on the medical history and clinical appearance of the lesion. Biopsy and histological evaluation of the lesion may be considered when patient's HIV status is unknown. *In situ* hybridisation techniques used on the cytological specimen taken from the lesion confirm the association of EBV with OHL.

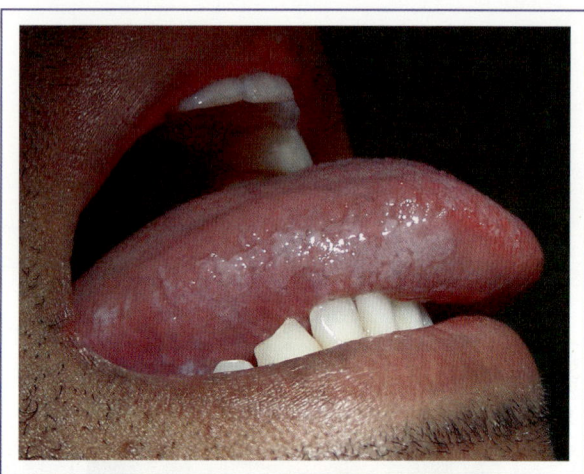

Figure 37.6 Oral hairy leukoplakia of the lateral surface of the tongue. *Courtesy*: Jeffrey Hill.

Management in the majority of patients does not require any specific treatment because of its asymptomatic nature. OHL lesions disappear with the systemic use of antiviral agents (acyclovir 800 mg five times a day for two weeks) but tend to recur with cessation of treatment. For severe cases of OHL, local treatment includes podophyllin resin (25%) one to two applications on the affected areas, one week apart. Some severe lesions may require surgical excision. If OHL presents concurrently with oral candidiasis, the management also includes antifungal agents. OHL is not a potentially malignant lesion.

Primary and Secondary Herpes Simplex Virus

Herpes simplex virus (HSV-1) infections may be either primary (acute) or secondary (recurrent). The prevalence of HSV-1 infection varies between 10% and 35% in HIV-infected adults and children. The presence of HSV infection for more than one month is regarded as an AIDS-defining condition. HSV-2-associated oral manifestations are less common.

Clinical features of primary HSV infection in adults present most often as pharyngitis and tonsillitis (acute herpetic pharyngotonsillitis). Fever, malaise, headache and sore throat, as well as cervical lymphadenopathy, may be present. Acute herpetic gingivostomatitis, marked by vesicular lesions of the oral mucosa, especially the gingiva, is the primary HSV-1 infection that occurs in children. It is seen less often as the primary presentation in adults. Sometimes, primary HSV infection in HIV-infected patients may be resistant to acyclovir.

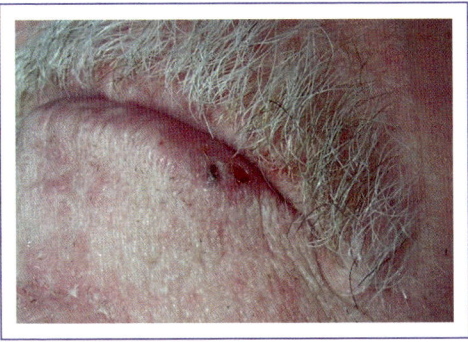

Figure 37.7 Herpes labialis of the lower lip vermillion border.
Courtesy: Jeffrey Hill.

In the most common secondary form of HSV infection, vesicles appear on the vermillion borders and perioral skin. This condition is called herpes labialis (Figure 37.7). Vesicles rupture and leave painful ulcers. Recurrent intraoral HSV lesions may also occur and are more frequently encountered in HIV-infected patients than the general population. These lesions appear as crops of vesicles on the hard palate and/or attached gingiva (keratinised mucosa).

Diagnosis is based on the medical history and clinical examination. Cytology for cytopathic effects of the virus on epithelial cells and serological evaluation of antibody titres during the acute and convalescent periods of the primary infection are useful.

Management with antiviral agents [acyclovir 800 mg per oral (PO), four hourly for 10 days for adults] is recommended. Treatment is more effective during the prodromal period. Patients taking acyclovir should be instructed to drink plenty of fluids. Foscarnet 24 to 40 mg/kg PO eight hourly is used for resistant herpetic infections in adults. Topical antiviral medications are useful for labial and perioral herpetic lesions.

Herpes Zoster (Shingles)

Primary infection of the varicella-zoster virus causes chickenpox. This is common in children and young adults. In adults who have had chickenpox in the past, varicella-zoster virus can remain latent in the semilunar ganglion at the base of the skull. When reactivation of this virus occurs (due to immunosuppression, stress or age more than 65 years), herpes zoster (also called shingles) is the result.

- Oral herpes zoster lesions are unilateral and appear as multiple painful vesicles on the face, lips and oral mucosa.
- These lesions follow the distribution of the maxillary and/or mandibular branches of the trigeminal nerve (Figure 37.8) without crossing the midline.

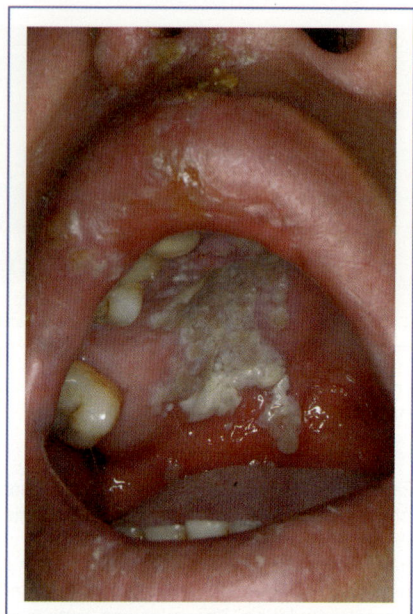

Figure 37.8 Intraoral lesions of herpes zoster (shingles).
Courtesy: Nagamani Narayana.

- Prodromal symptoms with itching, burning and redness are common.
- Skin lesions rupture and form crusts, whereas oral vesicles rupture and form ulcers. Oral lesions are most often found on the gingiva.
- Complications of shingles may include postherpetic neuralgia.

Diagnosis is based on the history and the distribution/clinical appearance of the lesions. Serology is useful in confirming the clinical diagnosis.

Management with antiviral agents (acyclovir 800 mg five times a day for 7 to 10 days) is effective in limiting the duration of the lesions. Pain management is also important.

Human Papillomavirus-Associated Oral Warts

The incidence of human papillomavirus (HPV)-associated oral warts in persons with HIV infection has increased considerably since the introduction of the highly active antiretroviral therapy.

Oral warts in HIV-infected patients include condyloma acuminatum, verruca vulgaris and squamous papilloma. HPV types 2, 4, 6 and 11 have been found to be aetiologically associated with these benign lesions.

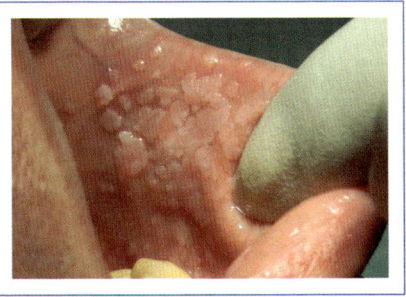

Figure 37.9 Oral condyloma acuminatum on the buccal mucosa.
Courtesy: Jeffrey Hill.

Condyloma Acuminatum (HPV Types 2, 6 and 11)

- Condyloma acuminatum, also known as venereal wart, is common in the anogenital region. This can spread to the mouth as a result of autoinoculation or oral sex.
- Oral condylomata are characterised by multiple soft, pink or white papillomatous growths with a sessile base (Figure 37.9) and appear most commonly on the buccal mucosa and soft palate.

Verruca Vulgaris (HPV Types 2 and 4)

- Verruca vulgaris generally appears on the keratinised surfaces of the skin but is also seen less commonly in the oral cavity.
- The lesions are usually solitary and found most often on the keratinised surfaces of the gingiva and palate. Less commonly, lesions may also be seen on other mucosal surfaces.
- Clinically, warts appear as sessile, circumscribed, rough papular or nodular lesions (Figure 37.10), with pointed surface projections and pink to whitish colour.

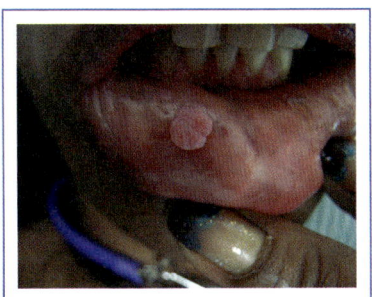

Figure 37.10 Oral verruca vulgaris on the labial mucosa.
Courtesy: Jeffrey Hill.

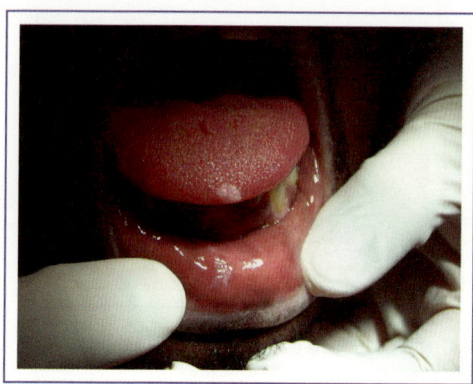

Figure 37.11   Oral squamous papilloma on the tongue.
Courtesy: Jeffrey Hill.

Squamous Papilloma (HPV Types 6 and 11)

- Squamous papillomas are the most common form of HPV-associated oral lesions.
- The lesions may be found on any mucosal surface but are most commonly seen on the tongue (Figure 37.11) and labial mucosa of the lips.
- Oral squamous papillomas have small, smooth finger-like projections and a light pink or whitish colour due to surface keratin.

Diagnosis is based on history and clinical examination. Biopsy is essential for histological diagnosis. The strain of HPV can be determined by immunofluorescence and immunoperoxide staining. It is not vital to clinically distinguish between verruca vulgaris and squamous papilloma, because the treatment for both types of lesions is the same.

Management includes surgical excision, carbon dioxide laser removal or cryosurgery. Chemical ablation is not very effective in the mouth because of the wet environment. Recurrences of oral warts are common.

NEOPLASMS

Kaposi's Sarcoma

- Kaposi's sarcoma (KS) is an angioproliferative neoplasm caused by KS-associated herpesvirus. KS is the most commonly found neoplasm in HIV-infected patients. KS-associated herpesvirus is also known as human herpesvirus 8 (HHV-8).

Clinical features of KS include brown or purple macular, papular, nodular or raised lesions, commonly located on the posterior lateral hard palate (Figure 37.12). Red to purple lesions may also be seen on the gingiva. KS lesions do not blanch on pressure.

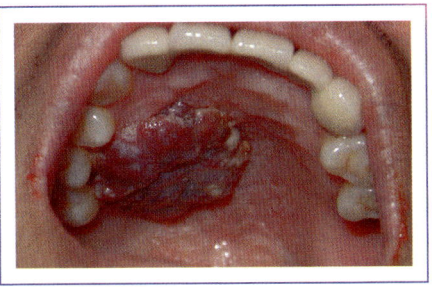

Figure 37.12 Kaposi's sarcoma of the hard palate (nodular form).
Courtesy: Jeffrey Hill.

Diagnosis is based on the medical history, clinical examination and histological evaluation of the lesion. Because of the clinical appearance similar to that of other vascular lesions, biopsy is essential to confirm the diagnosis.

Management of KS includes intralesional injections of chemotherapeutic agents (e.g., vinblastine sulphate) or surgical removal.

- For those with extraoral and intraoral involvement of KS, systemic chemotherapy is required.
- Early lesions may spontaneously regress with antiretroviral therapy.
- Oral hygiene should be emphasised for patients with gingival KS lesions.

Non-Hodgkin's Lymphoma

- Non-Hodgkin's lymphoma (NHL) is an AIDS-defining neoplastic lesion of B-cell origin.
- EBV is believed to be aetiologically associated with NHL.
- In the oral cavity, NHL is characterised by a large, painful, ulcerated mass on the palate or the gingival tissues (Figure 37.13). One-third of patients with NHL experience fever, weight loss, adenopathy, night sweats or hepatosplenomegaly.

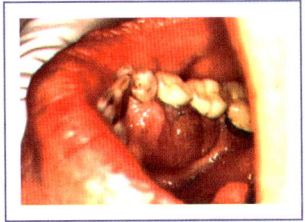

Figure 37.13 Lymphoma of the gingival tissues.
Reproduced with permission from: David Reznik. Available from: www. HIVdent.org

Diagnosis is based on the medical history, clinical appearance of the lesion, systemic findings and histological evaluation of the lesion.

Management of oral NHL includes treatment regimens containing chemotherapeutic agents such as doxorubicin. Referral of the patient to an oncologist is essential.

NONSPECIFIC LESIONS AND CONDITIONS

Recurrent Aphthous Ulcers

- Recurrent aphthous ulcers (RAUs) occur in about 1% to 7% of HIV-infected patients. RAUs are painful and have a site predilection for the nonkeratinised mucosa. Severe RAUs occur when the CD4+ cell count is less than 100 cells/μl. Although the exact cause of RAUs is unknown, these are reported to be associated with cell-mediated immune defects.

Clinical features of RAU include three presentations of ulcers: minor, major and herpetiform:

- Minor aphthous ulcers are less than 1 cm in diameter and are covered by a pseudomembrane and surrounded by a red halo (Figure 37.14 A). They usually heal leaving no scar.
- Major aphthous ulcers are larger in diameter (>1 cm) (Figure 37.14 B) and are more painful. They may interfere with mastication, swallowing and speaking. Major RAUs persist for weeks and heal with scarring. They may be mistaken for malignant ulcers.

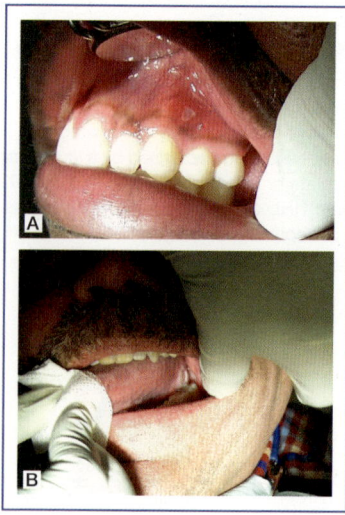

Figure 37.14   (A) Minor aphthous ulcer on the alveolar mucosa and (B) major aphthous ulcer on the posterolateral surface of the tongue.
Courtesy: Jeffrey Hill.

- Herpetiform aphthous ulcers occur as crops of several small ulcers, 1 to 2 mm in diameter. They are found on the soft palate, tonsils, ventral and lateral tongue and/or buccal mucosa.

   Diagnosis is based on the history, clinical appearance and number of ulcers.

   Management of RAUs includes topical application of corticosteroids. Triamcinolone in carboxymethyl cellulose, 0.1% paste, is effective. Other agents include betamethasone phosphate (0.5 mg tablet dissolved in 10 mL mouthwash and ulcer rinsed four hourly), fluocinonide 0.05% (ointment applied on ulcer four hourly) and dexamethasone (0.5 mg/5 mL) elixir rinse and expectorate.

- Major aphthous ulcers usually require systemic corticosteroids. Prednisone starting at 40 to 60 mg PO daily for one week, which then tapers, is recommended for severe ulcers resistant to topical agents. Thalidomide 200 mg PO daily for two weeks is indicated when recurrences are frequent and severe. Thalidomide should not be used in women of child-bearing potential.
- Nutritional supplements and pain management may be necessary in severe cases.

Salivary Gland Disease

- Salivary gland disease, resulting in an increase in the size of the salivary glands (in particular, parotid glands) is often noted in HIV-infected patients. This is a common feature in children with HIV infection. There has been a reported increase in salivary gland disease in the era of highly active antiretroviral therapy. It is caused by a lymphocytic infiltration of the glands.
- Salivary gland enlargement in HIV-infected patients may resemble Sjögren's syndrome; however, lymphocytosis is characterised by CD8+ cells, and not CD4+ cells, as in Sjögren's syndrome.

   Clinical features include unilateral or bilateral enlargement of the parotid glands, with or without xerostomia. Enlarged glands are soft but not fluctuant.

   Diagnosis is based on history, clinical examination and gland biopsy.

   Management: Generally, salivary gland enlargement is left untreated. In extreme cases, patients may require systemic use of nonsteroidal anti-inflammatory agents, analgesics, antibiotics or corticosteroids. Surgical removal of the parotid glands may be necessary for aesthetic reasons.

Xerostomia

- Xerostomia, or dry mouth, is a common complaint among HIV-infected patients.
- Contributing factors include medications, salivary gland disease and smoking.
- Patients suffering from xerostomia are at increased risk for dental caries.
- Dry mouth is also a risk factor for oral candidal infections.

Clinical features include patients complaining of thick, ropey saliva, difficulty in eating and swallowing, altered taste sensation, burning or tingling sensation and bad breath.

Diagnosis is based on history and clinical examination. On palpation, the gloved finger sticks to the oral mucosa. Quantitative and qualitative assessments of saliva may be necessary for those with severe xerostomia.

Management of xerostomia includes sucking on sugar-free hard candies, chewing sugar-free gum and the use of oral moisturisers. Frequent sips of water are recommended. Consumption of sugary and acidic foods and beverages should be minimised.

- For severe xerostomia, systemic use of pilocarpine 5 mg PO eight hourly before meals is effective. Oral hygiene should be stressed in these patients and topical fluoride preparations should be encouraged to prevent or control dental caries.
- Mouth rinses with high alcohol content should be avoided due to their drying effect.

Drug-Induced Pigmentation

- Antiretroviral drugs can give rise to changes in mucosal pigmentation. Patients receiving zidovudine, for example, frequently present with oral mucosal pigmented lesions. Brown-coloured patches on the oral mucosa are common (Figure 37.15) and may clinically resemble normal physiological pigmentation. These patches require no treatment.

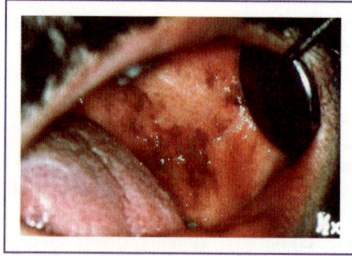

Figure 37.15 Brown pigmentation of the buccal mucosa in an HIV-infected patient receiving zidovudin.
Reproduced with permission from: David Reznik. Available from: www. HIVdent.org

LESS COMMON ORAL LESIONS AND CONDITIONS

Oral Lesions Due to Cytomegalovirus (HHV-5) Infections

Cytomegalovirus is one of the members of the herpes virus family (HHV-5). In patients with advanced HIV infection, cytomegalovirus infection can cause gastrointestinal and ocular lesions. Oral lesions are uncommon, but when present, they cause painful ulcers. Oral lesions respond to intravenous ganciclovir.

Oral Lesions of Histoplasmosis and Cryptococcosis

Histoplasmosis is an infection caused by the fungus *Histoplasma capsulatum*. This is an important infectious disease among patients with AIDS. Oral lesions of histoplasmosis may appear as ulcers with ill-defined margins and a granulomatous surface.

Cryptococcosis is caused by the fungus *Cryptococcus neoformans*. Oral lesions of cryptococcosis are rare. When present, they appear as ulcers.

Oral lesions in histoplasmosis and cryptococcosis can be treated with antifungals such as amphotericin B and itraconazole.

Oral Lesions of Tuberculosis

Tuberculosis (TB) is caused by the acid-fast bacillus *Mycobacterium tuberculosis*. Among patients with HIV/AIDS, pulmonary TB is common. Oral involvement of TB is rare. When present, oral TB lesions are secondary to the systemic infection (e.g., pulmonary TB). Oral involvement may present as persistent ulcers or granulomatous lesions. Oral lesions resolve with the treatment of systemic infection.

Mucosal Ulcerations in Neutropaenia

Mucosal ulcerations due to neutropaenia can occur when absolute granulocyte counts are less than 800 µL. These ulcers can occur on the keratinised as well as nonkeratinised mucosa. Ulcers are large and very painful.

Diagnosis is based on the medical history and clinical examination of the ulcers that cannot be otherwise identified. Complete blood count showing neutropaenia is confirmatory.

Management includes granulocyte colony-stimulating factor treatment, followed by systemic or local topical corticosteroid therapy, depending on the number, size and location of neutropaenic ulcers. Careful oral hygiene is essential to prevent the secondary infection of gingival lesions.

Mucosal Haemorrhages

Mucosal haemorrhages can occur in HIV-infected patients because of thrombocytopaenia. These may be seen in the form ecchymoses or haematoma. Patients may complain of spontaneous bleeding from the gingiva or blood in the mouth on waking. Patients may also complain of bleeding in other mucosal sites.

Diagnosis is based on the history and haematological findings. Blood tests, including platelet counts, should be performed before carrying out other diagnostic measures.

SUGGESTED READINGS

Greenspan D. Oral manifestations of HIV. *HIV InSite Knowledge Base Chapter*. San Francisco: University of California; 1998. Available from: http://hivinsite.ucsf.edu/insite?page=kb-04-01-14

Johnson NW. The mouth in HIV/AIDS: markers of disease status and management challenges for the dental profession. *Aust Dent J*. 2010;55(1 suppl):85–102.

Prabhu SR. Oral lesions in HIV/AIDS: In: Prabhu SR, editor. *HIV/AIDS in Dental Practice: An Illustrated Handbook for Caribbean Dental Practitioners*. Trinidad and Tobago: University of the West Indies; 2006. pp. 145–78.

Chapter 38

Oral potentially malignant disorders I: Leukoplakia and erythroplakia

S. Warnakulasuriya

TERMINOLOGY OF ORAL LESIONS WITH A MALIGNANT POTENTIAL

The development of cancer in precursor lesions or conditions is a well-recognised process of carcinogenesis. Many examples of precursor conditions are known to physicians and pathologists, such as cervical dysplasia (precancerous change in the lining of the cells of uterus cervix), colon polyps and Barrett's oesophagus. These carry an increased risk of malignancy. It has been known for over a century that oral cancer may develop in the areas of preexisting mucosal pathology found in the oral cavity. In the literature, these disorders were known by terms such as 'pre-cancer', 'premalignant conditions' and 'intraepithelial neoplasia'. Recently, a more precise term 'potentially malignant disorders' was adopted by the World Health Organization Collaborating Centre, as there is no certainty that all 'precancerous' lesions will eventually develop into oral cancer.[1] The term 'oral potentially malignant disorders' or OPMD also embraces both precancerous lesions and conditions that were included in the previous classification of the World Health Organization.[2]

Oral leukoplakia and erythroplakia are presented in this chapter, and other OPMDs have been described in Chapter 39 (Oral potentially malignant disorders II: Oral lichen planus, oral lichenoid lesions, oral graft-versus-host disease and oral submucous fibrosis).

ORAL LEUKOPLAKIA

Definition/Description

Over the past few decades, oral leukoplakia has been defined in several ways. The most recent definition in use refers to leukoplakia as 'a predominantly white plaque of questionable risk, having excluded (other) known diseases or disorders that carry no increased risk for cancer'.[2] Other benign white lesions that should be excluded so as to arrive at the diagnosis of oral leukoplakia are listed in Table 38.1, under white patches.

Table 38.1 Differential diagnosis of oral leukoplakia and erythroplakia: other common reactive or inflammatory disorders of the oral mucosa that appear white or red

White patches	Red patches*
White sponge naevus	Carcinoma
Frictional keratosis	Oral candidiasis
Morsicatio buccarum	Erosive lichen planus
Chemical injury	Lichenoid reactions
Acute pseudomembranous candidiasis	Lupus erythematosus
Leukoedema	Tuberculosis
Hairy leukoplakia	Histoplasmosis
Smokers' palate (nicotina stomatitis)	Psoriasiform mucositis
	Kaposi's sarcoma
	Purpura
	Haemangioma
	Lingual varices
	Erythema migrans

*Adapted from Reichart PA, Philipsen HP. Oral erythroplakia: a review. *Oral Oncol*. 2005;41:551–61.

Epidemiology and Aetiology

The global prevalence of oral leukoplakia[3] has been reported to be between 1% and 5%. However, people from South Asia and South-East Asia and migrants from South Asia have been found to have higher-point prevalence rate, with male preponderance. Wide geographical variations are due to harmful lifestyles (e.g., tobacco, alcohol and betel quid use) specific to the population, country or region.

More than 75% of oral leukoplakias have been reported to be aetiologically associated with tobacco use (e.g., smoking, chewing and snuff dipping), betel quid use and excessive alcohol consumption over and above the recommended guidelines. In those who do not smoke, drink or chew betel quid, a small percentage of leukoplakias has been reported to be associated with human papillomavirus infection (mostly, but not exclusively, types 16 and 18)[4] or could be considered idiopathic.

Clinical Features

Oral leukoplakias may be asymptomatic or display a benign clinical appearance, making it difficult for the clinician to sometimes differentiate them from common reactive or inflammatory disorders of the oral mucosa (Table 38.1).

- Leukoplakias are usually diagnosed after the fourth decade of life. They are more common in men and are about six times more common among smokers than nonsmokers. Excessive alcohol consumption and betel quid use are independent risk factors.
- Common sites of involvement in western industrialised populations include the lateral margin of the tongue and the floor of the mouth. However, among Asian people, buccal mucosa and lower buccal grooves are commonly affected due to placement of betel quid at these locations; smokeless tobacco is often placed under the lip

(upper or lower). Leukoplakia of the labial mucosa or labial gingivae is seen in regular users of these products (e.g., toombak users in the Sudan and snus users in Sweden).

- Two main clinical types of leukoplakia are encountered in clinical practice: homogeneous and nonhomogeneous leukoplakias. The distinction is based on surface colour and morphological (thickness and texture) characteristics.
  - ◆ Homogeneous leukoplakias are uniformly flat and thin (Figure 38.1).
  - ◆ Nonhomogeneous varieties comprise three clinical types:
    - − Speckled: Mixed, white and red (also termed erythroleukoplakia) (Figure 38.2) but are predominantly white.
    - − Nodular: Small polypoid outgrowths, with rounded red or white excrescences.
    - − Verrucous or exophytic: Wrinkled or corrugated appearance of the surface (Figure 38.3).
- Generally, most leukoplakias are asymptomatic and are found during a routine visual examination by a practitioner.

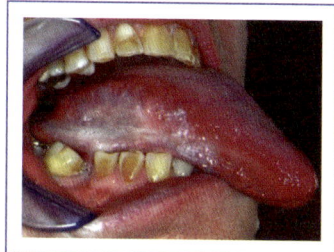

Figure 38.1   Homogeneous leukoplakia of the tongue with uniformly flat and thin white surface.
Courtesy: Saman Warnakulasuriya.

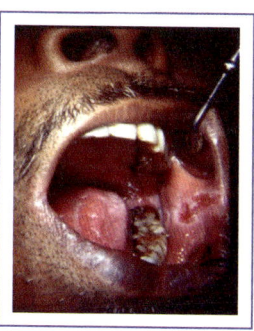

Figure 38.2   Speckled leukoplakia (erythroleukoplakia) of the buccal mucosa with mixed white and red surfaces.
Courtesy: Saman Warnakulasuriya.

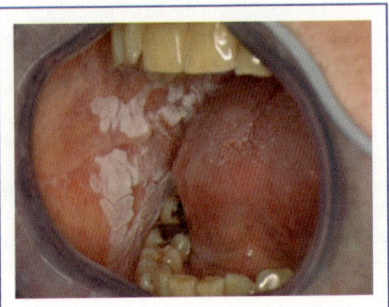

Figure 38.3 Verrucous (exophytic) leukoplakia of the buccal mucosa with wrinkled white surface.
Courtesy: Saman Warnakulasuriya.

- A red component in leukoplakia (erythroleukoplakia) indicates possible colonisation by *Candida* species and an increased risk of dysplasia and/or malignancy.
- When widespread or multiple patches of leukoplakia are noted, the term 'proliferative verrucous leukoplakia' is used. This is a distinct entity that carries a higher risk for malignant transformation and is fortunately rare.
- A provisional diagnosis of leukoplakia is made for a white patch after checking that it cannot be scraped off (with the dental mirror), and when the white colour does not disappear after stretching the tissue, with due consideration given by the clinician to exclude other conditions that clinically appear white in colour.

Malignant Transformation of Leukoplakia

The natural history of the disease suggests that the risk of malignant transformation in oral leukoplakia ranges from 0.9% to 17.5%.[5] These findings emphasise the importance of early detection of oral leukoplakia, the recognition of patients and lesions at risk and their appropriate management to reduce the future risk of malignant transformation.

ORAL ERYTHROPLAKIA

Definition/Description

Oral erythroplakia has been defined as 'a fiery red patch that cannot be characterised clinically or pathologically as any other definable disease'.[1] Examples of other red patches that need to be differentiated from erythroplakia are given in Table 38.1, under red patches.

Erythroplakia is much less common than leukoplakia. The global prevalence is in the order of 0.2% to 0.5%. Two common examples often mistaken by practitioners as erythroplakia are erythematous candidiasis and erythema migrans.[6]

Aetiology

Aetiology and predisposing factors associated with the development of oral erythroplakia are similar to those of leukoplakia; key risk factors are tobacco and excessive alcohol use.

Clinical Features

- Erythroplakia clinically appears as an entirely red patch with a velvety or a granular surface and presents with well-circumscribed clinical margins (Figure 38.4).
- Lateral margin of tongue and palate are predominantly affected.

Malignant Transformation of Erythroplakia

A very high proportion (up to 90%) of erythroplakias demonstrates severe dysplasia or can even represent early carcinoma at presentation.

Diagnosis of Leukoplakia and Erythroplakia

- A provisional diagnosis of leukoplakia or erythroplakia is made after excluding any other (similar) conditions (Table 38.1), and a definitive diagnosis is assisted by undertaking a biopsy for microscopical evaluation by a pathologist.
- The pathologist, however, is unable to confirm the diagnosis of leukoplakia or erythroplakia, as these conditions do not have pathognomonic microscopical features.
- Having excluded any other known pathology in the biopsy tissue, the pathologist can, however, remark that the microscopical features are consistent with the clinical diagnosis of either leukoplakia or erythroplakia.
- Therefore, the definitive diagnosis of leukoplakia and erythroplakia is made after a biopsy, usually an incisional biopsy.

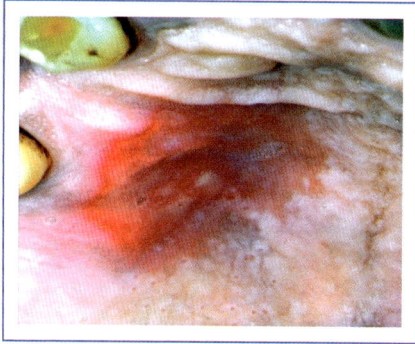

Figure 38.4 Erythroplakia of the hard palate with well-circumscribed margins.
Courtesy: Saman Warnakulasuriya.

- The biopsy should be taken at the most clinically suspicious area, if any, such as redness, an area of surface thickening or a symptomatic area. Particularly, in the case of a nonhomogeneous leukoplakia, an incisional biopsy may not be representative unless the red areas are included in sampling.
- In small leukoplakias, (e.g., <2 cm), an excisional biopsy may be considered.
- A biopsy of leukoplakia or erythroplakia is strongly recommended for the following reasons:
  ◆ To exclude any other specific disorder.
  ◆ To assess the absence or presence and, if present, grade of epithelial dysplasia.
  ◆ To check for the presence of candidal hyphae (as their presence increases the risk).
  ◆ To exclude carcinoma in situ or frank squamous cell carcinoma.
- When submitting an oral biopsy, it is important to submit all the essential clinical information about the patient and the lesion to the pathology laboratory.
- The risk evaluation of leukoplakia cannot be made on clinical grounds alone. However, three clinical features are the salient features of risky lesions: (a) presence of a red/ulcerative component, (b) anatomic location, particularly lateral tongue and floor of mouth and (c) pain arising in a previously asymptomatic plaque.
- A biopsy allows a pathologist to observe microscopical changes that offer clues about the degree of risk. The degrees of epithelial dysplasia that can be seen and to some extent quantified. The features could be broadly categorised as changes to the architecture (strata) of the epithelium and those that manifest as cellular atypia; the more prominent or numerous they are, the more severe the grade of dysplasia.
- A high proportion of leukoplakias does not show any epithelial dysplasia, while those that do, can be graded as mild, moderate or severe.[7] On the contrary, severe dysplasia is a feature of erythroplakia. The presence of dysplasia generally indicates a higher risk of malignant transformation.

Screening the Oral Cavity for Detection and Risk Evaluation

At least 50% of oral cancers are presumed to originate from oral potentially malignant disorders (OPMD). It is, therefore, important for clinicians to have an easy, noninvasive and a rapid method for identifying leukoplakia and erythroplakia during an oral examination. Most anatomical regions (subsites) of the oral cavity are easily accessible and can be visualised by using a proper illumination system. Therefore, systematic clinical visual examination is recommended to detect new lesions in clinical practice.

Adjuncts to conventional methods of detection are available through commercial manufacturers. These agents and techniques include the following:

1. **Toluidine blue (TBlue®)**: The use of this dye as a mouth rinse or topical (swab) application has been utilised as an aid for the diagnosis of OPMD.

- Leukoplakia and erythroplakia, when present, take up the dye.
- The binding with the dye stains abnormal tissue with a blue colour, which contrasts with adjacent normal mucosa.
- The stained area is usually well-demarcated by dark-blue staining. Pale-blue staining, if noted, is considered as an equivocal test result.
- To avoid false positives caused by inflammatory or traumatic oral lesions, the manufacturer recommends to wait for 10 to 14 days after initial screening with TBlue® and to repeat the test after simple therapies.
- TBlue® may increase the possibility of case detection and accelerate the need for a biopsy. However, some training is needed before a practitioner undertakes TBlue® staining, as interpretation of the stain result may be challenging at times.

2. **Autofluorescence method** of detection of potentially malignant oral lesions is carried out by using a hand-held device called Visually Enhanced Lesion Scope (VELscope®).

3. **Chemiluminescence technique** of detection also involves hand-held devices called Vizilite™ and MicroLux/DL™ systems. Detailed description of the techniques employed is beyond the scope of this chapter. Details of the detection techniques can be found in the manufacturer's brochures.

All three techniques outlined above are useful adjuncts to clinical visual examination by aiding in the visualisation of lesions.[8–10] TBlue® has been suggested to pick up altered mucosa, which is missed in a clinical examination,[11] and high-risk lesions.[12] However, Lingen et al., in a review, could not agree that any adjunctive test was superior to the clinical visual examination performed by a trained clinician.[13]

For clinicians in primary care settings, specific training is required for correct application of the test and correct interpretation of the results. The sensitivity and specificity of these techniques are outlined in a recent systematic review.[14]

Brush biopsy (OralCDx®): This technique was developed in the U.S. and has been advocated for assessing the risk status of oral leukoplakias.[15] The technique involves taking a transepithelial biopsy by using a cytospin brush. A sample of cells obtained with the help of the brush is used for reporting cellular atypia by computer-assisted diagnosis.

Results from a brush biopsy are classified as positive, atypical, negative or inadequate. The method has not received wide acceptance in Europe because of false-negative results. Therefore, it is necessary to perform a surgical biopsy for tissue diagnosis in most instances, when atypical cells are found in a brush biopsy.

Referral

Many dental and medical practitioners are unable (not equipped) to perform a biopsy in their clinical practice.

- For oral leukoplakia and erythroplakia, microscopical evaluation is mandatory to confirm the clinical diagnosis. Therefore, consultation with a specialist is advisable for any patient who is suspected to have leukoplakia or erythroplakia.

- The level of priority should be stated in the referral, which may vary, particularly depending on how red/speckled the lesion appears.
- For those presenting with red or red-white surface characteristics, particularly if these are accompanied with other symptoms, an urgent referral is recommended in the U.K. (under NICE guidelines). These guidelines vary within Europe and the practitioner needs to be aware of the local guidelines, if any.
- Homogeneous white lesions (homogeneous leukoplakia) are sent as routine referrals. Other benign white lesions (e.g., frictional keratoses) of candidiasis should be managed in primary care.
- The referral letter should include the following:
  - ♦ Patient information
  - ♦ Social history (tobacco, alcohol, betel quid use, both frequency and duration)
  - ♦ Clinical details, such as:
    - – Location (anatomical subsite)
    - – Size (widest diameter)
    - – Colour (red, white or mixed)
    - – Surface features (ulcerated, fissured, smooth or verrucous)
    - – Elevation (none or thickened)
    - – Results of any adjunctive tests undertaken should be preferably included, and it is good practice to send a copy of the photographical record of the lesion.

After initial investigations by the specialist, the high-risk patients may enter a 'shared care pathway' and those with low risk should be returned to the practitioner for further management. All patients detected with oral leukoplakia should be asked to consult again with the specialist if any changes are encountered: e.g., increase in redness, ulceration or pain.

Management

- For high-risk oral leukoplakia (with moderate or severe dysplasia), the most commonly used treatment modalities consist of cold-knife excision or CO_2, Nd:YAG or Er:YAG laser excision.[16,17] There is no strong preference for either of the modality mentioned above.
- Excision has the advantage of providing a specimen for additional histopathological evaluation. Excision of leukoplakia is known to reduce the risk of malignant transformation but does not completely eliminate that risk.[18] Local recurrences (10%–30%) are common after the excision of oral leukoplakia.
- Chemoprevention has been tried to reduce malignant transformation. Vitamin A and related carotenoids (in particular, β-carotene), vitamin C and lycopene appear to be particularly protective against most epithelial cancers and their precursor lesions, and much of the effect is attributable to their antioxidant activities. However, none of the randomised control trials using various chemoprevention agents have shown any significant benefits.[19] The latest trial using β-carotene (10 mg/day) and vitamin C (50 mg/day) given for a year to a Japanese population did not

show any significant benefit in the resolution of leukoplakia (over a two-year follow-up period) or cancer prevention (during a five-year follow-up period).[20]

- Erythroplakia needs to be immediately treated (excised) because of its high risk of malignant transformation. Besides, most erythroplakias are symptomatic and often exhibit severely dysplastic tissue or even focal areas of carcinoma *in situ*. Surgical excision with a clear margin, either by cold knife or by laser, is the recommended treatment modality. In planning excision, staining with toluidine blue (TBlue® and OraBlu™) may help in margin identification.

Guidelines for the management of OPMDs for oral medicine specialists are provided by the European Association of Oral Medicine in their protocol for further management.[21]

Prevention

Aspects of prevention of oral leukoplakia have been presented in detail by Warnakulasuriya.[22] Essential points are highlighted as follows:

- The identification of oral leukoplakia and erythroplakia at an early stage has significant benefits to both the patient and the practitioner.
- Their early detection may help to identify high-risk subjects, thus allowing the clinician to initiate appropriate intervention measures in order to reduce the risk of later malignancy.
- Missing any potentially malignant disorders that masquerade focal areas of malignancy may lead to future medico-legal issues.
- As stated earlier, more than 75% of leukoplakia and erythroplakia lesions are attributable to smoking or excessive alcohol consumption over and above the recommended guidelines. For patients with these lifestyles, cessation of smoking and moderation of alcohol consumption remain the most important first steps in the management of oral leukoplakia and erythroplakia.
- It is important for a dental and medical practitioner to learn the skills of tobacco cessation to help patients encountered with potentially malignant disorders. Methods of assisting in smoking cessation using the 5A scheme and practical details, including pharmacotherapy, are given elsewhere.[23]
- Cessation of tobacco use is expected to reduce the risk for oral cancer, but it may take a decade or so for an ex-smoker to demonstrate a substantial decrease in the risk ratio.
- Advice should include moderation of daily alcohol intake and appropriate referral for persons with a history of hazardous, harmful or dependent drinking.
- Consumption of adequate amounts of antioxidants may help in the prevention of leukoplakia and erythroplakia. It is recommended to eat five portions of fresh fruits or vegetables a day.[24]

Follow-Up and Surveillance

- Follow-up of oral leukoplakia is valuable to assess whether cancer would arise during surveillance and to provide access for the patient at the earliest opportunity, if any changes are noted. For this purpose, sequential photographical records are useful tools to judge any changes.

- Most patients with recurrent disease (following any excision) are identified in follow-up clinics; however, some present with new symptoms between follow-up appointments.
- Changes to the size and surface colour (e.g., a red area in an existing white patch, ulceration, lump, induration or even pain in a previously asymptomatic white patch) should arouse concern for reevaluation.
- Repeat biopsies should only be undertaken if there are good indications to do so. Re-staining with toluidine blue may help in the surveillance.
- There are no scientific data about the optimal intervals of follow-up visits for either untreated leukoplakias or after the treatment of leukoplakia; nevertheless, most specialists would adopt an individualised scheme based on the initial (or most recent) risk assessment to follow up their patients at 3, 6 or 12 months' intervals. The same protocol is also applicable to erythroplakia.
- Follow-up studies indicate that malignant transformation may occur more frequently within the first two years of detection of a leukoplakia.[25,26]
- Regular follow-up provides an opportunity to detect cancers at an early stage.[27]
- The period between routine follow-up appointments can be increased with each year after the initial consultations.
- Regular follow-up helps to monitor and predict the clinical evolution, particularly in the case of high-risk patients.
- Maintaining detailed records (with outline diagrams and digital photographs) allows the practitioner to assess the clinical evolution and the nature of any changes. The objective is to intervene at the earliest point if malignancy is suspected and to reduce the risk of transformation by managing the risky lifestyles that contribute to carcinogenesis.

REFERENCES

1. Warnakulasuriya S, Johnson NW, van der Waal I. Nomenclature and classification of potentially malignant disorders of the oral mucosa. *J Oral Pathol Med*. 2007;36:575–80.

2. WHO Collaborating Centre for Oral Precancerous Lesions. Definition of leukoplakia and related lesions: an aid to studies on oral precancer. *Oral Surg Oral Med Oral Pathol*. 1978;46:518–39.

3. Petti S. Pooled estimate of world leukoplakia prevalence: a systematic review. *Oral Oncol*. 2003;39:770–80.

4. Feller L, Lemmer J. Oral leukoplakia as it relates to HPV Infection: a review. *Int J Dent*. 2012;2012:540561.

5. Warnakulasuriya S, Ariyawardena A. Malignant transformation of oral leukoplakia: a systematic review. *J Oral Pathol Med*. 2016;45:155–66. doi: 10.1111/jop.12339.

6. Reichart PA, Philipsen HP. Oral erythroplakia: a review. *Oral Oncol*. 2005;41:551–61.

7. Warnakulasuriya S, Reibel J, Bouquot J, Dabelsteen E. Oral epithelial dysplasia classification systems: predictive value, utility, weaknesses and scope of improvement. *J Oral Pathol Med*. 2008;37:127–33.

8. Awan K, Morgan P, Warnakulasuriya S. Evaluation of an autofluorescence based imaging system (VELscope™) in the detection of oral potentially malignant disorders and benign keratoses. *Oral Oncol*. 2011:47:274–7.

9. Awan K, Morgan P, Warnakulasuriya S. Utility of chemiluminescence (ViziLite) in the detection of oral potentially malignant disorders and benign keratoses. *J Oral Pathol Med*. 2011;40:541–4.

10. Awan K, Yang Y-H, Morgan P, Warnakulasuriya S. Utility of toluidine blue in the detection of potentially malignant disorders of the oral cavity. *Oral Diseases*. 2012;18:728–33.

11. Warnakulasuriya S, Johnson NW. Sensitivity and specificity of OraScan toluidine blue mouth rinse in the detection of oral cancer and precancer. *J Oral Pathol Med*. 1996;25:97–103.

12. Zhang L, Williams M, Poh CF, Laronde D, Epstein JB, Durham S, et al. Toluidine blue staining identifies high-risk primary oral premalignant lesions with poor outcome. *Cancer Res*. 2006;65:8017–21.

13. Lingen MW, Kalmar JR, Karrison T, Speight PM. Critical evaluation of diagnostic aids for the detection of oral cancer. *Oral Oncol*. 2008;44:10–22.

14. Rashid A, Warnakulasuriya S. The use of light-based (optical) detection systems as adjuncts in the detection of oral cancer and oral potentially malignant disorders: a systematic review. *J Oral Pathol Med*. 2015;44:307–28.

15. Sciubba JJ, for the US Collaborative OralCDX Study Group. Improving detection of precancerous and cancerous oral lesions. *JADA*. 1999;130:1445–57.

16. Thomson PJ, Wylie J. Interventional laser surgery: an effective surgical and diagnostic tool in oral precancer management. *Int J Oral Maxillofac Surg*. 2002;31:145–53.

17. Suter VG, Altermatt HJ, Dietrich T, Reichart PA, Bornstein MM. Does a pulsed mode offer advantages over a continuous wave mode for excisional biopsies performed using a carbon dioxide laser? *J Oral Maxillofac Surg*. 2012;70:1781–88.

18. Mehanna HM, Rattay T, Smith J, McConkey CC. Treatment and follow-up of oral dysplasia-a systematic review and meta-analysis. *Head and Neck*. 2009;31:1600–9.

19. Lodi G, Sardella A, Bez C, Demarosi F, Carrassi A. Interventions for treating oral leukoplakia (review). *Cochrane Database Syst Rev*. 2008;CD001829.

20. Nagao T, Warnakulasuriya S, Nakamura T, et al. Treatment of oral leukoplakia with a low-dose of beta-carotene and vitamin C supplements: a randomized controlled trial. *Int J Cancer*. 2015;136:1708–17.

21. Diz P, Gorsky M, Johnson NW, et al. Oral leukoplakia and erythroplakia: a protocol for diagnosis and management. Available from: http://www.kcl.ac.uk/dentistry/about/acad/oral-leukoplakia-and-erythroplakia.pdf

22. Warnakulasuriya S. Squamous cell carcinoma and precursor lesions: prevention. *Periodontol 2000*. 2011;57:38–50.

23. Ramseier CA. Tobacco use prevention and cessation. In: Warnakulasuriya S, Tilakaratne WM, editors. *Oral Medicine &*

Pathology: A Guide to Diagnosis and Management. New Delhi, India: Jaypee Brothers Medical Publishers; 2014. pp. 541–51.

24. Warnakulasuriya S. Food, nutrition and oral cancer. In: Wilson M, editor. *Food Constituents and Oral Health: Current Status and Future Prospects*. Cambridge: Woodhead Publishing Ltd; 2009. pp. 273–95.

25. Silverman S, Jr. Gorsky M, Lozada, F. Oral leukoplakia and malignant transformation. A follow-up study of 257 patients. *Cancer*. 1984;53:563–8.

26. Warnakulasuriya S, Kovacevic T, Madden P, et al. Factors predicting malignant transformation in oral potentially malignant disorders among patients accrued over a ten-year period in South East England. *J Oral Pathol Med*. 2011;40:677–83.

27. Ho MW, Field EA, Field JK, et al. Outcomes of oral squamous cell carcinoma arising from oral epithelial dysplasia: rationale for monitoring premalignant oral lesions in a multidisciplinary clinic. *Br J Oral Maxillofac Surg*. 2013;51:594–9.

Oral potentially malignant disorders II: Oral lichen planus, oral lichenoid lesions, oral graft-versus-host disease and oral submucous fibrosis

K. Thongprasom, V. G. A. Suter
and S. Warnakulasuriya

ORAL LICHEN PLANUS

Definition/Description

Oral lichen planus (OLP) is a chronic inflammatory disease of the skin and oral mucosa. It commonly affects middle-aged women and rarely occurs in children or adolescents. Symptomatic OLP patients may present with oral soreness or a burning sensation, particularly at meal times, but they are often asymptomatic, or the patient may be unaware of its presentation. The condition may be first noted by a dentist during a screening examination.

Aetiology

- The aetiology of OLP remains unclear. Lichen planus is a muco-cutaneous inflammatory disease of unknown origin; however, the disease mechanism involves dysregulation of the cell-mediated immune response to an unidentified antigen.[1]
- Many studies have demonstrated that in OLP lesions, activated CD8+ T lymphocytes are present within the stroma and adjacent to damaged basal cell keratinocytes. The basal keratinocyte degeneration in OLP is attributed to cytotoxic CD8+ T lymphocytes.
- Proinflammatory cytokines and other factors are involved in the immunopathogenesis of OLP, such as interferon-γ, tumour necrosis factor-α, chymase, matrix metalloproteinases and tryptase. These factors can induce an inflammatory process, resulting in chronic OLP lesions.

Clinical Features

The clinical presentation of lichen planus varies from subject to subject. The oral manifestations of OLP can be divided into several clinical types: reticular, papular, plaque, atrophic and ulcerative.[2] However, rare clinical presentations of OLP such as bullous or pigmented types also occur.

- Reticular type is the most common type encountered in the clinical practice. The lesions usually present as bilateral keratotic white striae on the buccal mucosa and appear as interlaced raised lines, forming a latticework (Figure 39.1). Sometimes, the striae could just have a linear or annular presentation. Reticular type of OLP can be found on the mucobuccal fold, gingiva, lateral margins of tongue, labial mucosa, lips and palate.
- Papular type presents as small white raised papules that the clinician must differentiate from Fordyce granules (Figure 39.2).
- Plaque type closely resembles leukoplakia (Figure 39.3); however, keratotic white striae may be found at the lesion periphery

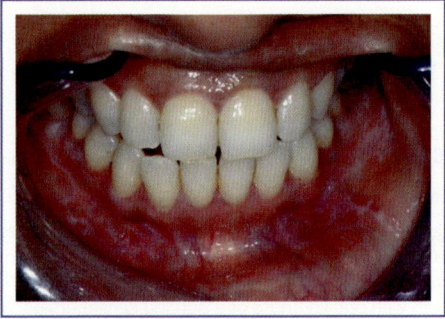

Figure 39.1   Reticular type of oral lichen planus of the buccal sulcus.
Courtesy: Saman Warnakulasuriya.

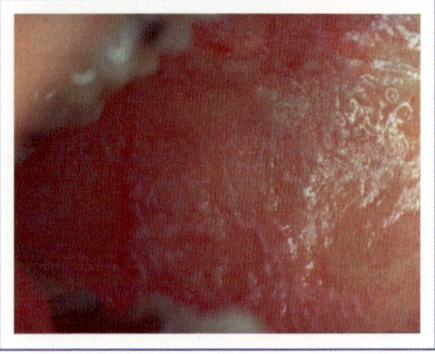

Figure 39.2   Papular form of oral lichen planus of the buccal mucosa.
Reproduced with permission from: Kobkan Thongprasom.

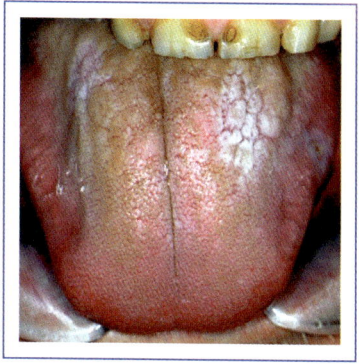

Figure 39.3 Plaque-type lichen planus on dorsal tongue.
Courtesy: Saman Warnakulasuriya.

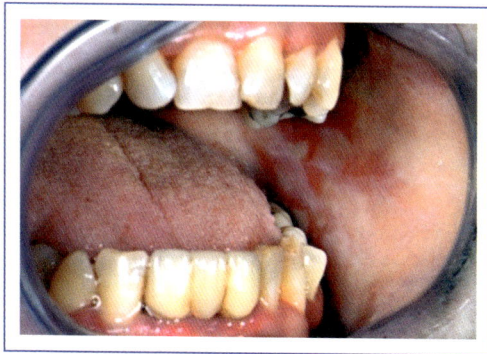

Figure 39.4 Atrophic and ulcerative types of oral lichen planus of the buccal mucosa.
Courtesy: Saman Warnakulasuriya.

or elsewhere in the mouth. These white patches can present with or without erythematous areas, and the clinician must differentiate plaque-type OLP from leukoplakia or lupus erythematosus.

- Atrophic erosive and ulcerative types may present as erythematous areas or with frank ulceration (Figure 39.4). Often, keratotic white striae are seen at the margins. Ulcerated patients typically complain of soreness or a burning sensation when eating hot or spicy food. When atrophic OLP presents on the gingivae, it can be seen as desquamative gingivitis (Figure 39.5).
- Bullous type is rare and tends to recur. It is important to differentiate this type from pemphigus or mucous membrane pemphigoid.
- Dark-skinned persons may develop dark-brown or black pigmented areas around the striae, often during the resolution of OLP.

CHAPTER 39 Oral potentially malignant disorders II: Oral lichen planus, oral lichenoid lesions, oral graft-versus-host disease and oral submucous fibrosis

333

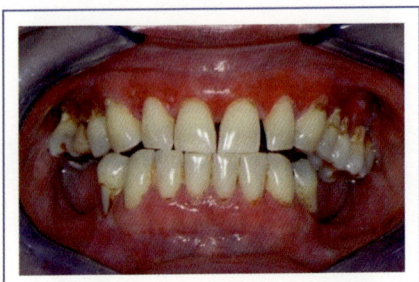

Figure 39.5 Atrophic type of oral lichen planus presenting as desquamative gingivitis.
Courtesy: Saman Warnakulasuriya.

Diagnosis

- Lichen planus is usually diagnosed clinically. Its bilateral distribution and the presence of the classic reticular forms with keratotic white striae are helpful for chairside diagnosis.
- Lichen planus should be distinguished from lichenoid reactions, as these have an underlying cause.[3]
- Atypical presentations could mimic discoid lupus erythematosus or mucous membrane pemphigoid and should be considered in the differential diagnosis.
- Biopsy and histopathological examination are recommended to make a definitive diagnosis.
- Histological findings are the same, regardless of the areas involved or the type of clinical presentation. Microscopy also aids to identify the presence of epithelial dysplasia, on rare occasions. Direct immunofluorescence studies do not aid the diagnosis of lichen planus but could assist to rule out discoid lupus erythematosus or mucous membrane pemphigoid.
- Histological features include hyperkeratosis or parakeratosis in reticular and plaque types; flattening of the epithelium in atrophic types, saw tooth appearance of rete pegs seen sometimes, destruction (liquefaction) of basal cells (apoptosis) and compact band-like subepithelial inflammatory infiltrate (CD8+ lymphocytes) hugging the basement membrane.
- OLP may last for several years, with periods of symptoms and remission. In patients with the ulcerative type of OLP, sclerotic fibrous bands may appear.

Premalignant Nature

- It is generally considered that OLP is associated with an increased risk of malignant.
- The malignant potential of longstanding OLP was reported to be approximately 0.5% to 2% over a five-year period.[4]

CHAPTER 39 Oral potentially malignant disorders II: Oral lichen planus, oral lichenoid lesions, oral graft-versus-host disease and oral submucous fibrosis

335

- Case studies have shown cancer development in OLP, and the condition is classified as a potentially malignant disorder; for this reason, refractory OLP should be closely followed up by the medical practitioner or by an oral medicine specialist.

Management

- Treatment is based on the presence and severity of symptoms. Various treatments have been tried to improve symptomatic OLP; however, complete remission is very difficult to achieve because of its chronic nature.
- Corticosteroids remain the mainstay in treating OLP.[5,6] Recommended therapies using corticosteroid preparations for symptomatic OLP are listed in Table 39.1.
- Figure 39.6 A and B illustrate a case before and after treatment with a topical corticosteroid. Topical corticosteroids such as clobetasol propionate 0.05%, fluocinonide 0.05%, fluocinolone acetonide 0.1% and triamcinolone acetonide 0.1% have been reported to control the symptoms of OLP, whereas systemic corticosteroids have been used for widespread lesions or unresponsive, severe cases.
- Systemic and topical forms of retinoids have been introduced to treat OLP; however, side effects and low remission rates have been reported.
- OLP lesions frequently recur after the discontinuation of retinoids.
- Calcineurin inhibitors such as cyclosporine have been reported to be effective. However, there have been reports of their varied

Table 39.1 Recommended therapies for symptomatic oral lichen planus

Preparation	Application	Recommended dose
Triamcinolone acetonide 0.1% (adcortyl in orabase)	Mucoadhesive paste	Apply after meals three to four times daily
Betamethasone sodium phosphate 500 µg tablets	Mouthwash	500 µg tablet dissolved in 10 mL water. Rinsed in mouth three times a day
Hydrocortisone 2.5 or 5 mg tablets	Mucoadhesive buccal tablets	2.5 or 5 mg tablet dissolved slowly in the mouth four times a day
Clobetasol 0.05% ointment	Topical use (mixed with plain Orabase paste, 50:50)	2 mL applied once or twice a day
Fluocinolone acetonide 0.1% orabase	Topical use	Applied thinly three times a day
Beclometasone 50 or 100 µg inhaler	Topical use as a spray over lesional area	Two puffs applied to lesions up to four times a day
Fluticasone spray 50 µg	Topical use as a spray over lesional area	Two puffs applied to lesions up to four times a day

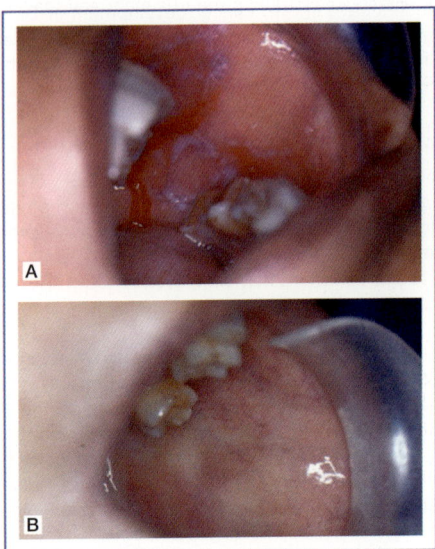

Figure 39.6 (A) Ulcerative oral lichen planus on the left buccal mucosa before and after treatment with fluocinolone acetonide 0.1% in orabase and (B) the lesion showed complete remission within three years.
Reproduced with permission from: Thongprasom K, Dhanuthai K. Steroids in the treatment of lichen planus: a review. *J Oral Sci*. 2008;50:377–85.

effectiveness, as well as side effects such as transient burning sensation, hypertension and nephrotoxicity. Because of the high cost of long-term treatment and the associated side effects, cyclosporine is not recommended for treating OLP.

- Tacrolimus and pimecrolimus are new potent immunosuppressive drugs that have been introduced for treating refractory OLP. These drugs have a rapid palliative effect; however, relapse of an OLP lesion is frequently found on follow up. One concern with these medications is that the Food and Drug Administration has warned about a possible increased risk of malignancies (squamous cell carcinoma and lymphoma) associated with their use. Moreover, a recent report on the topical use of tacrolimus 0.1% in a patient with OLP suggested that it caused the development of squamous cell carcinoma. Thus, treating OLP with tacrolimus needs to be carefully considered by experts.
- Photochemotherapy has been used in the severe forms of erosive OLP. However, this treatment has many side effects and its oncogenic potential is a concern.
- Laser excision may be useful in treating isolated ulcerative forms of OLP; however, lesion recurrence has been reported on follow up.

- The cost-effectiveness during the treatment and management of patients with recalcitrant OLP should be evaluated carefully. The treatment of OLP varies from individual to individual, and there are no conclusive treatment modalities because of patients' different genetic backgrounds. The management and treatment of OLP are very difficult to achieve because of the chronic nature of OLP and thus remain a challenge for clinicians.

ORAL LICHENOID LESIONS

Definition/Description

Oral lichenoid lesions (OLL) are intraoral white and red lesions with reticular striated appearances. These share the clinical features similar to those of OLP but have an underlying causative agent. Other term used for OLL is oral lichenoid reactions (OLR).

- OLL/OLR can be classified into three types:
  1. In topographical relationship with dental restoration, often mercury and amalgam, OLL is also named as oral lichenoid contact lesions or reactions.
  2. Drug-induced OLL/OLR: Some examples of drugs that induce OLL/OLR are shown in Table 39.2.
  3. OLL/OLR found in association with chronic graft-versus-host disease (GVHD). Oral aspects of chronic GVHD are presented in a separate section later in this chapter.

Causes

- OLL/OLR in direct topographical relationship with dental restorations, particularly amalgam fillings, represents an allergic type IV hypersensitivity reaction, occurring in a group of susceptible persons.[7]
- Studies have shown that the replacement of the causative restoration with another material may lead to the resolution of the lesions.
- OLL/OLR may also be a side effect of certain regular medications. A large list of medications can provoke lichenoid reactions (Table 39.2), most commonly nonsteroidal anti-inflammatory drugs and angiotensin-converting-enzyme inhibitors.[8]

Table 39.2 Some examples of drugs that can induce oral lichenoid reactions

Nonsteroidal anti-inflammatory drugs
Angiotensin-converting-enzyme inhibitors
β-blockers
Oral antidiabetic drugs
Antimalarials
Antibiotics (metronidazole, penicillins, tetracycline and sulphonamides)
Some tricyclic antidepressants
Allopurinol
Carbimazole

CHAPTER 39 Oral potentially malignant disorders II: Oral lichen planus, oral lichenoid lesions, oral graft-versus-host disease and oral submucous fibrosis

337

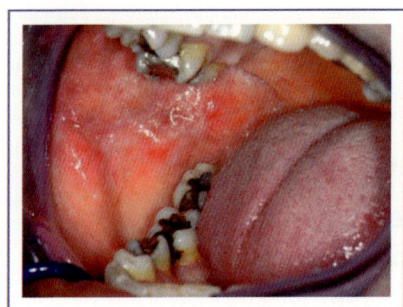

Figure 39.7 Oral lichenoid lesion in close association with dental restorations.
Courtesy: Saman Warnakulasuriya.

Clinical Features

- OLL/OLR presents as white or mixed white and red lesions, sometimes with additional ulceration.
- The pathognomic clinical signs present are white reticular, linear or annular striae and/or white plaque-like patches.
- Red and mixed lesions appear as erythematous atrophic patches, often with some ulceration of the oral mucosa, known as erosive type of OLL/OLR. The differentiation from OLP may be clinically difficult in some cases.
- OLL/OLR due to hypersensitivity to dental restorations is, however, often localised to the site in contact with the allergenic material (Figure 39.7), whereas OLP has a bilateral and widespread presentation.
- OLL/OLR induced due to a reaction to drugs shows various clinical features, with a certain tendency of being unilateral and erosive.

Diagnosis

- When OLL or OLP is suspected to be a reaction to dental material, performing a skin patch test, in particular to dental metals and synthetics, may be helpful in identifying the material responsible for the hypersensitivity reaction.
- This test is undertaken with the European baseline (standard) series and an additional group of other contactants, including a group of dental materials.
- These materials are applied in Finn chambers® on Scanpor® (Hermal, Reinbeck, Germany), pasted on the back of each patient with hypoallergen tape (Hypafix®, BSN medical GmbH, Hamburg, Germany) and left for 48 hours. The results are read on the day of patch removal and ideally also after 72 hours and 96 hours for later reactions.
- The skin patch test is, however, not reliable in all cases, as there may be some false-negative or false-positive reactions. A combination of a close clinical association of OLL/OLR with a specific dental material, together with a positive patch test result, is known

CHAPTER 39 Oral potentially malignant disorders II: Oral lichen planus, oral lichenoid lesions, oral graft-versus-host disease and oral submucous fibrosis

339

to be a good predictive factor for healing after replacement of the restoration.

- The diagnosis of OLP or OLL should be ascertained by biopsy and histopathological examination.[9]
- However, the distinction between OLL/OLR and OLP is often difficult when examined under the microscope, and there is no universal agreement among pathologists to distinguish between these two entities. As a result, the diagnosis of OLL/OLR is mostly based on history, clinical examination, a patch test, when indicated, and histopathology.
- For OLL/OLR suspicious to be drug-induced, the history of any correlation between the beginning of the intake of the medication and first symptoms may also be informative, even though reactions can occur several weeks or months after the prescription.

Premalignant Nature of Oral Lichenoid Lesions or Oral Lichenoid Reactions

- The malignant transformation of OLL/OLR varies between 0% and 6.5% in the literature.
- In one study, OLL/OLR group with an atypical OLP appearance had higher number of transformations reported than in the OLP group.[10] The problem is that many previous studies did not differentiate OLL/OLR from OLP, and there is still a debate on the possible malignant transformation of dental restorations-associated OLL/OLR.
- The mechanisms of cancer development in OLL/OLR are yet to be researched; however, in general, chronic inflammation is recognised as a mediator in carcinogenesis.
- There is also some speculation that irritants from metal restorations or other carcinogens may easily penetrate the eroded or ulcerated mucosa of OLL/OLR and act directly or indirectly as a trigger for malignancy.

Management

- The management of OLL/OLR significantly differs from that of OLP, because causes can be found for some of these reactions.
- For OLL/OLR in close association with a dental material, ideally confirmed by a patch test, it is advisable to replace the restorative material in question. There is good evidence to suggest that OLL/OLR may resolve after this procedure.[11]
- For drug-induced OLL/OLR, it is prudent to withdraw the medication and replace it with an alternative medication that has no cross-reactivity to the former.

ORAL CHRONIC GRAFT-VERSUS-HOST DISEASE

Definition/Description

Oral GVHD is a complication arising in recipients of allogenic haematopoietic stem cells or bone marrow transplantation. Chronic GVHD is a systemic condition with a wide variety of signs and symptoms and affects many organ sites. The oral cavity is one of the most frequently affected sites. In one report, 80% of chronic GVHD patients had oral mucosal GVHD.

Aetiology

- Oral GVHD is characterised by lichenoid inflammation and appears to be due to the reaction of donor T lymphocytes to the expression of tissue antigen by the recipient cells.

Clinical Features

- Oral GVHD can be widespread in the mouth. The primary symptom relates to soreness at mealtimes.
- The disease presents with keratotic striations, white plaques or erosive and ulcerative areas of the oral cavity (Figure 39.8). Typically, buccal mucosa and lateral tongue are involved. The dorsum of the tongue may show papillary atrophy.
- Other clinical features include xerostomia, and patients may develop recurrent mucoceles on labial and buccal mucosae, tongue or soft palate.

Diagnosis

- The knowledge of the history of bone marrow transplant is mandatory and relevant to diagnose oral GVHD.
- The clinical appearance is similar to OLP or OLL. There are no specific tests for oral GVHD, and histology is nonspecific.
- A recent study has indicated that a labial biopsy may demonstrate CD8[+] T-cell predominance surrounding ductal epithelium in oral GVHD.[12]

Association of Chronic Graft-Versus-Host Disease with Cancer

- The incidence of secondary neoplasms for cancer of the oral cavity,[13] oesophagus or thyroid gland in patients with previous haematopoietic stem cell transplant is four to seven times that in the

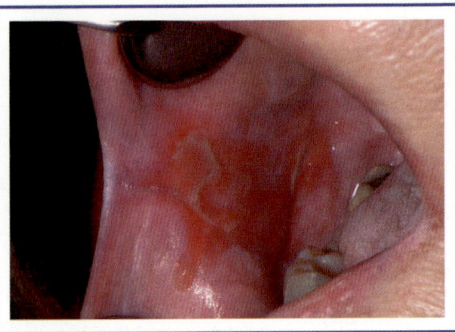

Figure 39.8 Classical appearance of oral graft-versus-host disease with widespread erosion and ulceration.
Courtesy: Valerie Suter.

general population, with men having a significantly higher risk than women and arising most often five years or more after the transplant.

- There are some indications that oral GVHD is a condition that could favour malignant transformation.
- Because of potential malignant transformation, it is recommended to monitor patients with oral GVHD in an oral medicine clinic.

Management

- The management of oral GVHD is mainly by intensive topical corticosteroid therapy.
- Mouth rinses are used for generalised disease and gels, creams and ointments are recommended for focal areas of ulcerations.
- Following are recommended to be used as mouth rinses:
  - ◆ Dexamethasone solution 0.5 mg/5 mL: swish 5 mL for five minutes and spit, two to four times per day
  - ◆ Clobetasol 0.05% solution
  - ◆ Budesonide mouthwash (3 mg/10 mL) or tacrolimus 0.1% solution.
- For focal disease (e.g., solitary painful ulcers), it is recommended to use fluocinonide 0.05% gel, two to four times per day; clobetasol 0.05% gel, two to four times per day or tacrolimus 0.1% ointment, two to four times per day.
- For recalcitrant cases (particularly on lips), use of intralesional triamcinolone injection is recommended; 0.2 mL to 0.4 mL of 40 mg Kenalog (depot preparation) is injected at the base of the ulcer, which may help in rapid resolution.
- Topical tacrolimus 0.1% has been shown to be effective. For patients on tacrolimus, serum levels are measured to monitor any absorption.
- Those on topical corticosteroids may develop secondary candidiasis, a common side effect that should be monitored and treated with topical and systemic antifungal agents in parallel.
- Topical thalidomide 20 mg gel qds has been tried for cases recalcitrant with corticosteroid use.

ORAL SUBMUCOUS FIBROSIS

Definition/Description

Oral submucous fibrosis (OSF) is a chronic, insidious disease that affects the lamina propria of the oral mucosa, and as the disease advances, it involves tissues deeper in the submucosa of the oral cavity, with resulting loss of fibroelasticity.[14]

Aetiology

- Recent studies have confirmed areca nut as the major (and the only) risk factor of OSF, among people who probably have a genetic predisposition to the disease.[15]
- Sufficient evidence on its aetiological role based on epidemiological, animal and *in vitro* studies has been assembled by the International Agency for Research on Cancer.

CHAPTER 39   Oral potentially malignant disorders II: Oral lichen planus, oral lichenoid lesions, oral graft-versus-host disease and oral submucous fibrosis

341

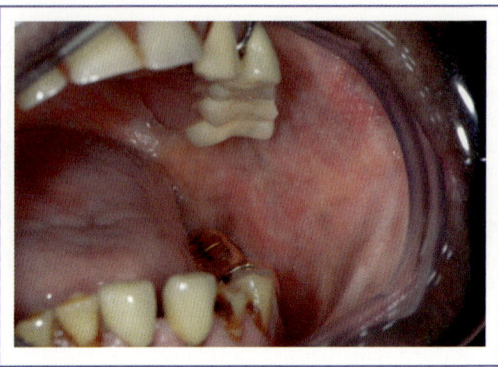

Figure 39.9 Early submucous fibrosis with blanching; a fibrous band is present on the anterior aspect.
Courtesy: Saman Warnakulasuriya.

- Arecoline, the main alkaloid of areca nut appears to be involved in the pathogenesis of OSF, causing fibroblastic proliferation and increased collagen formation.

Clinical Features

A workshop held in Kuala Lumpur, Malaysia,[16] recommended the following criteria for the diagnosis of OSF:

- Presence of palpable fibrous bands (Figure 39.9)
- Leathery mucosal texture
- Blanching of mucosa
- Loss of tongue papillae
- Burning sensation on eating spicy food
- Rigidity of the tongue

Progressive limitation of mouth opening is a hallmark feature of this disease.

Diagnosis

- While the above clinical features are diagnostic of the condition, biopsy and histopathological examination are recommended to confirm the diagnosis.
- Microscopy also helps to identify epithelial dysplasia, if present, as a part of the risk assessment.

Malignant Transformation

- Long-term follow-up studies indicated premalignant nature of this disorder. Jens Pindborg has outlined the basis on which its premalignant nature was determined.[17]

Management

- There is no effective medical management of OSF.[18]
- Habit intervention (e.g., advice to quit areca nut use) is an essential step to control the disease.
- Use of a zinc mouth rinse may reduce mucositis and improve mouth opening by 3 to 4 mm.
- Physical exercise with the help of mouth openers has been tried.
- For advanced cases, surgical excision of fibrous bands and various grafting procedures have reported limited rates of success.

REFERENCES

1. Bascones-Martínez A, García-García V, Meurman JH, Requena-Caballero L. Immune-mediated diseases: what can be found in the oral cavity? *Int J Dermatol*. 2015;54:258–70.
2. Al-Hashimi I, Schifter M, Lockhart PB, et al. Oral lichen planus and oral lichenoid lesions: diagnostic and therapeutic considerations. *Oral Surg Oral Med Oral Pathol Oral Radiol Endod*. 2007;103(suppl S25):e1–12.
3. van der Waal I. Oral lichen planus and oral lichenoid lesions; a critical appraisal with emphasis on the diagnostic aspects. *Med Oral Patol Oral Cir Bucal*. 2009;14:E310–4.
4. Fitzpatrick SG, Hirsch SA, Gordon SC. The malignant transformation of oral lichen planus and oral lichenoid lesions: a systematic review. *J Am Dent Assoc*. 2014;145:45–56.
5. Thongprasom K, Carrozzo M, Furness S, Lodi G. Interventions for treating oral lichen planus. *Cochrane Database Syst Rev*. 2011;CD001168. doi: 10.1002/14651858.CD001168.pub2.
6. Thongprasom K, Dhanuthai K. Review of steroids in the treatment of oral lichen planus. *J Oral Sci*. 2008;50:377–85.
7. McParland H, Warnakulasuriya S. Oral lichenoid contact lesions to mercury and dental amalgam: a review. *J Biomed Biotechnol*. 2012;2012. doi: 10.1155/2012/589569.
8. Firth NA, Reade PC. Angiotensin-converting enzyme inhibitors implicated in oral mucosal lichenoid reactions. *Oral Surg*. 1989;67:41–4.
9. Thornhill MH, Sankar V, Xu XJ, et al. The role of histopathological characteristics in distinguishing amalgam-associated oral lichenoid reactions and oral lichen planus. *J Oral Pathol Med*. 2006;35:233–40.
10. van der Meij EH, Mast H, van der Waal I. The possible premalignant character of oral lichen planus and oral lichenoid lesions: a prospective five-year follow-up study of 192 patients. *Oral Oncol*. 2007;43:742–8.
11. Issa Y, Brunton PA, Glenny AM, Duxbury AJ. Healing of oral lichenoid lesions after replacing amalgam restorations: a systematic review. *Oral Surg Oral Med Oral Pathol Oral Radiol Endod*. 2004;98:553–65.
12. Prochorec-Sobieszek M, Nasiłowska-Adamska B, Szumera-Ciećkiewicz A, et al. The significance of oral labial biopsy in hepatic graft-versus-host disease diagnosis in patients following allogenic haematopoietic stem cell transplantation: a preliminary report. *Ann Transplant*. 2012;17:85–92.
13. Mawardi H, Elad S, Correa ME, et al. Oral epithelial dysplasia and squamous cell carcinoma following allogeneic hematopoietic stem cell transplantation: clinical presentation and treatment outcomes. *Bone Marrow Transplant*. 2011;46:884–91.
14. Warnakulasuriya S. Semi-quantitative clinical description of oral submucous fibrosis. *Ann Dent*. 1987;46:18–21.

CHAPTER 39 Oral potentially malignant disorders II: Oral lichen planus, oral lichenoid lesions, oral graft-versus-host disease and oral submucous fibrosis

343

15. Tilakaratne WM, Klinikowski MF, Saku T, Peters TJ, Warnakulasuriya S. Oral submucous fibrosis: review on aetiology and pathogenesis. *Oral Oncol*. 2006;42:561–8.

16. Zain RB, Ikeda N, Gupta PC, et al. Oral mucosal lesions associated with betel quid, areca nut and tobacco chewing habits: consensus from a workshop held in Kuala Lumpur, Malaysia, November 25–7, 1996. *J Oral Pathol Med*. 1999;28:1–4.

17. Pindborg JJ. Oral submucous fibrosis: a review. *Annal Acad Med*. 1989;18:603–7.

18. Kerr AR, Warnakulasuriya S, Mighell AJ, et al. A systematic review of medical interventions for oral submucous fibrosis and future research opportunities. *Oral Dis*. 2011;17(suppl 1):42–57.

Oral carcinoma and other malignant lesions of the mouth and jaws

N. W. Johnson

ORAL SQUAMOUS CELL CARCINOMA

The majority of malignancies that arise in the mouth — more than 85% — are squamous cell carcinomas (SCCs), with origin in the mucous membranes of the lip vermillion, the anterior two-thirds of the tongue, the hard and soft palate, the gingivae and the lining mucosae of the oral vestibule and floor of mouth (Figure 40.1). Collectively, these may be referred to as 'oral cancers'. It is important to distinguish these SCCs from those arising in the oropharynx, viz the tonsil, posterior third or base of tongue and posterior wall of the oropharynx, and the hypopharynx, because these have a different mix

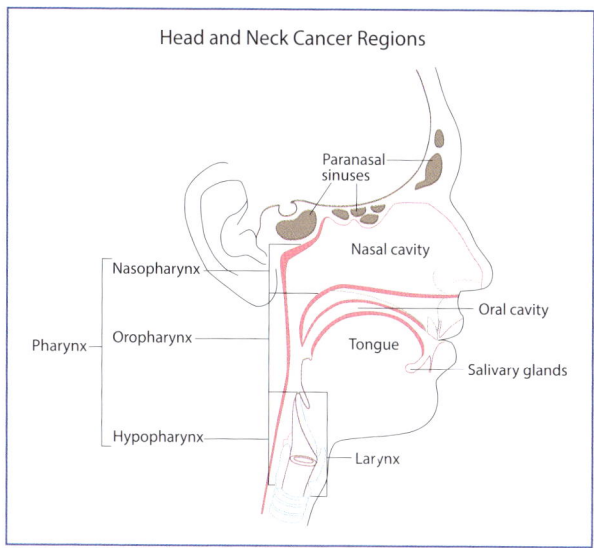

Figure 40.1   Head and neck cancer regions. Here, we are dealing predominantly with lip, tongue and oral cavity.
Illustration: Aniruddha De.

of risk factors and behaviours. Likewise, nasopharyngeal carcinomas are a distinctly different disease, most being driven by Epstein-Barr virus, with a predilection for Chinese ethnicity. In addition, because the naso-, oro- and hypopharynx require endoscopy for satisfactory visualisation, approaches that are not commonly performed in the primary care, this chapter is restricted to those sites and lesions that can be examined by direct vision. Details of the aspects mentioned briefly in this chapter can be found in several recent textbooks, such as the one by Shah and Johnson[1] and by Kuriakose.[2]

The author regards oral squamous cell carcinoma (OSCC) as a systemic disease. The cancer arises at a particular site of the mouth, but much of the upper aerodigestive tract is likely to be damaged — a 'field of change' in which molecular lesions or predisposition have accumulated over time. Further, it is possible that the patient's host response or immune system is failing to recognise the neoplasm as 'non-self' and so has not effectively prevented malignancy or rejected an early lesion. Systemic diseases are not cured by local treatment; the whole patient and his or her family require to be managed.

In the Western world, most oral cancers are diagnosed late in their natural history, usually without the patient or a clinician being aware of a long-standing preexisting lesion. In much of Asia, oral potentially malignant disorders (OPMD) with visible lesions, such as leukoplakia, erythroplakia or submucous fibrosis, usually precede the cancer, often for many years. OPMD provide an opportunity for the prevention of malignant transformation, principally by encouraging cessation of dangerous habits and perhaps by excision or ablation of the lesion. OPMDs have been discussed in Chapter 38 (Oral potentially malignant disorders I: Leukoplakia and erythroplakia) and Chapter 39 (Oral potentially malignant disorders II: Oral lichen planus, oral lichenoid lesions, oral graft-versus-host disease and oral submucous fibrosis).

Epidemiology: Global Scenario, Incidence, Mortality and Trends Over Time

Globally, in 2012, an estimated 300,365 cases and 145,328 deaths were caused from OSCC, a major public health problem. This burden is projected to grow to 450,870 cases by 2030. Oral cancer is the 12th most common cause of cancer-related mortality among women and 16th among women. However, there is marked geographical variation (Figures 40.2, 40.3 and 40.4). For example, in Sri Lanka, oral cancer is the leading cancer among men, sixth among women and second overall. The overall death-to-registration ratio of 0.48 is consistent with an average 5-year survival rate of less than 50%; however, cases do much better if diagnosed while the lesion is small and if strong multidisciplinary teams are responsible for patient care. Sadly, in much of the world, this is not the case. Around the world, with the exception of human papillomavirus (HPV)-related cancers, oral and other head and neck cancers occur predominantly in the poor.

Risk Factors

The risk factors associated with OSCC are summarised in Table 40.1. Risk is dominated by tobacco and alcohol, both in a dose-dependent

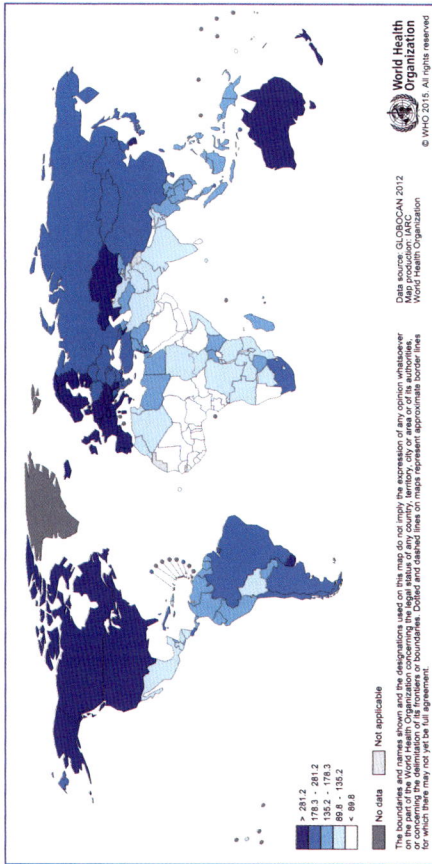

Figure 40.2 Incidence rates for oral cancer in men, expressed as cases per 100,000 population per annum, age-standardised, so that countries are comparable. The highest rates are in South Asia, Melanesia, Europe and Russia. High rates in the U.S. and Australia are influenced by lip cancer and are common in predominantly fair-skinned populations because of exposure to ultraviolet light.

Reproduced with permission from: Ferlay J, Soerjomataram I, Ervik M, et al. GLOBOCAN 2012 v1.0, Cancer Incidence and Mortality Worldwide: IARC CancerBase No. 11 [Internet]. Lyon, France: International Agency for Research on Cancer; 2013. Available from: http://globocan.iarc.fr [accessed 2015 Nov 26]

CHAPTER 40 **Oral carcinoma and other malignant lesions of the mouth and jaws**

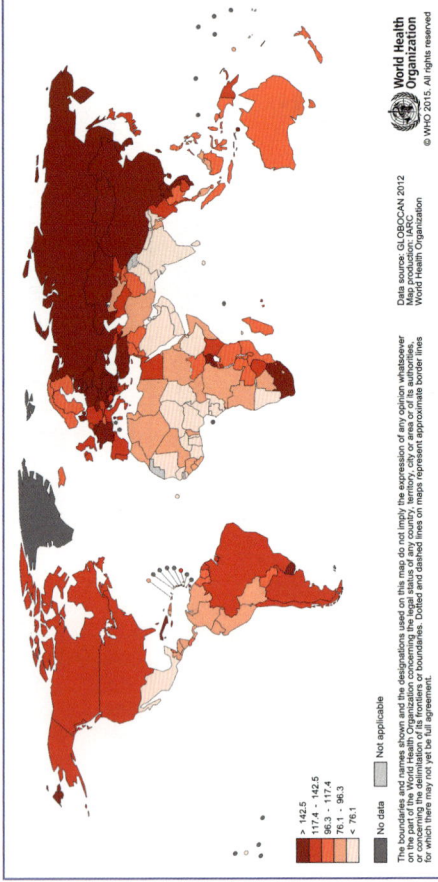

Figure 40.3 Mortality rates for oral cancer in men, expressed as cases per 100,000 population per annum, age-standardised, so that countries are comparable. The U.S. and Australia have dropped in the rankings, because lip cancer is relatively easily treated. South Asia, Eastern Europe and Russia remain as carrying the highest burden.

Reproduced with permission from: Ferlay J, Soerjomataram I, Ervik M, et al. GLOBOCAN 2012 v1.0, Cancer Incidence and Mortality Worldwide: IARC CancerBase No. 11 [Internet]. Lyon, France: International Agency for Research on Cancer; 2013. Available from: http://globocan.iarc.fr [accessed 2015 Nov 26]

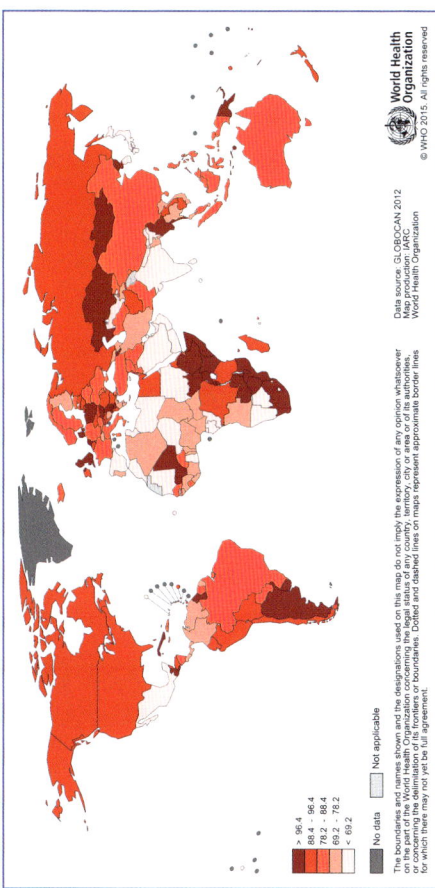

Figure 40.4 Mortality rates for oral cancer in women, expressed as cases per 100,000 population per annum, age-standardised, so that countries are comparable. The U.S. and Australia now drop in the rankings because lip cancer is relatively easily treated. South Asia, Eastern Europe and Russia remain as carrying the highest burden.

Reproduced with permission from: Ferlay J, Soerjomataram I, Ervik M, Dikshit R, Eser S, Mathers C, et al. GLOBOCAN 2012 v1.0, Cancer Incidence and Mortality Worldwide:IARCCancerBaseNo.11[Internet].Lyon,France:InternationalAgencyforResearchonCancer;2013.Availablefrom:http://globocan.iarc.fr[accessed2015 Nov 26]

CHAPTER 40 **Oral carcinoma and other malignant lesions of the mouth and jaws**

Table 40.1 Summary of risk factors for oral cancer

Nonmodifiable	Modifiable	Emerging	Factors with limited evidence (controversial)	Factors with limited scientific evidence
Age	Tobacco smoking	Human papillomavirus infection (unsafe sexual practices)	Poor oral hygiene and dentition	Heredity
Gender	Tobacco chewing	Mate† drinking	Indoor air pollution	Cannabis use
Ethnicity	Snuff* use	Immunosuppression		Khat†† chewing
Socioeconomic status	Areca nut chewing			Nicotine replacement therapy
	Excessive alcohol consumption			Human immunodeficiency virus infection
	Diet poor in fruits and vegetables			Alcohol-containing mouthwashes
	Exposure to sunlight (lip cancer only)			

*Oral snuff: Ground tobacco held in place in the mouth and sucked. Snuff can be loose or in a ready-to-use sachet.

†Mate: Mate is the caffeinated beverage made from Yerba mate plant, which is used as a stimulant to relieve mental and physical tiredness. Mate is very popular in Brazil, Paraguay and Argentina.

††Khat: Khat is a recreational drug made from a plant called *Catha edulis*. The leaves and stem of *Catha edulis* are chewed by people in East Africa and the Arabian countries to elevate mood.

fashion, and the combined effect is supermultiplicative. Importantly, OSCC is a preventable disease. Counselling on tobacco cessation and limited alcohol consumption are the duties of every health professional. Tobacco is consumed in many forms. While smoking of cigarettes, cigars and pipes, including a current fashion for hookah or water pipes, is familiar to most, the so-called smokeless tobaccos (ST) are a major cause of cancer in the world. For example, in the Indian subcontinent, people chew ST or use forms of snuff more often than smoke. ST is frequently used as a component of betel quid or paan, the other major ingredient of which is areca nut (often erroneously called betel nut); areca in all its forms is now regarded as a Class 1 human carcinogen. With the exception of cases putatively caused by certain strains of HPV, oral cancer is predominantly a disease of the poor and dispossessed worldwide. Diets with inadequate intake of red, green or yellow fruits and vegetables predispose to all cancers. This is because such essential foods provide vitamins and minerals, responsible for the scavenging of DNA-damaging free radicals in the body.

There is a real but small genetic predisposition related to polymorphisms in carcinogen-metabolising enzymes, but there is no strong hereditable component such as found with familial breast cancer or many colon cancers. Chronic trauma to oral soft tissues from sharp teeth or dentures and heavy microbial load in the mouth due to poor oral hygiene are reemerging as contributory factors. Mate is a herbal beverage, taken hot and frequently, particularly in Brazil. Marijuana is usually smoked with tobacco, making it difficult to separate the effects. Both indoor and outdoor air pollution by aromatic hydrocarbons affect some populations.

Very importantly, an epidemic of HPV-related head and neck cancer is emerging. Oncogenic or 'high-risk' strains, predominantly HPV-16 and HPV-18, are associated with approximately 30% of head and neck SCC, particularly in the tonsil and base of tongue. The same strains drive most cancers of the uterine cervix and anal and penile cancer, and their association with cancers of the mouth and pharynx is related to orogenital sexual practices. Such cancers are more common in the West — patients tend to be younger and of higher socioeconomic status than those with 'traditional' alcohol and tobacco-related cancers. Fortunately, such cases respond well to radiation, permitting deescalation of treatment intensity and less-severe side effects.

These are the same risk factors that underlie risk for an oral potentially malignant disorder (OPMD). Should such a disorder, or a lesion associated with such disorders, be suspected, referral to a specialist in oral medicine or other experienced oral surgeon or physician is indicated.

Clinical Features and Diagnosis

The clinical signs of OPMD have been described in detail in Chapter 38 (Oral potentially malignant disorders I: Leukoplakia and erythroplakia) and Chapter 39 (Oral potentially malignant disorders II: Oral lichen planus, oral lichenoid lesions, oral graft-versus-host disease and oral submucous fibrosis). For overt OSCC, any ulcer that has been present for two or more weeks without a clear cause, such as trauma, is cancer, until proved otherwise. The common signs are ulceration, frequently with rolled borders, induration, fungation (exophytic swelling) and, in mobile tissue areas, fixation (Figure 40.5 A). However, the signs are often much more subtle (Figure 40.5 B). Cancers produced by areca nut and ST are typically large and slow-growing (Figure 40.6). Symptoms are often imprecise. Lesions can be painless for many months unless

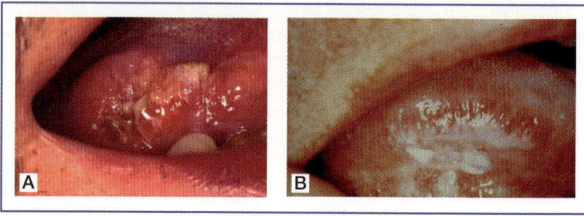

Figure 40.5 (A and B) Two examples of squamous cell carcinomas presenting on the lateral border of the tongue — the most common site for oral squamous cell carcinoma in the Western World. In Figure 40.5 A, the lesion is red due to increased vascularity and depressed, with limited fungation and ulceration. It was hard to palpation. In Figure 40.5 B, the major sign is leukoplakia (white plaques because of hyperkeratosis). Note the angiogenesis along the upper border. The lesion was indurated. Both showed deeply invasive squamous cell carcinoma on biopsy, including infiltration of muscle. In both of these cases, the patient had become aware of the lesion only in recent months.
Courtesy: Newell Johnson.

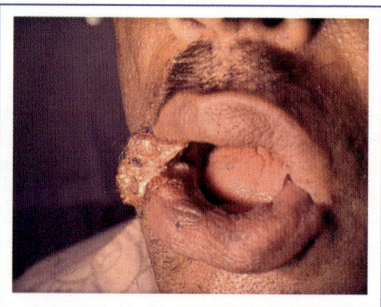

Figure 40.6 Typical oral squamous cell carcinoma of the right buccal mucosa and commissure in a chronic chewer of betel quid containing areca nut and smokeless tobacco. This patient was also a heavy smoker of beedis — raw tobacco wrapped in a tembhurni leaf, commonly used in south Asia. Typically, these cancers arise out of longstanding white, red or speckled oral potentially malignant disorders. They are diagnosed at a later stage. Such large lesions are difficult to treat without creating disfigurement.
Courtesy: Newell Johnson.

and until ulcerated or secondarily infected. Awareness and surveillance of high-risk patients is necessary; that is, people who smoke, use ST or areca and drink more than two standard measures of alcohol per day should have careful visualisation of every oral mucosal surface at every dental visit, and failing this, they should get a check-up done at six-month intervals by a family physician. Oral self-examination (just like breast self-examination) can play a role, but choosing and instructing individuals in whom the potential benefit outweighs the disadvantages of anxiety and inaccuracy or false reassurance requires judgement.

Clinical diagnosis requires good lighting, with white light, retraction of the cheeks and manipulation of the tongue, to ensure all surfaces are visually scrutinised and palpated. The lymphatic chain of the face and neck must also be skilfully palpated for enlargement in every patient suspected with oral cancer. Cervical lymphadenopathy may be inflammatory or reactive but is usually a sign of metastatic cancer. Lymph node metastases are a sign of poor prognosis; as a simplification, the more the node groups that are involved and the lower in the neck they occur, the worse the prognosis. Sophisticated imaging will be performed by specialists as a part of patient workup.

Early diagnosis is important and leads to better treatment outcomes, because it is easier to excise a small lesion and/or to irradiate the primary neoplasm, with minimal damage to the adjacent tissues. Conceptually, however, it is important not to equate lesion size with the length of time for which malignant transformation has been present. Size is a product of time and growth rate — a small and slow-growing neoplasm may have been present for many months; however, some neoplasms can grow and spread very fast. In general, the smaller the lesion, the less likely the neck metastases.

Prognostic Factors, Treatment Modalities and Outcomes

As with every disease, prognosis is a product of the aggressiveness of the disease process itself and the nature and efficacy of the host response. Thus, there are overall patient-related factors and factors within the neoplasm itself that influence the prognosis. These are listed in Table 40.2.

Surgery remains the mainstay of the treatment and may be sufficient for small lesions. Involved lymph nodes must be excised by neck dissection. Treatment of the so-called N0 neck, viz where there is an oral SCC but no clinical or imaging evidence of nodal metastases, remains controversial. Some centres would dissect the neck in high-risk patients or those with a high-risk primary cancer in the knowledge that a proportion of such patients will prove to have positive neck nodes on microscopical examination. Others would first seek the confirmation of the nodal status, for example, by excision and histopathology of a 'sentinel' node, viz detection of the major draining node(s) by injection of dye or radioactive tracer into the primary site.

Radiotherapy by external beam, in some centres, brachytherapy by the insertion of radioactive wires, may be used as sole treatment modality. This is possible for small neoplasms not closely related to bone or major salivary glands and can affect cure and

Table 40.2 Prognostic factors for oral cancer

Patient characteristics

- Age (younger patients do better).
- Gender (women usually do better).
- Relationship status (married and cohabiting patients do better).
- Comorbidities (cardiovascular and respiratory diseases are common in oral cancer patients, often due to the common risk factors of smoking and alcohol abuse).
- Integrity and efficacy of immune system (patients can become anergic towards their neoplasm).

Characteristics of the primary growth

- Site (advanced tongue cancers can have bilateral neck metastases, and more posterior lesions tend to metastasise to lower lymph nodes; lip cancer has a good prognosis because squamous cell carcinomas are usually less aggressive and are more easily treated).
- Size or volume (used as a crude indicator of age and duration of the neoplasm). T stage correlates with survival. Velocity of tumour growth is a strong indicator.
- Degree of histological differentiation; mitotic activity; and nuclear and cellular pleomorphisms.
- Induced angiogenesis.
- Intensity of cell-mediated immune inflammatory infiltrate (in most cases, this is protective; however, local cytokine production can enhance the growth of the neoplastic cell population).
- Vascular and lymphatic invasion; perineural permeation; and extent of spread to surrounding tissues, especially the mandible or maxilla.

Characteristics of regional lymphatics (N stage correlates with survival)

- Number of lymph nodes with metastatic deposits.
- Extent of lymphatic chain(s) involved.
- Penetration of capsule; extracapsular spread to adjacent tissues, including, on occasion, the external jugular vein.

Presence of blood-borne metastases

- Most oral squamous cell carcinoma patients die with disease still above the clavicle. Causes of death are usually cachexia, pneumonia and organ failure. Distant metastases are becoming more common, with better locoregional control, and may involve lung, bone and brain.

cause fewer functional complications. In contemporary best practice, however, surgery and adjunctive radiotherapy are used, especially intensity-modulated radiotherapy. For extensive lesions, chemo-therapy may be added. All of these modalities are aggressive and damage normal as well as neoplastic tissues.

We have now entered 'the age of personalised medicine' in which the molecular and biochemical dependencies of each patient's cancer are investigated. Drugs or other biotherapies are then targeted to aberrant pathways in the particular cancer of a particular patient. These approaches are making strides in leukaemias and cancers such as breast and colon cancers, but the only approved biotherapy of oral and head and neck SCC in 2015 is the use of monoclonal antibodies against epidermal growth factor receptor molecules on the surface of the malignant epithelial cells. Before employing anti-epidermal growth factor receptor drugs, it is essential to establish that the patient does indeed have significant overexpression of these molecules. Research into targeted biotherapies is intensive.

Management of patients with oral cancer, along his or her entire 'cancer journey', demands multidisciplinary teams comprising dentists; head and neck or maxillofacial surgeons; medical oncologists; radiation oncologists; specialist nurses; speech, swallowing and language therapists; dieticians; and those able to provide social and spiritual support. Best practice guidelines are published by many bodies, such as the British Association of Head and Neck Oncologists and the National Comprehensive Cancer Network in the U.S.[3,4] The Cochrane Oral Health Group has published systematic reviews on all aspects of current management.

SALIVARY GLAND NEOPLASMS

Salivary gland neoplasms are important, though much less common than SCC from lining mucosae. Detailed classifications are arcane but relevant for treatment planning and prognosis by specialists. Benign neoplasms are more common than malignant varieties in the major glands: parotid, submandibular and sublingual; albeit that the most common of all are pleomorphic adenomas, especially of the parotid gland, which show a range of intermediate behaviours. Most neoplasms of the major glands are benign, whereas most arising from the minor (intraoral) glands are malignant. Among the latter, adenoid cystic carcinomas are most to be feared; they infiltrate widely, have a renowned propensity for perineural permeation and recurrence after surgery with or without radiotherapy. They are most common on the hard palate, and the base of skull often becomes involved, with very poor prognosis.

Differential diagnoses must be considered at the outset: these are principally retention and extravasation cysts, chronic sialadenitis, lymphoid neoplasms and acute infections.

LYMPHOMAS AND ORAL MANIFESTATIONS OF LEUKAEMIAS

There are large amounts of lymphoid tissue in and around the mouth. Components of Waldeyer's ring are the lingual tonsils, the palatine tonsils and the adenoids in the oropharynx. There is lymphoid tissue within major and minor salivary glands. All forms of primary lymphoid neoplasm can occasionally arise in these tissues, and they can be involved in multifocal lymphoid diseases such as Hodgkin's and non-Hodgkin's lymphomas.

Leukaemias have significant and early oral signs and are thus of diagnostic importance to primary care clinicians. These are principally infiltration of gingival tissues (Figure 40.7). All forms of leukaemia will produce oral signs, which should trigger haematopathology investigation and lead to the earliest possible diagnosis. Changes tend to be most severe in acute lymphoblastic leukaemia, at whatever age the disease develops, and in chronic myeloid leukaemias. Good professional dental care and good personal oral hygiene are essential.

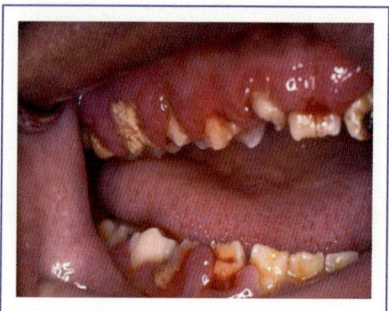

Figure 40.7 Oral and dental changes in a patient with acute lymphocytic leukaemia. The free and attached gingival tissues (the gums) are extremely swollen and erythematous. This results from neoplastic leukocytes spilling from the blood stream into the connective tissues. There is associated inflammation in response to microbial biofilm on tooth and gingival surfaces, and some of this biofilm has calcified to produce dental calculus/tartar. There may be pallor of mucous membranes of the cheeks and tongue (secondary to the associated anaemia) and ecchymoses (secondary to the associated thrombocytopaenia). Developmental hypoplasia of several teeth is also evident in this patient.
Courtesy: Newell Johnson.

TUMOURS OF THE JAW BONES

These do not represent anything like the major public health problem of epithelial neoplasms of the head and neck. Epidemiological clarity is limited. They may be 'odontogenic tumours', that is, they arise from tooth-forming tissues, or may be one of a range of primary bone 'tumours'. Most odontogenic growths are benign, even hamartomatous. A concise summary of the situation with odontogenic tumours is given in the World Health Organization's (WHO's) 'Blue Book'.[5] Most primary bone neoplasms, especially in children and adolescents, are malignant.

There has long been an impression that odontogenic tumours are more common in Africa and Africans than any other country and people, perhaps because so many advanced lesions come late to diagnosis in much of that continent. Ameloblastoma is the most common benign odontogenic tumour worldwide.

Osteosarcomas account for 40% to 60% of the primary malignant bone tumours, and approximately 10% of these occur in the head and neck region, mostly in the jaws. They carry a grave prognosis.

OTHER SOFT TISSUE MALIGNANCIES

Any tissue of the mouth and jaws can give rise to a malignant neoplasm. Thus, lymphomas, sarcomas, neurosarcomas and vascular neoplasms are seen regularly in oral medicine, oral pathology and oral surgical practice. Referral is the best approach when such lesions are suspected in primary care.

METASTASES TO THE MOUTH AND JAWS

Tumours metastatic to the head and neck region from distant sites are comparatively rare, representing about 1% of oral neoplasms. Most lesions are found in patients between the fifth and seventh decades of life. They affect the jaws more commonly than soft tissues, in a ratio of 2:1. The most common primary malignancies metastatic to the jaws are breast (20%), lung (13%), kidney (8%), adrenal (8%), bone (7%), colorectal (6%), prostate (5%) and liver (5%) malignancies.

Quality of Life Issues

Malignancy involving the face and mouth is devastating. Apart from the fear and reality of early demise, patients have to suffer pain, disfigurement and loss of function, including taste, mastication, swallowing and speech. This affects the whole family. High-quality treatment centres mostly use one of the several internationally evaluated Quality of Life instruments to monitor the difficulties their patients experience.

Oral mucositis and xerostomia after irradiation of major salivary glands and the mouth, and also after some chemotherapy regimens for distant malignancies, can be devastating for patients. Paraneoplastic pemphigus may present with oral ulcers or bullae. Referral to specialist oral medicine units, where available, is desirable. Unfortunately, most treatments are of limited efficacy, but there is active research led by the Multinational Association of Supportive Care in Cancer, whose website contains current best practice guidelines. Benzydamine mouthwash is safe and available from pharmacies. Where associated pain is severe, patient-administered morphine is in order. Use of recombinant human keratinocyte growth factor 1 and palifermin, cryotherapy to the mouth and low-level laser therapy needs experienced hands.

For dry mouth, frequent sips of water are safest. Many pharmacies carry proprietary formulations of animal-derived or synthetic mucins and specially formulated toothpastes and mouthwashes. It is important to minimise sugars in the diet and to use a fluoride rinse and fluoride-containing toothpaste to reduce the risk of production of severe dental caries.

REHABILITATION AND FOLLOW-UP

Regular screening of patients suffering from head and neck cancer is mandatory to check for recurrence. A high proportion of patients with oral SCC will develop a second primary malignancy, especially if smoking or other risk factors persist. Counselling and support in tobacco and areca nut cessation are critical. Alcohol should be consumed in moderated quantities, except in the terminally ill, when it may be enjoyed.

Rehabilitation requires the ideal comprehensive head and neck cancer care team to have all the specialty skills mentioned above, including diet and nutrition; swallowing and speech therapy;

physiotherapy, in case shoulder damage has resulted from nerve damage during neck dissection or functional damage to a graft donor site; and psychotherapy, as indicated.

Palliative Care

Patients with head and neck cancer are in physical pain, psycho-logical pain, social pain and spiritual pain. All need management by appropriately skilled carers. The easiest of these maladies to manage is the physical pain because analgesics can be stepped up a ladder from simple drugs, such as paracetamol, through var-ious grades and formulations of opioid; there are many interna-tional and national guidelines on their use. Primary care physicians have a key role because they understand the whole context of their patient. In some countries, the specialty of palliative med-icine is well-developed and the hospice movement, founded by Dame Cicely Saunders, now exists in many countries and provides excellent end-of-life care.

Essential Role of Primary Prevention and Public Policy

The risk factors for OSCC are clear. Control of tobacco use in all its forms and areca nut consumption and the value of a healthy diet and good oral hygiene are a part of standard health promotion across the globe. Messages need to be clear, simple and integrated into the rest of health promotion, for these are the risk factors common to many diseases. This 'bottom-up' approach needs constant effort, must be in appropriate languages and be culturally sensitive. Social mar-keting via print, radio and television needs continuous reinvention. Current social media (Facebook, Twitter and special apps) are being used to advantage in some parts of the world (e.g., in India). To bring the current global epidemic of HPV-related head and neck cancer under control, public education about the importance of sexual hygiene is necessary. Again, messages are common and hold value for the prevention of cervical cancer in women across the globe, where rates in less-developed countries continue to be a serious concern, and for the prevention of genital and anal cancers in men, especially men who have sex with men (though in the latter case, the need for targeted messaging is clear). The roll-out of HPV vaccina-tion programmes in many countries is proving an effective primary prevention against cervical cancer. Evidence is beginning to accu-mulate around reduced head and neck cancer rates; for this to be truly effective, vaccination of young men, as well as of young women, will be necessary.

Primary care clinicians have a vital role to play. For example, there is strong evidence that brief advice from a medical practitioner achieves a small percentage of successes in smoking cessation, and this is very cost-effective.

Government actions and regulations, that is, 'top-down' approaches, are also necessary. The success of the WHO Framework Convention on Tobacco Control in reducing smoking prevalence around the world gives hope. Some of us are currently pressing for a Framework Convention on Areca Nut. We know that bans on smoking in public places and restaurants, plain packaging and large warning notices on cigarette and other tobacco packets have a measurable effect.

Limited Role of Secondary Prevention, Viz., Screening

Evaluation of cancer-screening programmes is a complex and often controversial science. These are only effective where the cancer is common, a diagnostic test with good sensitivity and specificity for detecting small or early lesions is available and there is an effective treatment intervention. Thus, screening programmes for breast and cervical cancers are commonplace; bowel cancer programmes are mostly still research entities and population screening for prostate cancer is not recommended.

There is a considerable recent literature regarding screening for oral cancer. Because of low prevalence in the West, population screening is not advised (see the relevant Cochrane review). However, in high-prevalence or high-risk populations, such as in South Asia, such screening can be cost-effective and save lives,[6] and we have recently shown the validity of a simple algorithm to identify high-risk subjects in Sri Lanka, who then go into a diagnostic and care pathway.[7] There may be a role of encouraging mouth self-examination (akin to breast self-examination) in suitable patients, viz, those at high risk and where it is judged that the balance of risk and psychological harm is reasonable.

The Role of Primary Care Practitioners

The role of primary care practitioners is important and clear. They should follow the following steps:

- Counsel patients on healthy lifestyle: ask, assess, advise, assist (to quit) and arrange follow-up for all addicted clients (Royal Australian College of General Practitioners).
- Examine the head, neck and mouth of the adult patients routinely.
- Establish clear referral pathways.

REFERENCES

1. Shah J, Johnson NW. *Textbook of Oral Cancer*. 2nd ed. London, U.K.: CRC Press, Taylor & Francis Group; 2016.
2. Kuriakose MA, editor. *Oral Cancer: A Comprehensive Approach*. 1st ed. New York: Springer; 2015.
3. British Association of Head and Neck Oncologists. *BAHNO Standards 2009*. West Sussex, U.K.: BAHNO; 2009. Available from: http://bahno.org.uk/wp-content/uploads/2014/03/BAHNO-STANDARDS-DOC09.pdf
4. Cochrane Oral Health Group. *Treatment Methods for Oral Cancer and the Value of Screening Programmes*. Manchester, U.K.: Cochrane Oral Health Group. Available from: http://ohg.cochrane.org/-updates-reviews-and-protocols
5. Barnes L, Eveson JW, Reichart P, Sidransky D. *World Health Organization Classification of Tumors: Pathology and Genetics of Head and Neck Tumours*. Lyon: IARC Press; 2005. pp. 221–4.

6. Sankaranarayanan R, Ramadas K, Subramanian S, Amarasinghe H, Johnson NW, Subramaniam S. Prevention, early detection, and treatment of oral cancer. In: Sankaranarayanan R, Jha P, Gelband H. *The Cancer Volume of the Disease Control Priorities Network*. Available from: http://www.dcp-3.org/chapter/1138/prevention-early-detection-and-treatment-oral-cancer

7. Amarasinghe HK, Johnson NW, Lalloo R, Kumaraarachchi M, Warnakulasuriya S. Derivation and validation of a risk-factor model for detection of oral potentially malignant disorders in populations with high prevalence. *Br J Cancer*. 2010 27;103:303–9. doi: 10.1038/sj.bjc.6605778.

Chapter 41

Oral complications of cancer therapy

S. R. Prabhu

CANCER THERAPY AND THE MOUTH

Cancer survival rate has increased in the last three decades because of advances in cancer treatment. Patients with head and neck cancers are treated with surgical resection, external beam radiotherapy and/or brachytherapy and chemotherapy, depending on the location, clinical stage, histological grade of the tumour and clinical condition of the patient.[1,2] Patients with haematopoietic malignancies who are treated with haematopoietic stem cell transplantation (HSCT) and those with cycled chemotherapy, with or without targeted therapies for nonoral solid tumours, can develop oral complications. Oral complications of cancer therapy may present as acute or chronic symptoms. Acute complications occur during cancer therapy, whereas chronic complications occur after the completion of therapy and may persist for several years.[3]

ORAL COMPLICATIONS ASSOCIATED WITH SURGICAL TREATMENT OF ORAL CANCER

The long-term complications associated with surgical treatment of oral and oropharyngeal cancers include speech limitations, masticatory problems, swallowing problems, neurological problems, chronic fistulas, trismus and delayed wound healing.

ORAL COMPLICATIONS ASSOCIATED WITH CHEMOTHERAPY

Oral complications of chemotherapy depend on the types of chemotherapeutic drugs used and their dose and duration. These complications also relate to mucosal integrity and oral and systemic status of the patient.

Complications arise from the direct cytotoxic effects of chemotherapeutic drugs on oral tissues and/or from the indirect effects of myelosuppression caused by the effects of drugs. Range of oral complications associated with chemotherapy for cancer include oral mucositis, oral infections, intraoral bleeding, alterations in taste, pain, xerostomia and dental developmental abnormalities in children receiving chemotherapy. The following subsections provide a brief description on each of these complications.

Oral Mucositis

Oral mucositis is an acute complication of chemotherapy characterised by inflammation and painful ulceration of the oral mucosa. Usually, these complications have an onset around the 7th through the 11th day after the start of chemotherapy. Reported incidence of oral mucositis ranges from 75% to 99%.[4] Symptoms may persist until the effect of chemotherapy last.

Buccal mucosa, labial mucosa, the ventral surface of the tongue, the floor of the mouth and soft palate are the common sites of mucositis. Severity of mucositis may range from erythema to ulceration and haemorrhage. Mucosal burning sensation is common. As the condition progresses, eating, swallowing and talking become increasingly difficult.

Oral Infections

Chemotherapy-related oral infections contribute significantly to the morbidity and mortality in cancer patients. Infections from *Candida* species, thus causing pseudomembranous or erythematous candidiasis, are common. *Candida* species and staphylococcal species are also associated with angular cheilitis of the mouth.

Viral infections of the oral mucosa include herpes simplex virus, varicella-zoster virus and cytomegalovirus infections.

Intraoral Bleeding

Mucosal bleeding associated with chemotherapy can be spontaneous or traumatically induced. Bleeding can also be due to thrombocytopaenia secondary to myelosuppression.

Alteration in Taste (Dysgeusia)

After the administration of chemotherapeutic agents, patients may complain of alteration in taste. Chemotherapy-related dry mouth also contributes to the loss of taste sensation. This is usually a transient feature.

Pain

In the absence of any detectable dental cause, patients may complain of pain mimicking toothache. This is often constant and bilateral. This phenomenon is common in those receiving chemotherapy with vincristine or vinblastine.

Xerostomia

Patients on cancer therapy complain of decreased or thickened saliva. Duration of xerostomia depends on the length of chemotherapy and the use of other prescribed medications. Dry mouth may lead to rampant caries and render the mucosa to pain, infections and irritation.

Dental Developmental Abnormalities in Children

In children receiving chemotherapy, dental developmental anomalies such as enamel defects, delayed eruption and malformed roots may occur.

ORAL COMPLICATIONS ASSOCIATED WITH RADIOTHERAPY

Oral complications associated with radiotherapy are common in those who receive radiotherapy for head and neck cancers. Orofacial tissues affected by radiotherapy may include salivary glands, taste buds, mucous membranes, jaw bones, teeth, temporomandibular joint and related musculatures of the head and neck region.

Oral complications associated with radiotherapy are categorised as acute and chronic types. The acute complications usually develop in the early phase of the treatment period and may persist for two to three weeks after the completion of radiation treatment. Chronic (late) complications may become evident any time after the completion of radiation treatment, ranging from weeks to years.[5]

It has been reported that 90% to 100% of patients receiving radiotherapy for the oral region develop oral complications.[6]

Acute oral complications associated with radiotherapy include xerostomia, taste disturbances, mucositis, including ulceration, and infection. Chronic complications include xerostomia or salivary gland dysfunction, radiation caries, trismus, temporomandibular joint disorders, osteoradionecrosis and developmental abnormalities of teeth and jaws. Factors that influence intensity and duration of radiation-associated oral complications include total dosage of radiation, rate of radiation delivery, fraction size, field of radiation, radiation source, previous surgical interventions, oral hygiene and dental status, medical and nutritional status of the patient and tobacco and alcohol use.[7]

Salivary Gland Dysfunction or Xerostomia

Salivary glands within the field of radiation may be permanently damaged during radiation therapy. This leads to reduced salivary flow, thus causing xerostomia. Salivary dysfunction occurs shortly after the initial exposure to radiation and persists thereafter. For patients whose major salivary glands are in the radiation fields, the prevalence of xerostomia is reported to range from 94% to 100%.[8]

Saliva becomes thick, scanty and viscous, and patients may experience pain, discomfort and difficulty in chewing, speech and swallowing. Dryness of the oral mucosa may put the patient at a higher risk of oral infections and dental caries. Because of the reduced salivary flow, taste sensation for sweet, salty, sour and bitter is also altered. Taste disturbances are reversible within two to four months after radiation therapy.[9]

Mucositis

Mucositis is the most common acute complication of radiation therapy. Mucosal erythema can develop within one week after the start of radiation and would intensify with the continued treatment. Mucosa exposed to radiation may become denuded, ulcerated and intensely painful. Mucositis is accompanied by dysphagia and painful swallowing. Radiation-induced mucositis persists two to three weeks after the completion of radiation therapy and 90% to 95% of patients show complete resolution by the fourth week.[10]

Infection

Candidiasis is a common fungal infection of the oral mucosa in patients receiving radiation therapy. Patients are also susceptible to a wide range of bacterial and viral infections. These are the secondary infections caused due to radiation-associated xerostomia and mucosal damage.

Radiation Caries and Tooth Demineralisation

Radiation caries and tooth demineralisation occur when the major salivary glands are included in the field of radiation. Saliva in these patients becomes more acidic, making cariogenic bacteria to thrive. In addition, xerostomia also contributes to the development and progression of dental caries and demineralisation of tooth substance.

Osteoradionecrosis

Osteoradionecrosis is a chronic oral complication, whose incidence ranges from 1% to 37.5%. The range of symptoms and signs of osteoradionecrosis range from small exposed parts of the jaw bone to a foul-smelling necrotic bone with or without suppuration.[5] Mandible is commonly affected in osteoradionecrosis.

Temporomandibular Joint Disorders

Patients who have received radiation therapy for head and neck cancer may experience trismus, which is characterised by gradual reduction and inability in mouth opening because of fibrosis of the temporomandibular joint and muscles of mastication. It has been reported that about 5% to 38% of patients who have received radiation therapy to the head and neck region develop trismus.[11] Limited mouth opening may interfere with oral hygiene, dietary intake and use of dental prosthesis and may restrict access to dental care and general anaesthesia.[7]

Developmental Abnormalities in Children

Children who receive radiation to the head and neck region during their formative years are likely to develop developmental abnormalities of the teeth and jaw bones.

ORAL COMPLICATIONS ASSOCIATED WITH HAEMATOPOIETIC STEM CELL TRANSPLANTATION

In general, haematopoietic stem cell transplantation and conventional chemotherapeutic treatment have comparable risk of complications. Patients are at a high risk of developing bacterial, fungal and viral infections. Graft-versus-host disease (GVHD) is the most important complication of allogenic transplantation for cancer. Acute oral complications of GVHD include desquamative painful oral lesions. Chronic oral complications of GVHD include mucosal erythema, desquamative gingivitis, loss of lingual papillae, lichenoid reactions and xerostomia.

MANAGEMENT OF ORAL COMPLICATIONS

Pain Management

Mucositis is managed in medical practice with pain management and by providing encouragement to eat. 'Magic mouthwash' is very effective with this regard. This mixture is composed of diphenhydramine, viscous lidocaine, bismuth salicylate and corticosteroids.[12] Magic mouthwash relieves the acute pain and reduces the inflammation, making oral consumption of food easier. Systemic analgesics such as acetaminophen or ibuprofen may be taken for pain. Intense mucositis-related pain can be relieved by using opioids. Application of ice chips to the mouth every 30 minutes for the prevention and treatment of oral mucositis is also useful. Low-level laser therapy has proved to be useful for the prevention of mucositis.[13]

Management of Oral Infections

Localised bacterial infections of the oral mucosa can be treated with a combination of penicillin and metronidazole. Oral hygiene practice is important in these patients. Patient should be advised to use soft-bristle toothbrush and dental floss. Antimicrobial mouthwash containing chlorhexidine is also recommended.

For fungal infections, nystatin rinses are recommended. Systemic use of fluconazole (100–200 mg/day for two weeks) may be used for moderate to severe fungal infections. Itraconazole capsules (200 mg/day for two to four weeks) are recommended for fluconazole-resistant cases.

For viral infections, acyclovir and valacyclovir are effective in the prevention and treatment of herpes simplex virus infections. Oral hairy leukoplakia can develop in those undergoing chemotherapy for myelogenous leukaemia, acute lymphocytic leukaemia and multiple myeloma. High doses of valacyclovir may be used effectively for these patients. Topical treatment of 25% podophyllin resin alone or in combination with acyclovir may also be considered for patients with oral hairy leukoplakia.

Management of Xerostomia

Patients with xerostomia should be advised to take sips of water every 10 minutes and melt ice chips in the mouth frequently for comfort. The use of artificial saliva spray and mouth-moisturising gels is also effective. The lips may be lubricated with petroleum jelly. Patients should be advised to minimise the intake of coffee, tea, soft drinks with caffeine and alcohol, and mouth washes containing alcohol should be avoided. In cases of severe dry mouth, saliva-stimulating medications are recommended.

Management of Disturbances in Taste Sensation (Dysgeusia)

Supplementing diet with zinc and vitamin D has been reported to improve taste sensation. Patients are advised to drink plenty of fluids during meals in order to enable the dissolution of taste components in the food to reach taste buds.[14] Patient should be advised to chew food slowly in order to release more flavours and stimulate saliva production.[7]

Management of Trismus and Temporomandibular Joint Disorders

Radiotherapy to the muscles of mastication and the temporomandibular joint may cause severe pain and limited mouth opening. Conservative nonsurgical treatment and referral of the patient for physical therapy is recommended.

Management of Oral Hygiene and Patient Self-Care Procedures[1–14]

The patient should adopt the following practices for the management of oral hygiene:

- After every meal and at bedtime, the patient should brush the teeth and tongue with an extra-soft nylon-bristle toothbrush. If pain is intense, mouth may be rinsed with a topical local anaesthetic before brushing.
- Plaque may be wiped from the oral tissues with gauze moistened in baking-soda-saline solution.
- Dental floss should be used daily.
- The mouth should be kept moist. Alcohol-based over-the-counter mouthwashes should not be used.
- Daily fluoride-containing gel application in custom-made gel applicator trays is recommended.
- If patient suffers from mucositis or ulceration, he or she should avoid wearing removable prosthesis. Dentures must be soaked in an antimicrobial denture-soaking solution. When out of the mouth, dentures should be stored in clean water. Denture adhesives should not be used.
- Tobacco use is contraindicated.
- Diet should be as bland and soft as possible. Straws can be used to drink liquids.

Medical and health professionals should refer the patients to dentist for instruction on oral hygiene and management of dental problems.

REFERENCES

1. Hancock PJ, Epsein JB, Sadler GR. Oral and dental management related to radiation therapy for head and neck tumor. *J Can Dent Assoc*. 2003;69:585–90.
2. Epstein JB Thariat J, Benasdoum RJ, et al. Oral complications of cancer and cancer therapy: from cancer treatment to survivorship. *CA Cancer J Clin*. 2012;62:400–22.
3. Epstein JB, Gilneri P, Barasch A. Appropriate and necessary oral care for people with cancer: guidance to obtain the right oral and dental care at the right time. *Support Care Cancer*. 2014;22:1981–8. doi: 10.1007/s00520-014-2228-x.
4. Sonis ST, Elting S, Okeefe D, et al. Perspectives on cancer therapy-induced mucosal injury: pathogenesis, measurement, epidemiology, and consequences for patients. *Cancer*. 2004;100:1995–2015.

5. Scuibba JJ, Goldenburg D. Oral complications of radiotherapy. *Lancet Oncol*. 2006;7:175–83.

6. Herrstedt J. Prevention and management of mucositis in patients with cancer. *Int J Antimicrob Agents*. 2000;16:161–3.

7. Barker GJ, Barker BF, Gier RE. *Oral Management of the Cancer Patient: a Professional Guide for the Management of Patients Undergoing Chemotherapy and Head and Neck Radiation Therapy*. 6th ed. [Biomedical PCommunications]. Kansas, MO: UMKC School of Dentistry; 2000.

8. Hughes PJ, Scott PM, Kew J, et al. Dysphagia in treated nasopharyngeal cancer. Head Neck. 2000;22:393–7.

9. Conger AD. Loss and recovery of taste acuity in patients irradiated to the oral cavity. *Radiation Res*. 1973;53:338–47.

10. Million RR. The effect of radiation on normal tissues of the head and neck. In: Cassisi NJ, editor. *Management of Head and Neck Cancer: A Multidisciplinary Approach*. Philadelphia, PA: J P Lippincott; 1984.

11. Steelman R, Sokol J. Quantification of trismus following irradiation of the temporomandibular joint. *Mo Dent J*. 1986;66:21–3.

12. Chan A, Ignoffo RJ. Survey of topical oral solutions for the treatment of chemo-induced oral mucosits. *J Oncol Pharm Pract*. 2005;11: 139–43.

13. Silva GB, Mendonca EF, Bariani C, Antunes HS, Silva MA. Prevention of induced oral mucositis with low level laser therapy in bone marrow transplantation patients: a randomised clinical trial. *Photomed Laser Surg*. 2011;29:27–31.

14. Wong HM. Oral complications and management strategies for patients undergoing cancer therapy. *Sci World J*. 2014;2014. Available from: http://dx.doi.org/10.1155/2014/581795

Index